The Lacrimal System

The Lacrimal System

Editor

Jeffrey Jay Hurwitz, M.D., F.R.C.S.(C)
Professor, Department of Ophthalmology
Director, Oculoplastics Program
University of Toronto Faculty of Medicine;
Ophthalmologist-in-Chief
Mount Sinai Hospital; and
Consultant Ophthalmologist
Sunnybrook Health Sciences Centre Toronto
The Hospital for Sick Children
The Toronto Bayview Cancer Clinic
Central Hospital, Toronto
Toronto, Ontario, Canada

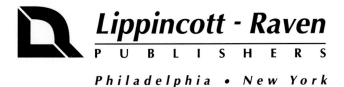

Lippincott - Raven
P U B L I S H E R S

Philadelphia • New York

Lippincott-Raven Publishers, 227 East Washington Square, Philadelphia, Pennsylvania 19106–3780

Made in the United States of America

Library of Congress Cataloging-in-Publication Data
The Lacrimal system/Jeffrey Jay Hurwitz.
  Hurwitz, Jeffrey Jay.
     p. cm.
  Includes bibliographical references and index.
  ISBN 0-7817-0334-4
    1. Lacrimal apparatus—Diseases.   2. Lacrimal apparatus—Surgery.
    3. Lacrimal apparatus—Physiology. I. Title.
    [DNLM: 1. Lacrimal Apparatus Diseases—diagnosis. 2. Lacrimal
Apparatus Diseases-therapy.   3. Lacrimal Apparatus Diseases—physiology.
WW 208 H967L 1995]
RE201.H87 1995
617.7'64—dc20
DNLM/DLC
for Library of Congress   95-17719
                                                     CIP

9 8 7 6 5 4 3 2 1

To my wife, Evelyn; my children, Cary, Michael, and Gillian; and to our parents, Lillian and Nathan Hurwitz and Patricia Main.

Contents

Section III. Clinical Presentation and Management

Section IV. Surgery of Lacrimal Drainage

Contributing Authors

Chidambaram R. Ananthanarayan, M.D., F.R.C.P.C.   *Consultant Anesthesiologist, Mount Sinai Hospital, 600 University Avenue, Toronto, Ontario M5G 1X5, Canada; and Assistant Professor, Department of Anesthesia,   University of Toronto Faculty of Medicine, 1 King's College Circle, Toronto, Ontario M5S 1A8, Canada*

Oleh H. Antonyshyn, M.D., F.R.C.S.C.   *Assistant Professor, Department of Surgery, Division of Plastic Surgery, University of Toronto Faculty of Medicine, Sunnybrook Hospital, 2075 Bayview Avenue, Toronto, Ontario M4N 3M5, Canada*

Kris Conrad, F.R.C.S., F.R.C.S.(C), F.A.C.S.   *Co-Director, Facial Plastic Surgery Unit, Department of Otolaryngology, Mount Sinai Hospital, 600 University Avenue, Toronto, Ontario M5G 1X5, Canada; and Assistant Professor, Department of Otolaryngology, University of Toronto Faculty of Medicine, 1 King's College Circle, Toronto, Ontario M5S 1A8, Canada*

David Cowen, M.D.   *Director, Oculoplastics Program, and Clinical Associate Professor, Department of Ophthalmology, University of Kentucky College of Medicine, 800 Rose Street, Lexington, Kentucky 40536-0084; Fellow in Oculoplastic Surgery, University of Toronto (July 1992– December 1993)*

Jeremy L. Freeman, M.D., F.R.C.S.C., F.A.C.S.   *Consultant Otolaryngologist, Mount Sinai Hospital, 600 University Avenue, Toronto, Ontario M5G 1X5, Canada; and Professor, Department of Otolaryngology, University of Toronto Faculty of Medicine, 1 King's College Circle, Toronto, Ontario M5S 1A8, Canada*

Michael Hawke, M.D., F.R.C.S.C.   *Professor, Departments of Otolaryngology and Pathology, University of Toronto Faculty of Medicine, 1 King's College Circle, Toronto, Ontario M5S 1A8, Canada; and Otolaryngologist-in-Chief, St. Joseph's Hospital, Toronto, Ontario, Canada; and Associate Scientific Staff, Mount Sinai Hospital, 600 University Avenue, Toronto, Ontario M5G 1X5, Canada*

Ernest M. Hew, M.D., F.R.C.P.C.   *Consultant Anesthetist, Mount Sinai Hospital, 600 University Avenue, Toronto, Ontario M5G 1X5, Canada; and Associate Professor, Department of Anesthesia, University of Toronto Faculty of Medicine, 1 King's College Circle, Toronto, Ontario M5S 1A8, Canada*

David J.C. Howarth, M.D.   *Ophthalmic Pathologist, Departments of Pathology and Ophthalmology, Mount Sinai Hospital, 600 University Avenue, Toronto, Ontario M5G 1X5, Canada; and Assistant Professor, Department of Pathology, University of Toronto Faculty of Medicine, 1 King's College Circle, Toronto, Ontario M5S 1A8, Canada*

Cary Hurwitz, B.A.   *Research Assistant, Department of Ophthalmology, University of Toronto, Faculty of Medicine, 1 King's College Circle, Toronto, Ontario M5S 1A8, Canada (July–August 1994)*

Jeffrey Jay Hurwitz, M.D., F.R.C.S.(C)   *Professor, Department of Ophthalmology, Director, Oculoplastics Program, University of Toronto Faculty of Medicine, 1 King's College Circle, Toronto, Ontario M5S 1A8 Canada; and Consultant Ophthalmologist, Sunnybrook Health Sciences Centre Toronto, The Hospital for Sick Children; and Consultant Ophthalmologist, The Toronto Bayview Cancer Clinic and Central Hospital, Toronto; and Ophthalmologist-in-Chief, Mount Sinai Hospital, 600 University Avenue, Toronto, Ontario M5G 1X5, Canada*

Nasir M. Jaffer, M.D., F.R.C.P.C. *Consultant Neuroradiologist, Mount Sinai Hospital, 600 University Avenue, Toronto, Ontario M5G 1X5, Canada; and Assistant Professor, Department of Medical Imaging, University of Toronto Faculty of Medicine, 1 King's College Circle, Toronto, Ontario M5S 1A8, Canada*

Edward E. Kassel, M.D., D.D.S., F.R.C.P.C. *Radiologist-in-Chief, Department of Medical Imaging, Mount Sinai Hospital, 600 University Avenue, Toronto, Ontario M5G 1X5, Canada; and Associate Professor, Department of Medical Imaging, University of Toronto Faculty of Medicine, 1 King's College Circle, Toronto, Ontario M5S 1A8, Canada*

Joel C. Kirsch, M.D., F.R.C.P. (C) *Head, Division for Nuclear Medicine Program, Mount Sinai Hospital, 600 University Avenue, Toronto, Ontario M5G 1X5, Canada; and Assistant Professor, Department of Medical Imaging, University of Toronto Faculty of Medicine, 1 King's College Circle, Toronto, Ontario M5S 1A8, Canada*

Paul La Pierre *Oculoplastic Fellow, Mount Sinai Hospital, 600 University Avenue, Toronto Ontario M5G 1X5, Canada (July–December 1994)*

Per G. Liavaag, M.D. *Assistant Clinical Professor, Department of Otolaryngology, University of Bergen, Haukeland Hospital, N-5020 Bergen, Norway; Fellow in Otolaryngology, Mount Sinai Hospital (July 1994–January 1995)*

Robert C. Pashby, M.D., F.R.C.S.C. *Consultant Oculoplastic Ophthalmologist, Mount Sinai Hospital, 600 University Avenue, Toronto, Ontario M5G 1X5, Canada; Hospital for Sick Children, Toronto; and Assistant Professor, Department of Ophthalmology, University of Toronto Faculty of Medicine, 1 King's College Circle, Toronto, Ontario M5S 1A8, Canada*

Charles J. Pavlin, M.D., F.R.C.S.C. *Consultant Ophthalmologist, Director, Ultrasound Program, Princess Margaret Hospital, Toronto, Ontario; and Consultant Ophthalmologist, Toronto Hospital, Toronto, Ontario; and Associate Professor, Department of Ophthalmology, University of Toronto Faculty of Medicine, 1 King's College Circle, Toronto, Ontario M5S 1A8, Canada*

Raymond Stein, M.D. *Consultant Ophthalmologist, Director, Cornea and External Disease Program, Mount Sinai Hospital, 600 University Avenue, Toronto, Ontario M5G 1X5, Canada; and Lecturer in Ophthalmology, University of Toronto Faculty of Medicine, 1 King's College Circle, Toronto, Ontario M5S 1A8, Canada*

Ian J. Witterick, M.D., F.R.C.S.C. *Consultant Otolaryngologist, Mount Sinai Hospital, 600 University Avenue, Toronto, Ontario M5G 1X5, Canada; and Assistant Professor, Department of Otolaryngology, University of Toronto Faculty of Medicine, 1 King's College Circle, Toronto, Ontario M5S 1A8, Canada*

Foreword

How and by whom diseases of the lacrimal drainage apparatus should be managed are once again topical and pertinent questions. Technical developments in the use of endoscopes, fiber optics, lasers, and video cameras for functional sinus surgery have rekindled the interest of both nasal and ophthalmic surgeons in the endonasal approach to operations on the tear passages. This avenue had all but been abandoned in favor of the direct route described by Toti in 1904. His technique, refined by Dutemps and Bourget in 1921, continues to give predictable and highly successful results.

The outcome of lacrimal surgery depends not only on the location and etiology of the pathological process, but also on the technical skill of the surgeon, who must clearly understand the physiological processes involved in tear production and drainage, as well as have a comprehensive knowledge of the regional anatomy and its many variations.

Arriving at Moorfields Eye Hospital in London in 1973, Jeffrey Hurwitz, the new fellow in lacrimal and orbital surgery, impressed his mentors not only with his energy, capability, and enthusiasm for work but also with his capacity to involve himself in, and bring to fruition, research projects both of a clinical and basic science nature. The somewhat "laid back" image that he presented to the world in those days—casually attired in jeans and cowboy boots—certainly belied the dynamo that lay beneath the shoulder-length hair!

Returning to his native Canada in 1975, Dr. Hurwitz first worked at Sunnybrook Hospital and later at the Mount Sinai Hospital and The Hospital for Sick Children in Toronto. There he directed his tireless energy to accumulating a vast knowledge of lacrimal surgery enjoyed by only a handful of practitioners in the world. As a clinical teacher his expertise is renowned, and the positions on his residency and fellowship programs are coveted by international applicants. In addition to his clinical and teaching commitments, Dr. Hurwitz continues to make regular and important contributions to the scientific literature on the subject.

Uniquely armed with his vast surgical and research experience, there is no one better qualified than Jeffrey Hurwitz to document the theoretical and practical facts available and to put in perspective the relevance of the new developments in the field. He and his contributors have given us a textbook with a uniformity of style that comprehensively covers the subject. It will become an essential part of the armamentarium of any surgeon operating on the tear passages well into the next millennium.

Richard Welham
Director, Lacrimal Unit
Moorfields Eye Hospital
London, England
1971–1993

Preface

Patients with disorders of the lacrimal system comprise a high percentage of those presenting to the ophthalmologist. These patients may also present to the otolaryngologist, plastic surgeon, dermatologist, general practitioner, or dentist. The symptoms may be distressing and very important to the patient, and a satisfactory diagnosis and subsequent rational management is desirable.

The care of these patients has often been less than ideal, falling somewhere between the purvue of ophthalmology, otolaryngology, dentistry, dermatology, and plastic surgery. Although much has been written on the treatment of patients with lacrimal problems, the relationship between the diagnostic and the subsequent therapeutic modalities has been confusing.

Many years have passed since the initial descriptions of the classical operations we perform today. There have been numerous publications describing the use of more modern technology in an attempt to improve the success rate of these procedures and to decrease the morbidity. In order to determine the long-term efficacy of these procedures, a large volume of patients must be available, and long-term follow-up is mandatory.

We have been extremely fortunate in Canada to have a comprehensive universal health care system whereby all patients have access to medical care. With the advent of subspecialization, a system of rational triaging of patients to centers of excellence has evolved. Therefore, it becomes possible to establish a "lacrimal unit," where a high volume of patients can be assessed using clinical, radiological, and other modalities, and treatment can be undertaken with a dedicated team experienced in lacrimal surgery. Such a unit also sets the stage for research endeavors and the possibility for external funding of these important projects. With this large population base, one can ultimately determine with some statistical significance which procedures work and which procedures do not work. Such a unit also has the opportunity of becoming a teaching unit for medical students, residents, and postresidency fellows.

There has been no single-authored work on the lacrimal system in over 20 years. This book formulates a uniform outlook with a particular approach to patients with lacrimal system disorders. Because of the multidisciplinary nature of these patients, key chapters have been co-authored by members of the lacrimal team including otolaryngology, head and neck oncology, ophthalmic pathology, anesthesia, radiology, nuclear medicine, cranio-facial plastic surgery, and, within ophthalmology, cornea and external disease. In addition, because lacrimal disorders affect children as well as adults, there is a designated chapter describing lacrimal disorders in children.

Whenever one describes a uniform approach to a subject, there will undoubtedly be some areas that will be controversial, and some with which others may disagree. The approach outlined in this book may appear to be, in some ways, conservative. However, after one has been in practice for 20 years, one tends to be less enthusiastic about newer and not yet proven techniques, and err on the side of making sure that whatever techniques are utilized have withstood the test of time.

With over 1,500 patients per year presenting to our lacrimal clinic, and with over 450 lacrimal drainage procedures being performed each year, one is able to establish a "game-plan" for the investigation and management of these patients as is outlined in this book.

Jeffrey Jay Hurwitz

Acknowledgments

The Lacrimal Unit was established at Sunnybrook Health Sciences Centre in Toronto in 1975. I would like to thank Dr. John Speakman for helping make this possible by bringing together Ophthalmology with Otolaryngology (Dr. Julian Nedzelski and Dr. Derek Birt), Radiology (Dr. Don MacRea and Dr. Perry Cooper), Nuclear Medicine (Dr. Douglas Chenoweth), and Plastic Surgery (Dr. Ian Munro, Dr. Joseph Gruss, and Dr. Oleh Antonyshyn).

In 1985, Dr. Clive Mortimer, Chairman of Ophthalmology at the University of Toronto, in conjunction with the administration of Mount Sinai Hospital (Mr. Gerry Turner, Mr. Ted Freedman, and Mr. Joe Mapa), made available the opportunity for a multispecialist, multidisciplinary Oculoplastic Unit at Mount Sinai Hospital in Toronto. This regionalization and rationalization of services augmented the scope of the Lacrimal Unit and increased its reputation. The late Dr. Jack Crawford, a mentor and personal friend, was instrumental in the implementation of the program, which incorporated adult lacrimal diseases at Mount Sinai Hospital and pediatric lacrimal diseases at the Hospital for Sick Children. The success of this unit depends on the multidisciplinary collaboration with Otolaryngology (Dr. Jeremy Freeman and Dr. Ian Witterick), Radiology (Dr. Joel Kirsch, Dr. Ted Kassel, and Dr. Nasir Jaffer), Plastic Surgery (Dr. Oleh Antonyshyn), Ophthalmic Pathology (Dr. David Howarth and Dr. Godfrey Heathcote), and the Department of Anesthesia (Dr. Ernest Hew, Dr. Chidam Ananthanarayan, and others). In addition, the collaboration with cornea and external disease specialists, Dr. Raymond Stein at Mount Sinai Hospital and Dr. William Dixon at Sunnybrook Health Sciences Centre, is crucial.

Compilation of the myriad of articles written in this century on the lacrimal system has been a tremendous task. This has been undertaken and accomplished by my son, Cary Hurwitz, and I am indebted to him for the many hours spent in helping to prepare this publication. Thank you also to my son, Michael Hurwitz, for editing numerous chapters.

Lippincott-Raven Publishers and Vickie Thaw have been tremendously supportive throughout the duration of this project.

It would have been impossible to write this book without the tremendous secretarial support of Mrs. Rosemary Williams. Her many hours of wordprocessing during the day, at night, and on the weekends will never be forgotten. Also, I thank my office staff, Mrs. Linda Sheppard and Mrs. Rika Kerum, for keeping things in order during the time that it took to complete this work. The Medical Imaging Department at Mount Sinai—John, Irene, and Randy—have helped tremendously.

I am also indebted to the students, residents, and fellows who have stimulated and challenged me through the past 20 years.

Thank you very much to the many physicians who shared their patients with us at the Lacrimal Clinic. We are grateful for your confidence that, in spite of the fact that we would not be able to cure everyone, we would certainly do our best.

Finally, and perhaps most importantly, I would like to thank Professor Barrie Jones of Moorfields Eye Hospital in London, England, for allowing me the privilege to work under the guidance of Mr. Richard Welham, Director of the Lacrimal Clinic. Mr. Welham had the capacity to make sense of a very difficult and confusing topic. His many patients and students were the beneficiaries of his exceptional talents. I will always be indebted to him for his teaching, guidance, and friendship that he has shown me over the past 20 years.

The Lacrimal System

CHAPTER 1

Anatomy and Physiology of Tear Secretion

Raymond Stein and Jeffrey Jay Hurwitz

The optical quality and normal function of the eye depend on an adequate supply of fluid covering its surface. The anterior surface of the cornea is covered by the tear film, which is composed of three layers: an anterior lipid layer, a middle aqueous layer, and a posterior mucous layer (Fig. 1). The average thickness of the precorneal tear film is 6.5 to 7.5 μm, with the aqueous phase constituting the majority of the thickness.

The tear film is vital for normal corneal function. It has a number of important roles (Fig. 2):

1. moistens and lubricates the anterior surface of the globe
2. provides a smooth optical surface, which allows a sharp image to be focused on the retina
3. removes desquamated corneal cells and bacteria
4. contains antibacterial substances such as lysozyme, lactoferrin, beta-lysin, and immunoglobulin, which play an important role in maintaining the sterility of the ocular surface
5. bathes the cornea and conjunctival epithelial cells in a fluid medium necessary for their proper function and survival
6. provides a slight amount of nourishment to the corneal epithelium, although its glucose concentration is extremely low.

The maintenance of the tear layer depends on a secretory mechanism and a drainage or elimination mechanism (Fig. 3). Components of the secretory component include the lacrimal gland and accessory lacrimal gland tissue, as well as the sebaceous glands of the eyelids and the goblet cells and other mucin-secreting elements of the conjunctiva. The elimination of tears depends on the flow of tears across the eye, aided by the act of blinking, and a drainage system consisting of the lacrimal puncta, canaliculi, sac, and nasolacrimal duct.

The optical quality of the eye depends on the normal functioning of each of these two mechanisms, as well as on a proper balance between them. A disturbing excess of tear fluid may result from obstruction in the drainage system, or from an excessive secretion of tears despite a normal drainage mechanism. Conversely, normal comfort and hydration of the eye may exist with a relative impairment of the outflow mechanism, if this is accompanied by a decrease in tear secretion.

Under normal conditions, the tear fluid comes from the palpebral glands, the so-called basal secretion, which secretes about 1 to 2 μl liquid per minute. It has been estimated that an average secretion of 9.5 μl/day takes place (1). In cases of corneal irritation, emotional excitement, or irritation by foreign bodies, the tear secretion, mainly coming from the lacrimal gland, can increase 20 to 30 times.

The corneal epithelial surface is characterized by fine microvillae and microplicae, which increase the surface area and provide a greater area for attachment of the tear film. Corneal scars, dystrophies, or deposits may result in patches of localized corneal drying.

TEAR FILM LAYERS

Lipid Layer

The lipid layer is 0.1 μm thick and is secreted primarily by the meibomian glands located in the tarsal plates of the upper and lower lids (Figs. 4 and 5). The glands lie in a row at the edge of the upper and lower eyelids and their ducts open directly onto the inner margin of the eyelids. There are approximately 30 to 40 meibomian glands in the upper lid and 20 to 30 smaller glands in the lower lid.

R. Stein: Cornea and External Disease Program, Mount Sinai Hospital, Toronto, Ontario M5G 1X5, Canada.

J. J. Hurwitz: Oculoplastics Program, Mount Sinai Hospital; and Department of Ophthalmology, University of Toronto Faculty of Medicine, Toronto, Ontario M5S 1A8, Canada.

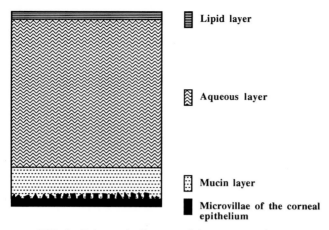

FIG. 1. Schematic diagram of the precorneal tear.

Each gland has an orifice that opens on the lid margin between the tarsal "gray line" and the mucocutaneous junction. The sebaceous glands of Zeis, located at the palpebral margin of the tarsus, and the apocrine glands of Moll, located at the roots of each eyelash, also secrete lipid that is incorporated into the tear film.

Meibum (the meibomian gland secretion) contains hydrocarbons, sterol esters, wax esters, triglycerides, free cholesterol, free fatty acids, and polar lipids (2,3). This layer increases the surface tension of the tear film and decreases its rate of evaporation.

The meibomian glands are located deep in the lid structure and can be visualized by transilluminating the lid. Their gross morphology can be appreciated by transillumination photography employing infrared film. The factors controlling excretion rates in meibomian glands are poorly understood. Extrapolating from what is known concerning the oil glands of the skin, it is probable that excretion of meibum from these glands is at least somewhat influenced by hormonal changes. In infections of the meibomian glands and/or dysfunctional conditions, there is a qualitative change in the excretion with an increase in free fatty acids.

The meibomian gland orifices normally are visible on the eyelid margin and as such are described as open.

When a meibomian gland orifice is not visible on the eyelid margin but oil can be expressed by gentle lid pressure, the orifice is described as "stenosed." If the orifice is not visible and oil cannot be expressed, it is termed "closed."

The meibomian glands are long sebaceous glands that, during their development, separate from the roots of the cilia or eyelashes. Their ducts terminate near the lid margin. The distal portion of the ducts is surrounded by muscle bundles that derive from the orbicularis oculi muscle of the lids. This distal muscle, which is known as Riolan's muscle, is able to squeeze the terminal portion of the ducts so that the meibomian material is secreted onto the lid margin, which results in an oily film over the moistened cornea after blinking. The meibomian glands are located within the tarsal plates, which otherwise consist of collagenous and elastic fibers surrounding the glands. The glands have a vertical orientation. Each consists of a central canal into which open numerous rounded appendages that secrete the sebum.

Meibomian glands consist of lobules or alveolar units of secretory cells that empty into a duct. As the cells move toward the duct, the endoplasmic reticulum develops, as do the lipid-containing droplets synthesized by the endoplasmic reticulum and stored in the cell. Secretion occurs by the degeneration of the lipid droplet–containing cells in the center of the lobule into the ducts.

During blinking, contraction of the pars palpebrae of the orbicularis oculi results in compression of the meibomian glands with resultant secretion occurring by relaxation of the pars marginalis muscles that surround the duct orifice, thus allowing the release of meibum accumulated in the duct (4). Between blinks, the pars marginalis muscles are in a contracted state, preventing the meibomian secretions from leaving the ducts and the pars palpebrae are relaxed, allowing secretions to move into the duct.

In rabbits, early studies suggested the meibomian gland secretion was under sympathetic control as sectioning of the cervical sympathetic nerves increase secretion. There may also be parasympathetic control of meibomian secretion as the nerves surrounding the gland are

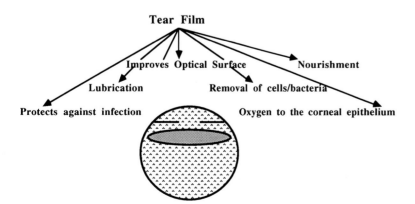

FIG. 2. Functions of the tear film.

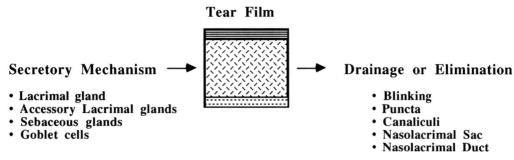

Tear Film

Secretory Mechanism →

- **Lacrimal gland**
- **Accessory Lacrimal glands**
- **Sebaceous glands**
- **Goblet cells**

→ **Drainage or Elimination**

- **Blinking**
- **Puncta**
- **Canaliculi**
- **Nasolacrimal Sac**
- **Nasolacrimal Duct**

FIG. 3. Tear film integrity depends on tears secreted vs. tears drained.

reactive for cholinesterase, and the anticholinesterase physostigmine, which prolongs the activity of acetylcholine (5). Thus, there may be a neuromechanism for meibomian gland secretion in addition to the mechanical effects of blinking.

The glands of Moll are considered specialized sweat glands, which differ from ordinary sweat glands in that their terminal portion is either straight or coiled. The duct length is normally 1.5 to 2 mm and open into the follicles of the eyelashes. The glandular cells produce a secretion rich in proteins and lipoproteins.

The glands of Zeis are small, rudimentary sebaceous glands, morphologically similar to the meibomian glands. They are located within the distal portion of the eyelids near the lid margin. Their ducts open at the lid margin or into the follicle of the eyelashes.

The lipids secreted by the meibomian glands are made up of a variety of lipid components, including waxy esters, nonpolar sterol, other esters, free sterols, triglycerides, and free fatty acids. Polar lipids are reported to account for approximately 15% of meibomian gland secretion. The meibomian lipid is secreted as a fluid. The lipid flows on to the aqueous precorneal tear film. This can be seen as visible streams coming from the meibomian orifices. The orientation of the lipid forming the outermost layer of the tear film is thought to be such that the polar components spread most rapidly with their charged polar groups oriented toward the aqueous phase.

The more slowly spreading nonpolar lipids quite cover the polar layer to form a thicker film.

The presence of an anterior lipid layer of the tear film has been suspected from biomicroscopic observation of interference patterns seen from the surface of the tear film. A uniform field biodifferential interference microscope has been developed that allows three patterns to be identified in the lipid layer:

1. an amorphous pattern
2. a marmoreal pattern
3. a flow pattern.

Other methods to study these lipid patterns include the use of a modified slit-lamp, specular microscopy, keratometry, and a grid pattern consisting of a noninvasive low illuminance reflection instrument that attaches to a slit-lamp and is known as a toposcope.

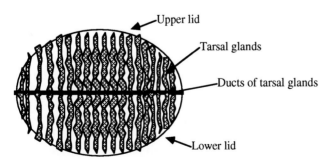

FIG. 4 Posterior view of the eyelids with the palpebral fissure nearly closed. Note the tarsal glands with their short ducts and orifices.

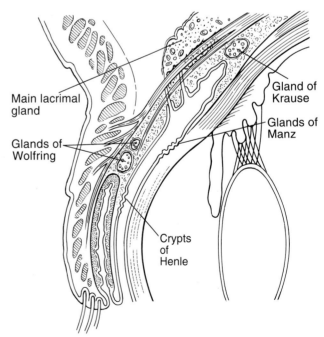

FIG. 5. The accessory lacrimal glands of the upper eyelid. (From Jones, ref. 9, with permission.)

During blinking, it is thought that the lipid layer undergoes a considerable compression and decompression.

Aqueous Layer

The aqueous layer is 0.8 μm thick and is secreted by the main lacrimal glands and by the accessory glands of Krause and Wolfring. This layer accounts for 90% of the tear volume and contains electrolytes, minerals, enzymes, and proteins. Exfoliated epithelial cells, lymphocytes, and remnants of cells are also found within the aqueous layer. Some of these proteins include albumin, lactoferrin, lysozyme, and immunoglobulins. The immunoglobulins come mainly from the conjunctiva and consist basically of IgA and IgG. Normally a serum protein deriving from the conjunctival vasculature does not penetrate into the lacrimal fluid, but it is found in cases of conjunctivitis, sicca syndrome, and other pathological situations. The aqueous layer's main function is to provide nourishment and wetting for the cornea.

The main lacrimal gland provides reflex secretion. This secretion may be in response to a number of different stimuli:

1. physical irritation of the trigeminal nerve (V1) fibers that originate from the conjunctiva, cornea, nasal mucosa, or eyelid margins
2. psychogenic stimulation
3. the effect of bright light on the retina.

The accessory glands of Krause and Wolfring provide basic secretion. There is no known stimulus for basic tear secretion or specific innervation to the basic tear secretory glands. The glands of Krause comprise two thirds of the accessory lacrimal glands and are located in the lateral part of the upper fornix proximal to the main lacrimal gland. A variable number of Krause glands are located in the lower fornix. The glands of Wolfring are located along the orbital margin of each tarsus. Normally there are two to five glands of Wolfring in the upper and two or three in the lower lid. The epithelium of the ducts is continuous with that of the conjunctiva.

The accessory lacrimal glands of Krause and Wolfring located in the conjunctival mucosa are small glands with the same structure as the main lacrimal gland. In humans, there are 4 to 42 accessory lacrimal glands in the upper conjunctival tissue and 6 or fewer in the lower conjunctiva (6). Their weight is about 10% of the weight of the main lacrimal gland.

By histochemical and immunohistochemical techniques the main and accessory lacrimal glands are virtually indistinguishable. Both types of glands contain the regulated secretory proteins lysozyme and lactoferrin and the constitute of protein secretory component (7). The immunoglobulins IgG, IgA, IgM, IgD, and IgE have similar localization in both types of glands (8). The only

recognized difference between the lacrimal and the accessory glands is that the main lacrimal gland stains positively with 4S-100, a marker for nervous tissues and cells of neurocrest origin, and the accessory glands do not (7).

It is thought that 95% of tears arise from the orbital and palpebral portions of the main lacrimal gland. The rest is thought to come from the accessory glands of Krause and Wolfring. Anatomic dissection of cadaver specimens has demonstrated that there is considerable variability in the number and size of accessory lacrimal gland tissue in normal subjects. This variability may account for the importance of the main lacrimal gland in providing adequate tear production in given individuals. The aqueous portion of the tears is secreted as an isotonic or slightly hypotonic solution. The flow of aqueous tears originates in the ductal openings of the main and accessory lacrimal glands in the superior fornix. This fluid flows into the forniceal spaces and flows over the exposed portions of the corneal and conjunctival surface. The flow direction of aqueous fluid is from the temporal to medial aspect of a globe.

This flow is driven by the action of the orbicularis oculi muscle, with the fluid being drawn into the punctal openings in a relaxation phase immediately subsequent to a blink. Some aqueous fluid is lost through evaporation and reabsorption to the conjunctival surface but the majority of fluid flows out through the punctal openings into the superior and inferior canaliculi, then into the common canaliculus, and out to the nasolacrimal duct, emptying out by the inferior meatus in the nasal cavity. There is, however, a considerable reabsorption of this fluid across the mucosa of the nasolacrimal duct during its passage.

When small samples of tears are collected from the marginal tear film and osmolarity is measured, normal subjects showed a value of 302+/−6 mosmol/L. This is approximately isotonic with saline. Earlier studies, however, have found a slightly lower osmolarity from tear samples obtained from the lower fornix. The aqueous tear volume can be studied using fluorimetry measuring the decay rates of concentration of fluorescein instilled in the tear film as a measure of tear film dilution by newly secreted tears. Employing this methodology, tear volume values of 6 to 8 μl have been reported.

The marginal strips have been reported to contain approximately 3.0 μl, precorneal tear film 1 μl, and the fornicial spaces approximately 3 μl. The flow of aqueous tears has been reported to be approximately 1.2 μl/min (range 0.5–2.2), the so-called basal rate of tear secretion occurs in the eye without any evidence of stimulation. With stimulation of tear flow, the volume can be increased 100-fold. The thickness of the tear film has been estimated by a variety of methods and it is reported to be about 6 to 7 μm.

It has been proposed by Jones (9) that aqueous tear secretion driven from both the main and accessory lacrimal glands be divided into "basic" (or "basal") secretion and reflex. He suggested that "basal" secretion can be measured by a Schirmer test following a drop of a topical anesthetic. Subsequent studies have demonstrated a 300% increase in tear turnover rate following lid margin stimulation in the anesthetized human eyes. In addition, tear flow rate in such eyes is found to be greater than that in anesthetized eyes after the testing stimulus was reduced. These data suggest that tear secretion is driven reflexively and that a Schirmer test performed after topical anesthesia is not a measure of "basal" tear flow. In fact, the existence of "basal" tear secretion has been called into question (10).

It is probable that aqueous tear secretion is driven by stimulus at all times. Supporting evidence for this hypothesis comes from the fact that under conditions of decrease in external stimuli, for example night sleep or general anesthesia, aqueous tear secretion diminishes. A similar reduction in salivation occurs during sleep.

Mucous Layer

The mucous layer is the thinnest. It is approximately 0.02 to 0.05 μm thick. It is secreted by the goblet cells of the conjunctiva and spreads directly over the microplicae of the corneal epithelial cells. This acts to decrease surface tension so that the aqueous component of the tears can spread over and absorb to the epithelial surface and make an intact tear film for 15 to 25 seconds between blinks. Abnormalities of the mucin layer or the epithelial surface would cause the tear film to break up rapidly into dry spots after a blink.

This layer is complex but consists mostly of mucous glycoproteins associated with a mixture of protein electrolytes and cellular material.

The goblet cells are unicellular, mucous-secreting glands found within the bulbar and palpebral conjunctiva. The topographic distribution of these cells is highly varied. The greatest density of these cells is found in the inferior palpebral conjunctiva, with approximately 25 to 40 cells/mm. The goblet cell density has been found to be similar in different age groups. However, there is a slight decrease in density in persons in the seventh decade of life or older. Histochemical studies have demonstrated goblet cells stained with Periodic Acid-Schiff (PAS) and alcian blue; these staining characteristics at a pH 1 to 2.5 are consistent with the presence of sulfated and sialoglycoproteins. Fluorescein-conjugated antibody studies against fractions of human tear mucous glycoprotein have demonstrated the presence of this material within the goblet cells.

Holly and Lemp (11) have demonstrated that tear mucous glycoproteins lower the tear surface tension from a level of about 70 dyne/cm to 40 dyne/cm. This is thought to be related to an interaction between mucin and the surface lipid layer. They proposed that the surface corneal epithelium is hydrophobic because of the lipid content of the cell wall and that mucin forms a loose coating that temporarily forms a new surface that is wettable by the overlying aqueous tear layer. This theory is based on a series of experiments in which the mucin layer was carefully wiped from the surface, presumably exposing the underlying epithelial cells. This exposed surface was found to be nonwettable by saline and artificial tear preparations containing proteins. When the surface was wiped by mucous plug, however, aqueous solutions spread over the surface. Subsequent investigators have criticized these experiments by suggesting that this method produced damage to the corneal surface and that the hydrophobicity noted was caused by this trauma.

EYELID MOVEMENT AND THE TEAR FILM

Eyelid movement is important in tear film distribution. As the eyelids close in a complete blink, the superior and inferior fornices are compressed by the force of the preseptal muscle, which is part of the orbicularis muscle, and the lids move toward each other, with the upper lid moving over the largest distance and exerting force on the globe. This force clears the anterior surface of debris and expresses sections from the meibomian glands. The lower lid moves horizontally in the nasal direction and pushes the tear film and debris toward the superior and inferior puncta. When the eyelids are opened, the tear film is redistributed in two steps. Initially, the upper lid attracts the aqueous phase of a tear film by capillary action; secondarily, the lipid layers spread slowly and upward over the aqueous phase.

Abnormalities in the quantity or quality of the tear film (mucin, aqueous, or lipid layer) or problems with the blink response that governs the distribution of tears can create problems.

Tear film osmolarity may be influenced by any disorder that increases evaporation or decreases tear secretion, including meibomian gland dysfunction, and lacrimal gland disease usually due to an autoimmune mechanism (12). In both cases, the surface disease that results is known as keratitis sicca and is characterized by decreased conjunctival goblet cell density and corneal glycogen levels, characteristic epithelial abnormalities, and rose bengal staining (13).

EVAPORATION OF TEARS

The evaporation rate of the normal tear film is low because of the protective oily surface. Approximately 10% to 25% of the total tears secreted are lost by evaporation. In the absence of the protective oily layer, the rate of evaporation is increased 10 to 20 times (11,14).

The tonicity of tears depends on the evaporation process and the rate of tear flow. When evaporation is prevented, the osmotic pressure of tears is equivalent to 0.9% sodium chloride solution. As tear flow increases, the effect of evaporation lessens.

When the eyes are closed, there is no evaporation of tears, and the precorneal tear film is in osmotic equilibrium with the cornea. With the eyes open, evaporation takes place, increasing the tonicity of the tear film and producing an osmotic gradient from the aqueous through the cornea to the tear film. This flow will continue as long as evaporation maintains the hypertonicity of the tear film.

pH OF TEARS

The pH of tears is on average 7.4 (usual range 7.3–7.7), which approximates that of blood plasma. The tear pH is lowest on awakening as a result of acid by-products associated with the relatively anaerobic conditions in prolonged lid closure. It increases with the loss of CO_2 as the eyes are open. Tear pH is characteristic for each individual, and the buffering mechanism maintains the pH at a relatively constant level during waking hours (15). When solutions with a pH level below 6.6 or above 7.8 are instilled into the conjunctival sac, subjective discomfort occurs.

ENZYMES IN TEARS

Lysozyme is a long-chain, high-molecular weight proteolytic enzyme produced by lysosomes. It can dissolve bacterial walls by enzymatic digestion of mucopolysaccharides. The concentration of lysozymes in human tears is greater than in any other body fluid (16). Lysozyme makes up 21% to 25% of the total protein in tears. Its concentration is high enough to be bactericidal only in white blood cells, nasal secretions, and tears. In the presence of epiphora, lysozyme is decreased in concentration. Lysozyme levels decrease with age, although not necessarily in proportion to the decrease in tear volume (17). The bactericidal action of lysozyme depends on pH. The optimum pH for lysis varies with the solubility of the bacterial proteins, but in general it lies between 6.0 and 7.4.

Beta-lysin is a nonlysozymal bactericidal protein that is found in tears and aqueous humor (18). It is derived mainly from platelets, but it is found in higher concentration in tears than in blood plasma. Beta-lysin acts primarily on the cellular membrane, whereas lysozyme dissolves bacterial cell walls.

Twelve enzymes, including lactate dehydrogenase, pyruvate kinase, malate dehydrogenase, and amylase, have been identified in tears. These are present in concentrations similar to those in the lacrimal gland but unlike serum concentrations (19).

PHYSIOLOGY OF TEAR PRODUCTION

Two types of tear secretion, basic and reflex, have been postulated (9). Basic secretion was felt to be a constant, slow secretion by glands such as the accessory lacrimal glands and the goblet cells, which were not known to have innervation. Reflex secretion was defined as an increased rate of secretion caused by neural stimulation and was thought to apply primarily to the main lacrimal gland. A general principle of homeostasis is that all cellular processes are regulated or controlled, and usually very tightly. It is unlikely that the three essential layers of tears from several different glands would not be regulated. Furthermore, even a gland not directly innervated may be subject to paracrine control (diffusion of stimulatory chemicals from a nearby nerve or endocrine cell) or hormonal control. Arguing against the concept of basic versus reflex secretion was a demonstration that tear flow declined and sensory input was decreased, suggesting that secretion by all the orbital glands probably regulated at some level (10). However, only secretion by the main lacrimal gland, the largest and most easily accessible of the orbital glands, has been studied in any detail.

Parasympathetic fibers are in close contact with acinar cells, duct cells, myoepithelial cells, and blood vessels of the lacrimal gland (20). Sympathetic nerves innervate the blood vessels and are in close contact with secretory and myoepithelial cells. The parasympathetic nerves are the major control of both electrolyte/water and protein secretion. Stimulation of the parasympathetic lacrimal nerve or intra-arterial injection of cholinergic agonist stimulates both types of secretion (21). In addition to containing the parasympathetic neurotransmitter acetylcholine, the parasympathetic nerve endings also contain at least one biologically active peptide, vasoactive intestinal peptide (VIP) (22). Intra-arterial injection of VIP stimulates lacrimal gland electrolyte, water, and protein secretion, as do cholinergic agonists (23).

VIP is present in the lacrimal gland as shown by immunochemistry (23). VIP can stimulate tear secretion as evidenced by a report of a patient with pancreatic cholera who had high serum VIP levels, tearing, and a significant Schirmer test, and significantly lower tear osmolarity values than normal controls (24).

In addition to acetylcholine, norepinephrine, and VIP, lacrimal gland nerves also contain other neurotransmitters, including substance P, a family of enkephalins, calcitonin gene-related peptide, and neuropeptide Y (24,25).

These peptides could be present in the sympathetic or parasympathetic nerves and be released with norepinephrine or acetylcholine. Of the peptides identified in the lacrimal gland, only the enkephalins have a known physiologic role: they inhibit protein secretions stimulated by cholinergic agonists or VIP (26). Stimuli of electrolyte and water secretion include cholecystokinin and porcine histidine isoleucine–containing peptide (27).

The accessory lacrimal glands together with the other glands located in the conjunctiva have traditionally been termed "basic secretors." They continuously secrete the protein, electrolytes, and water of the aqueous layer of the tear film and they are not thought to be controlled by nerves or other stimuli. It has not been determined whether the accessory lacrimal glands contain nerve terminals. Indirect evidence suggests that the accessory lacrimal glands can be stimulated to secrete fluid. In a dry eye model in the rabbit, the main lacrimal gland excretory duct was closed by cautery and a variety of tests performed. An increase in tear volume in response to topical application of stimuli has been interpreted as indicating an increase in accessory lacrimal gland secretion (28). There has been no research on the mechanism of water, protein, and electrolyte secretion by the accessory lacrimal glands, but it is likely the mechanisms are similar to those of the main lacrimal gland.

Goblet cells located on the surface of the conjunctiva are the primary secretors of the inner mucous layer of the tear film. The conjunctiva is innervated by sensory parasympathetic and sympathetic nerves. The nerves that innervate blood vessels are present in the subepithelial layers and partially in the epithelium. Nerve endings have not been seen in apposition to goblet cells. There are, however, other stimulatory mechanisms, including paracrine stimulation (release of stimulus from nearby nerve endings or other cells), autocrine stimulation (release of stimulus from self-stimulating goblet cells), and hormonal stimulation. Finally, compounds present in tears could also stimulate goblet cell secretion, for example, epidermal growth factors secreted by lacrimal duct cells into the tears.

NEUROPHYSIOLOGY OF TEAR SECRETION (Fig. 6) (9)

Afferent Pathways

1. *The fifth cranial nerve.* This is the reflex sensory afferent pathway. Any stimulation of the nerve will cause tearing. Fibers from the trigeminal nucleus reach the lacrimal nucleus in the pons. Ocular or nasal irritation via VI afferents may therefore reach the trunk of the fifth nerve to cause tearing.

2. *Ocular.* Retinal stimulation sends messages along fibers that leave the optic nerve, perhaps with pupillary fibers, and reach the lacrimal nucleus in the pons. Therefore, bright light may cause reflex tearing.

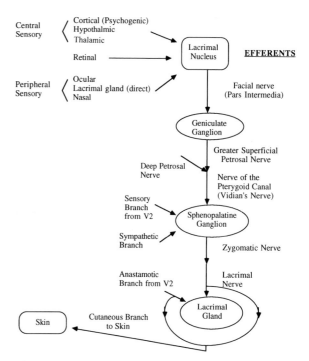

FIG. 6. Neurophysiologic pathways of lacrimal secretion.

3. *Higher levels.* Stimulation of the basal ganglion, thalamus, hypothalamus, cervical sympathetic ganglia, and frontal cortex (psychogenic or emotional crying) may cause an increased secretion of tears.

4. *Parasympathetic and sympathetic fibers* probably play a role in the afferent arc of tear secretion, but the exact mechanism has not been established.

5. *Direct lacrimal gland stimulation.* Certain substances, such as mecholyl, may stimulate the lacrimal gland cells to increase tear production. Thyroid disease may cause hypersecretion in a similar manner.

Efferent Pathways

The seventh nerve (facial nerve) is the efferent pathway for the fibers from the lacrimal nucleus that the afferent pathways ultimately reach. The lacrimal nucleus lies next to the facial nucleus in the pons. From the lacrimal nucleus, the fibers run in the pars intermedia to the geniculate ganglion and become the greater superficial petrosal nerve. The deep petrosal nerve joins the greater superficial petrosal nerve (Vidian's nerve) and travels to the sphenopalatine ganglion. Of note is the fact that parasympathetic fibers (from the zygomatic branch of V2) and sympathetic fibers (from around the sphenopalatine artery) are also present in the sphenopalatine ganglion.

The fibers (sensory, sympathetic, parasympathetic) pass from the sphenopalatine ganglion in the zygomatic nerve (V2). The zygomatic nerve branches into the lacrimal nerve, lying on the inferior surface of the lacrimal gland. Some branches from the lacrimal nerve and the accessory parasympathetic connection pass directly into the gland itself and some course together past the gland to end as a cutaneous branch to the skin.

SUMMARY

Tears are a three-layer structure that is stable and can respond to environmental challenges to protect the ocular surface. The orbital glands and epithelia secrete products including lipids, electrolytes, water, protein, and mucus. The secretion of electrolytes and water from the main lacrimal gland is well documented to be under neuroendocrine control. There is some evidence that secretion from the accessory lacrimal glands, the meibomian glands, and the goblet cells is under neuroendocrine regulation.

REFERENCES

1. Brand T, Fritsch E. Studies on tear secretion. *Acta Ophthalmol (Copenh)* 1967;45:166.
2. Baron C, Blough HA. Composition of the neutral lipids of bovine meibomian secretions. *J Lipid Res* 1976;17:373–376.
3. Tiffany JN. Individual variations in human meibomian lipid composition. *Exp Eye Res* 1978;27:289–300.
4. Linton RG, Curnow DH, Riley WJ. The meibomian glands: an investigation into the secretion and some aspects of the physiology. *Br J Ophthalmol* 1961;45:718–723.
5. Montagna W, Ellis RA. Cholinergic innervation of the meibomian gland. *Anat Rec* 1959;135:121–128.
6. Allansmith MR, Kajiyama G, Abelson MB, Simon MA. Plasma cell content of main and accessory lacrimal glands and conjunctiva. *Am J Ophthalmol* 1976;82:819–826.
7. Vigneswaran N, Wilk CM, Heese A, Hornstein OP, Naumann GOH. Immunohistochemical characterization of epithelial cells 1. Normal major and accessory lacrimal glands. *Graefes Arch Clin Exp Ophthalmol* 1990;228:58–64.
8. Gillette TE, Allan Smith MR, Greiner JV, Janusz M. Histologic and immunohistologic comparison of main and accessory lacrimal tissue. *Am J Ophthalmol* 1980;89:724–730.
9. Jones LT. The lacrimal secretory system and its treatment. *Am J Opthalmol* 1966;62:47–64.
10. Jordan A, Baum J. Basic tear flow, does it exist? *Ophthalmology* 1980;87:920–930.
11. Holly FJ, Lemp MA. Tear physiology and dry eyes. *Surv Ophthalmol* 1989;22:69–87.
12. Gilbard JP, Rossi SR, Gray KL. Mechanisms for increased tear osmolarity. In: Cavanagh D, ed. *The cornea: transactions of the World Congress on the Cornea III.* New York: Raven Press; 1988: 5–7.
13. Ralph RA. Conjunctival goblet cell density in normal subjects and in dry eye syndromes. *Invest Ophthalmol Vis Sci* 1975;14:299–302.
14. Mishima S. Some physiological aspects of the precorneal tear film. *Arch Ophthalmol* 1965;73:233.
15. Carney LG, Hill RM. Human tear pH. *Arch Ophthalmol* 1976;94:821.
16. Milder B, Weil BA. *The lacrimal system.* Norwalk, CT: Appleton-Century-Crofts; 1983.
17. Pietsch RL, Pearlman ME. Human tear lysozyme variables. *Arch Ophthalmol* 1973;90:94.
18. Ford LC, DeLange RJ, Petty RW. Identification of a nonlysozymal bactericidal factor (beta lysin) in human tears and aqueous humor. *Am J Ophthalmol* 1976;81:30.
19. Van Haeringen NJ, Glasius E. Enzymatic studies in lacrimal secretion. *Exp Eye Res* 1974;19:135.
20. Ichikawa A, Nakajima Y. Electron microscope study on the lacrimal gland of the rat. *Tohoku J Exp Med* 1962;77:136–149.
21. Botelho SY, Hisada M, Fuenmayor N. Functional innervation of the lacrimal gland in the cat. *Arch Ophthalmol* 1966;76:581–588.
22. Nikkinen A, Lehtosalo JI, Uusitalo H, Palkama A, Panula P. The lacrimal glands of the rat and guinea pig are innervated by nerve fibers containing immunoreactivities for substance P and vasoactive intestinal peptide. *Histochemistry* 1984;81:23–27.
23. Dartt DA. Signal transduction and control of lacrimal protein secretion: a review. *Curr Eye Res* 1989;8:619–636.
24. Gilbard JP, Dartt DA, Rood RP, Rossi SR, Gray KL, Donowitz M. Increased tear secretion in pancreatic cholera a newly recognized symptom in an experiment of nature. *Am J Med* 1980;85:552–554.
25. Lehtosalo J, Uusitalo H, Mahrberg T, Panula P, Palkama A. Nerve fiber showing immunoreactivities for proenkephalin A–derived peptides in the lacrimal glands of the guinea pig. *Graefes Arch Clin Exp Ophthalmol* 1989;227:455–458.
26. Cripps MM, Bennett DJ. Peptidergic stimulation and inhibition of lacrimal gland adenylate cyclase. *Invest Ophthalmol Vis Sci* 1990;31:2145–2150.
27. Dartt DA, Shulman M, Gray KL, Rossi SR, Matkin C, Gilbard JP. Stimulation of rapid lacrimal gland secretion with biologically active peptides. *Am J Physiol* 1988;254:300–306.
28. Gilbard JP, Rossi SR, Heyda KG, Dartt DA. Stimulation of tear secretion by topical agents that increase cyclic nucleotide levels. *Invest Ophthalmol Vis Sci* 1990;31:1381–1388.

CHAPTER 2

Embryology of the Lacrimal Drainage System

Jeffrey Jay Hurwitz

The embryology of the lacrimal system, in conjunction with the development of the nose and the eyelids, is important in the understanding of congenital abnormalities of the lacrimal drainage pathways. The understanding of this process is facilitated by dividing the embryology into three groups:

1. early embryology of the face
2. development of the upper end of the nasolacrimal passages
3. development of the lower end of the nasolacrimal passages.

EARLY DEVELOPMENT OF THE FACE

The first indication of the development of the nose, which is the key in the developing face, is in a 6.5-mm embryo as the development of the placodes (Fig. 1). Around each nasal placode three swellings develop: the maxillary process, the medial nasal process, and the lateral nasal process. In the 7-mm embryo there is an outgrowth of the placode via a nasal groove that forms between the medial and lateral elevations. The nasal pit then develops into the nasal tube. Within the lateral wall of the nasal tube, the lateral nasal process and maxillary process are separated by grooves at the lateral side (to become the face) and the medial side (to become the nasal lumen). The epithelial linings of the walls come into contact with each other and a double epithelial layer develops at these points of contact. The nasolacrimal duct develops from the lateral groove, which runs into the optic cup. The lower end of the nose develops from the medial one (1) (Fig. 2).

J. J. Hurwitz: Oculoplastics Program, Mount Sinai Hospital; and Department of Ophthalmology, University of Toronto Faculty of Medicine, Toronto, Ontario M5S 1A8, Canada.

The frontal nasal process, which had previously split into the medial and lateral nasal processes, gives rise to the upper lid bud, whereas the maxillary process gives rise to the lower lid bud. During the sixth week of development, the lateral nasal wall begins to develop grooves that will become the turbinates and the nasal meati. The maxillary process will develop into the beginnings of the inferior turbinate. Canalization in the area of the inferior meatus develops, but it does not form the nasolacrimal canal. The inferior turbinates begin as structures sitting against the lateral wall of the nose. With growth and elongation, they tend to move in a more medial and inferior direction, allowing for an opening to develop in the inferior meatus. However, the movement in the inferior and medial direction is variable. Potentially, fusion at the junction of the inferior turbinate and the lateral nasal wall might account for a bony obstruction that may develop between the nasolacrimal canal and the inferior meatus, or a nondevelopment of the nasolacrimal canal inferiorly. It may also account for the fact that, if the nasolacrimal canal is present at the floor of the inferior meatus but the inferior turbinate is abutting on the lateral wall of the nose, a fracturing of the inferior turbinate to open up the upper recesses of the meatus may be therapeutic.

DEVELOPMENT OF THE UPPER SYSTEM

The cells in the area of the lacrimal sac are thicker than cells elsewhere within the developing system. Canalization may occur within the lacrimal sac initially, and spread toward the canaliculi and toward the nasolacrimal duct (Fig. 3). However, canalization probably occurs fairly uniformly within the system (Fig. 4). As the epithelial buds grow toward the eyelids, they branch into two smaller buds, and these will become the canaliculi (Fig. 5). Because of the rapid growth of the maxilla compared

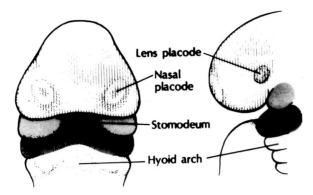

FIG. 1. Development of the nasal placode in a 6.5-mm embryo. (From Older, ref. 9.)

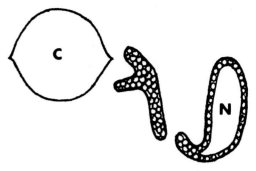

FIG. 3. The system begins to develop in the 6-week-old embryo. (From Duke-Elder and Cook, ref. 10.)

to the growth of the frontal bone, the migration laterally causes the inferior canaliculus to be pulled in that direction. For this reason, the inferior punctum comes to lie at a more lateral position than that of the superior punctum. The exaggerated lateral growth of the lower lid and canaliculus accounts for a fold of conjunctiva to develop at the inner canthus, which becomes the plica. There is also a plug of ectoderm that is pulled laterally to become the caruncle. Accessory canaliculi may develop if more than two cords stem superolaterally from the rudimentary lacrimal sac. They may grow toward the eyelids and represent true canaliculi. However, there may also, at a later date of embryogenesis, be outpouchings from the rudimentary canaliculi, which may themselves grow into the eyelid. These would represent side openings in the canaliculi. Accessory channels may develop and end not in the eyelids but below the caruncle on the skin. These have been referred to as "lacrimal anlage ducts" (2). These structures are really a form of lacrimal fistulae, with connections to the canaliculus or common canaliculus.

Canalization is usually complete at the puncta when the lids separate at about 7 months of gestation. How-

ever, some authors feel that the puncta are patent at 6 months of gestation, or even at 4 months in certain individuals (3). Therefore, an earlier maldevelopment (4–6 months of gestation) might produce a total absence of the punctum and papilla. A later maldevelopment when the eyelids separate (6–7 months) might produce a normal punctal papilla, with a small imperforate membrane overlying it.

At the same time as the canaliculi and puncta are developing, the orbicularis muscle is developing from the local mesenchymal tissue. The sphincter-like orbicularis can be seen to cover the entire anterior surface of the lids while the lids are fused. When the lids separate, the muscles separate as well and the medial canthal tendon is developed (4). The muscle usually surrounds the canaliculi by the time the eyelids separate. It is felt that if the punctum develops and there is a papilla, with an obstructing membrane over it, the musculature around the canaliculus and punctum is probably normal. The membrane may indeed be a failure of the conjunctiva that overlies the canaliculus to spontaneously perforate. There may be a hereditary predisposition for this abnormality. If there is total absence of the punctum and papilla, the canaliculi may either be imperforate (due to a lack of canalization of the canalicular cord) or may be totally absent (due to the nondevelopment of the cana-

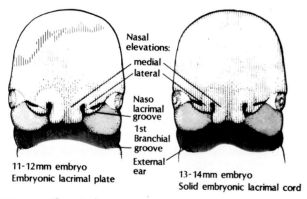

FIG. 2. The 11.5-mm embryo showing the development of the embryonic lacrimal plate. The 13.5-mm embryo showing the solid embryonic lacrimal cord. (From Older, ref. 9.)

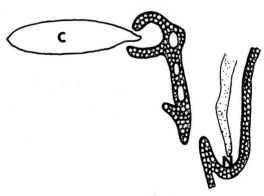

FIG. 4. The solid cord begins to develop a lumen at 12 weeks. (From Duke-Elder and Cook, ref. 10.)

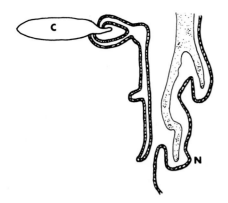

FIG. 5. Canalization begins through the duration of gestation. (From Duke-Elder and Cook, ref. 10.)

licular cord). These situations usually cannot be rectified surgically, and a bypass tube is usually necessary in the latter situation.

DEVELOPMENT OF THE LOWER END OF THE NASOLACRIMAL SYSTEM

Canalization seems to begin at approximately the fourth month of gestation, usually in the area of the lac-

rimal sac. The lacrimal sac epithelial cords are thicker, and therefore the sac, when it canalizes, has a larger diameter than the canaliculi or the nasolacrimal canal. If there is a defect in the optic end of the naso-optic fissure, congenital fistulae of the lacrimal sac may develop with communication to the skin. Usually there is some thickening of the skin around the fistulous opening. The nasolacrimal sac, and especially the nasolacrimal duct, may have many irregular outpouchings. These seem to decrease with development of the fetus and become less prominent. These diverticulae are quite common and of little significance.

Most of the abnormalities that occur within the lacrimal system do so after the fourth month of gestation. It is exceedingly rare to have a total maldevelopment of all the nasolacrimal passages, but this may occur in patients who have facial clefts, cyclops, and other rare conditions (5). Some authors have felt that there is a bud of cells from the inferior meatus that grows toward the lacrimal sac and eventually joins with the sac that is canalizing in an inferior direction. However, dissections of fetuses at various stages of development have shown that this is probably not true (3,6). It would seem that canalization of the nasolacrimal duct proceeds inferiorly until it strikes a membrane at the superolateral aspect of the in-

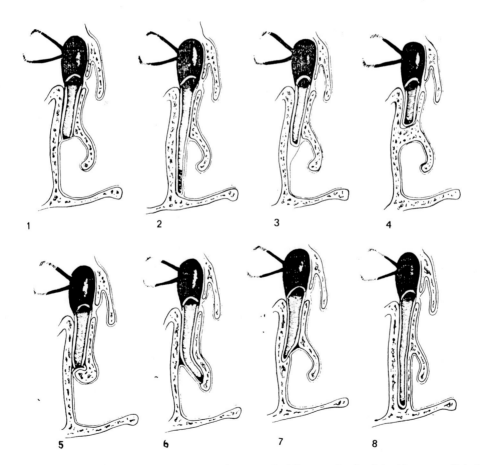

FIG. 6. The eight types of variations seen in a lower end of the nasolacrimal duct in congenital obstructions. (From Schaefer et al., ref. 11, with permission.)

TABLE 1. *Embryonic development of the lacrimal system and associated structures*

Gestational age	Embryonic size	Tissue differentiation
Day 21	4–5 mm	Sensory epithelium of the olfactory placode is present in the nasal area
		Visceral mesenchyme of the maxillary process is at the lower part of the eye, though not yet an eyelid fold
Day 24		The optic pit makes contact with the neural crest
Day 26	6–7 mm	The optic vesicle is sheathed with neural crest cells
		The nasal areas become depressed due to mesenchymal thickening
		The mesenchyme starts to form the extraocular muscles
Days 27–33		All recti and oblique muscles and their nerves develop
Day 32	8–9 mm	The frontonasal process becomes the medial and lateral nasal processes
		The maxillary process makes contact with the nasal processes
Day 36	9–12 mm	The mesenchyme condenses into the sclera
		Epithelial buds from the superior conjunctival fornix appear and the lacrimal gland bud begins
		Grooves appear on the lateral nasal wall, the inferior and middle meatuses begin
Day 45	16 mm	The maxillary process gives rise to the lower eyelid bud
	22 mm	The extraocular muscles insert onto the cartilaginous skeleton of the sphenoid
	22–30 mm	The dorsomedial aspect of the superior rectus muscle gives rise to the levator muscle
		The maxillary process overgrows, buries the surface ectoderm in the nasooptic fissure and fuses with the lateral nasal process
		Mesenchymal plates between the nasal sacs and mouth cavity become reduced and form the nasobuccal membranes
	25 mm	Invading nerve fibers and collagen fibrils are seen in the eyelids
		Paraxial mesenchyme gives rise to the upper eyelid bud beginning at the outer canthus
Day 48		Evagination of the nasal epithelium begins formation of the ethmoid sinus
	30 mm	Buried surface ectoderm in the nasooptic fissure sends two solid epithelial cords to the rims of the upper and lower lids
	32 mm	The eyelids begin to grow and meet. There is controversy as to whether they meet at the inner or outer canthus first
Month 3	35–37 mm	The eyelids fuse
	38–40 mm	The epithelial cords to the eyelids canalize
	40 mm	The lacrimal sac is outlined by a connective tissue sheath
	45 mm	Evagination of the ethmoid infundibulum gives rise to the maxillary sinus
		Desmosomes are present at the site of eyelid fusion
		The orbicularis muscle and eyelashes form
	52 mm	The conjunctival sac has mucus-secreting goblet cells
	60 mm	The recti tendons fuse with the sclera
		Motor fibers are seen in the orbicularis muscle
		The orbital walls differentiate
	80 mm	The meibomian glands appear as epithelial buds
		The apocrine glands of Moll start to develop
Month 4	90–100 mm	Sebaceous Zeiss glands develop and start producing lipid
	110–120 mm	The cilial canals keratinize
		The levator muscle is completed
		Canalization of the nasolacrimal duct system is occurring
Month 5	150–170 mm	The anterior surface of the eyelids separate
	170 mm	The meibomian glands keratinize
	180–200 mm	The posterior surface of the eyelids separate
		The levator palpebrae tendon begins to divide the lacrimal gland
		Evagination from the nasal chamber begins to form the ethmoid sinus
Month 6		Sensory nerve fibers are identifiable in the tarsus and eyelid skin
		Evagination from the nasal fossa fuses with the inferior nasolacrimal duct (reported but unlikely)
		The greater wing of the sphenoid ossifies and fuses
Month 7		The cellular plug of the raised lacrimal papillae detaches and the punctum open
		The eyelashes are shed and replaced twice
		Krause's corpuscles are seen in the subcutaneous tissues

From Kaplan, ref. 12, with permission.

ferior meatus. The nasolacrimal duct itself is often dilated before canalization occurs. Of note is the fact that the duct canalization proceeds toward the inferior meatus in a medial direction, and not in a straight line. This would suggest that probing of the nasolacrimal duct may cause a false passage with the probe directed too far laterally at the lower end (7). The opening of the nasolacrimal duct into the inferior meatus (at the valve of Hasner) depends on two factors: (a) the separation of the inferior turbinate from the lateral wall of the nose, and (b) the perforation of the fibromucous membrane at the junction of the soft tissues of the nasolacrimal duct and the mucous membrane of the inferior meatus.

It has been shown by Sevel (6) that in newborns approximately 60% to 70% of fetuses examined do not have an opening between the nasolacrimal canal and the inferior meatus, and there is an obstructing membrane at the mucosal level. Most of these membranes, however, will perforate spontaneously during the first month of life. Occasionally, the clump of cells in the nasolacrimal duct area will grow toward the skin rather than toward the inferior meatus and cause a fistulous opening through the skin (8). Jones and Wobig (2) described eight types of variations seen at the lower end of the nasolacrimal duct in congenital obstructions of this area (Fig. 6):

1. *The duct ends at or near the superior vault of the inferior meatus and canalization of the membrane does not develop.* This is the usual obstruction that one sees, and will most often resolve spontaneously. If not, it is the type of obstruction that can usually be cured with a high success rate by probing.

2. *The duct is located along the lateral wall of the nose and extends to the floor of the nose lateral to the nasal mucosa.* There is a mucosal membrane between the inferior meatus and the inferomedial aspect of the lacrimal duct. It is more difficult to cure this problem with probing, and perhaps fracturing the inferior turbinate away from the lateral wall might help to open up the obstructing membrane.

3. *The duct may extend midway down the lateral wall of the inferior meatus without an opening into it.* The mucosal obstruction might be cured spontaneously or by probing, perhaps in conjunction with fracturing of the inferior turbinate.

4. *The duct ends quite superior to the inferior meatus and there is a bony obstruction.* This may be seen with cleft abnormalities or if there is a fusion of the bone of the superior aspect of the inferior turbinate with the lateral wall of the nose. It is often impossible to cure these abnormalities with probing, and a dacrocystorhinostomy (DCR) may become necessary.

5. *Obstruction of the lower end of the duct at the superior aspect of the inferior meatus because of an impacted inferior turbinate.* An inferior turbinectomy might help, but, failing this, a DCR might be indicated.

6. *The duct ending blindly in the anterior end of the inferior turbinate.* This might open spontaneously or, if necessary, a probing possibly in conjunction with an outfracturing of the turbinate might be indicated.

7. *The duct ends blindly in the medial wall of the maxillary sinus.* Treatment will depend on whether there is mucosa and/or bone between the lower end of the duct and the inferior meatus. With a mucosal obstruction, spontaneous resolution may occur and, if not, a probing might be therapeutic. With a bony obstruction, a probing, possibly with tubes, might be useful. Failing this, a DCR would be indicated.

8. *The nasolacrimal canal is encased in bone to the floor of the lateral wall of the nose with no opening into the inferior meatus.* It would seem that this bony obstruction would be impossible to cure without a DCR.

SUMMARY

The development of the nasolacrimal system is complex and proceeds during virtually all phases of development of the embryo (Table 1). The system begins to develop in the 6-week-old embryo (Fig. 3). The solid cord begins to disintegrate at 12 weeks (Fig. 4), and canalization then begins through the duration of gestation (Fig. 5).

Abnormalities in the normal embryologic development of the nasolacrimal system can account for the various congenital abnormalities that we see clinically. An understanding of these abnormalities helps one in planning appropriate management.

REFERENCES

1. Vermeij-Keers C. *De facialismusculatuur en transformaties in het kopgebied.* Thesis. Leiden; 1967.
2. Jones LT, Wobig JL. *Surgery of the eyelid and lacrimal system.* Birmingham: Aesculapius; 1976:160.
3. Adenis JP, Lebraud T, Leboutet MJ, Loubet R, Loubet A. Étude embryologic des voies lacrymales chez l'homme. *J Fr Ophthalmol* 1983;6:351.
4. Sevel D. A reappraisal of the development of the eyelids. *Eye* 1988;2:123.
5. Mann I. *Developmental abnormalities of the eye.* Philadelphia: JB Lippincott; 1957:371.
6. Sevel D. Development and congenital abnormalities of the nasolacrimal apparatus. *J Pediatr Ophthalmol Strabismus* 1981;18:123.
7. Busse H, Muller KM, Kroll P. Radiologic and histologic findings of the lacrimal passages of newborn. *Arch Ophthalmol* 1980;9:528.
8. Lowe D, Martin F, Beckenham E, Williams B. Congenital lower nasolacrimal duct anomaly—a case report. *Austr N Z J Ophthalmol* 1986;14:65.
9. Older JJ. Congenital lacrimal disorders and management. In: Linberg JV, ed. *Lacrimal surgery.* New York: Churchill Livingstone; 1988:92.
10. Duke-Elder S, Cook C. Normal and abnormal development part I. Embryology. In: Duke-Elder S, ed. *System of ophthalmology,* vol 3. Chicago: CV Mosby; 1963.
11. Schaefer AJ, Campbell CB, Flanagan JC. Congenital lacrimal disorders. In: *Ophthalmic plastic and reconstructive surgery,* vol 2. Chicago: CV Mosby; 1987:943–944.
12. Kaplan LJ. Embryology of the bifunctional lacrimal system. *Adv Ophthal Plast Reconstruct Surg* 1984;3:1.

CHAPTER 3

Anatomy of the Lacrimal Drainage System

David Cowen and Jeffrey Jay Hurwitz

The anatomy of the lacrimal system can be divided into secretory, distributory, and excretory components. The secretory component of the lacrimal system comprises the lacrimal gland and the accessory lacrimal glands. The distributory portion can be divided into the tear film and the eyelids. The secretory system and the tear film of the lacrimal system have been included in Chapter 1. The eyelids and the excretory component of the lacrimal system provide a fascinating and intriguing study of both form and function. The specifics of function as pertaining to the dynamic elements of the lids and the excretory system are appropriately covered in Chapter 4. Understanding and increased knowledge of the anatomy of the lacrimal system has spanned well over 100 years (1,2). Recent developments further delineating the actual configuration and anatomy of the lacrimal system continue to add knowledge where previously there had been speculation (2). This review of the anatomy of the lacrimal system will present the anatomy of the eyelids, primarily their static features, and divide the lids generally into regions medial and lateral to the lacrimal puncta. The anatomy of the excretory system is divided into a review of the osteology and soft tissue components of the system. Nasal anatomy is presented in Chapter 5.

EYELID ANATOMY

The eyelids represent one of the most critical structures of soft tissue facial anatomy. Their normal development, configuration, and function are critical not only

to the visual apparatus but also to the proper functioning and maintenance of the lacrimal excretory system. Aberrations or malfunctioning of the eyelids from changes related to aging, trauma, or other elements of pathogenesis potentially affect the normal functioning and physiology of the lacrimal system. A proper understanding of normal eyelid anatomy and physiology is not only central to the evaluation and diagnosis of lacrimal excretory problems but is even more important when considering medical or surgical intervention in problems affecting the lacrimal system.

SUPERFICIAL EYELID ANATOMY

Human anthropometric studies have demonstrated wide variations in the normal soft tissue landmarks in the human. Farkas has characterized the variation of landmarks and measurements developmentally, between races, and between genders (3). In general, the adult palpebral aperture measures approximately 10 to 14 mm vertically and 28 to 32 mm horizontally. The normal resting position of the upper eyelid is to be found at the upper limbus in the pediatric and young adult population. In the absence of pathologic changes, the position is more frequently 1 to 2 mm lower in the adult. With few exceptions, the position of the lower eyelid is generally accepted to be at the lower limbus. In their resting positions, the lower eyelids make complete contact with the eye the full length of the arc of each eyelid, departing from their contact from the eye medially in the area of the caruncle and plica semilunaris. The horizontal relationship between the medial and lateral canthal regions varies according to race. The antimongoloid angulation describes the relative position of the medial canthus approximately 1 to 2 mm below that of the lateral. The reverse is seen in the mongoloid configuration of the canthi (3). The proper orientation and position of each of these superficial structures is critically important in

D. Cowen: Oculoplastics Program, Mount Sinai Hospital, Toronto, Ontario M5S1A8, Canada; and Department of Ophthalmology, University of Kentucky College of Medicine, Lexington, Kentucky 40536.

J. J. Hurwitz: Oculoplastics Program, Mount Sinai Hospital; and Department of Ophthalmology, University of Toronto Faculty of Medicine, Toronto, Ontario M5S 1A8, Canada.

the proper physiologic functioning of the lacrimal excretory system.

EYELID SUPPORTIVE STRUCTURES

The subcutaneous and supportive structures of the eyelid involve contributions from muscular and fibrous tissues. Each of these structures must be oriented and positioned correctly relative to each other and to the eye in order to insure normal physiologic function of the lacrimal system. The muscular structure of the eyelid lateral to the punctum comprises divisions of the orbicularis oculi muscle. Jones has elegantly demonstrated in his writings the divisions of the orbicularis muscles (4). The normal function of the preseptal and pretarsal orbicularis innervated by the seventh cranial nerve generates the normal blink response by contracture of the muscle and thereby closure of the eyelid. The fibrous components of each eyelid are represented by the tarsal plates and septum orbitale. The intimate relationship between the muscular and fibrous elements of the eyelid is critical for normal apposition to the globe and formation of the palpebral aperture. The lateral insertion of the muscular and fibrous components of the eyelids into the periosteum and bone at Whitnall's tubercle forms the normal lateral canthus. At their point of insertion posterior to the lateral rim, they draw the eyelids posteriorly and thereby place them in direct contact with the globe.

The anatomy of the lacrimal region becomes complex at the level of the upper or proximal portion of the lacrimal excretory system. At the level of the puncta, the pretarsal orbicularis muscle divides. The deep pretarsal heads of the orbicularis muscle insert on the posterior lacrimal crest and on the lacrimal fascia (Horner's muscle) (Fig. 1A). The deep portion of the preseptal orbicularis muscle inserts primarily on the lacrimal fascia. Between the deep and the superficial fibers of the orbicularis muscle are the lacrimal canaliculi and sac. The anterior and superficial fibers of the pretarsal orbicularis insert along the anterior lacrimal crest on the frontal process of the maxillary bone, and onto the frontal bone (Fig. 1B).

The positioning of these muscles is felt not only to contribute to the lacrimal pump mechanism, but also the appropriate anatomic positioning of the tissues of the medial canthal region relative to the globe. The attachments to the lacrimal fascia as described by Horner are felt to contribute directly to the functioning of the lacrimal pump (1). Aberration or loss of structural integrity in any of these structures as might be seen in lid laxity, entropion or ectropion from loss of insertion of the retractors, and especially malposition of a puncta can potentially result in symptomatic epiphora.

OSTEOLOGY

The bony anatomy of the lacrimal excretory system can be divided into proximal, orbital, and distal (nasal) components. The bones of the lacrimal excretory system begin at the fossa superiorly, continuing inferiorly as the nasolacrimal canal terminating laterally and inferiorly in the inferior meatus underneath the inferior turbinate of the nose.

The superior and proximal component is the lacrimal excretory fossa. This fossa contains the lacrimal sac and at times the proximal portions of the nasolacrimal canal.

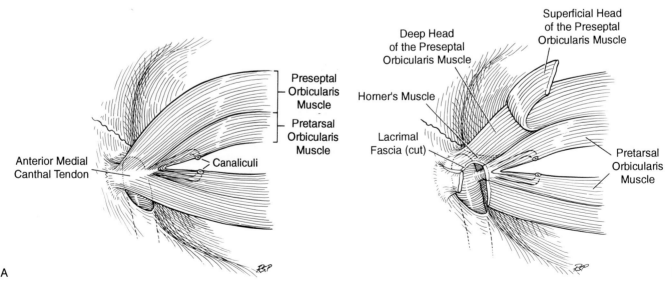

A

B

FIG. 1. A: Superficial pretarsal and preseptal orbicularis oculi musculature in relationship to lacrimal drainage pathways and lacrimal drainage structures. **B:** Preseptal and pretarsal orbicularis contributions to the lacrimal fascia. Cut-away fascia reveals underlying lacrimal excretory passages. (Courtesy of Richard Pennell, Lexington, KY.)

The position and configuration of the fossa varies considerably and, therefore, can dramatically affect surgery performed in this area. Approximate dimensions are 14 to 16 mm vertically, 4 to 8 mm anteroposteriorly, and 2 to 4 mm in depth (5). The bones comprising the lacrimal excretory fossa are the frontal process of the maxillary bone anteriorly, and the lacrimal bone posteriorly. In general, these bones form the anterior and posterior lacrimal crests, respectively. These two bones join in a vertical fashion at the lacrimal-maxillary suture (Fig. 2). The horizontal suture is encountered at the superior aspect of the fossa, where the nasal process of the frontal bone encounters the superior edges of each of these bones. Some have termed the suture between the nasal process of the frontal bone and frontal process of the maxillary bone the "sutura notha." This runs inferiorly just anterior to the anterior lacrimal crest. Elevation of the lacrimal sac from the fossa often reveals an arm of this suture as well as the frequent presence of a penetrating blood vessel.

The relative contributions of the maxillary and lacrimal bones affect the position of the lacrimal fossa and, therefore, the thickness of the bone encountered in the fossa. Regardless of the contribution of each bone, the fossa varies in all its dimensions ranging from a very shallow, superficial, and low-lying fossa to a very deep, almost entirely bone-encapsulated fossa (6). A lacrimal fossa characterized by a significant contribution from the frontal process of the maxillary bone will be characterized by a thick-boned fossa, potentially presenting considerable difficulty for the lacrimal surgeon performing an osteotomy.

As noted above, the anterior and posterior lacrimal crests are the location for the bony attachments of the

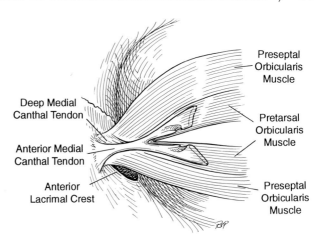

FIG. 3. The medial canthal tendon relative to the lacrimal sac and lacrimal fossa. (Courtesy of Richard Pennell, Lexington, KY.)

superficial and deep components of the medial canthal tendon (Fig. 3). Depending on the position of the fossa and the lacrimal sac relative to the medial canthal tendon structures, these may or may not be encountered at the time of dacryocystorhinostomy (DCR). The posterior and superior extensions of the medial canthal tendon should be respected as these are the primary supportive structures of the medial canthal tendon. The anterior extensions are less critical for support and are often sacrificed at the time of surgery. Loss of all supportive structures can, therefore, result in telecanthus.

The lacrimal sac fossa courses posteriorly, inferiorly, and laterally to develop into the nasolacrimal canal. The canal terminates in the inferior meatus beneath the inferior turbinate. The three bones that are found to contribute varying portions of the canal are the maxillary and lacrimal bones and, in some cases, the inferior turbinate. The anterior, posterior, and lateral walls of the canal are usually formed by the maxillary bone. The medial wall comprises the lacrimal bone superiorly (rarely the maxillary) and by an extension of the inferior turbinate inferiorly (7). Uncomplicated contribution of these bones creates a medial wall of the canal and fossa that, upon removal during osteotomy, allows access to the underlying nasal mucosa and, therefore, the nasal cavity. Significant variation occurs, however, depending on the anterior and inferior positioning of the anterior ethmoidal air cells. Extensive pneumatization of the lacrimal bone may result in intervening air cells between the lacrimal fossa and nasal bone and mucosa. Awareness of this variation is critical in surgical considerations during DCR. Studies by Whitnall demonstrate that in approximately 50% of individuals studied, the air cells extend at least to the lacrimal crest, with additional extension to the maxillary-lacrimal suture in 30% (8).

Nasal anatomy is described in Chapter 5. One must remember that the position and variation of the middle

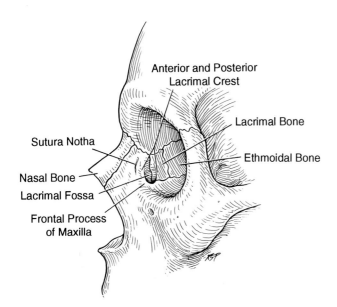

FIG. 2. Osteology of the lacrimal drainage system. (Courtesy of Richard Pennell, Lexington, KY.)

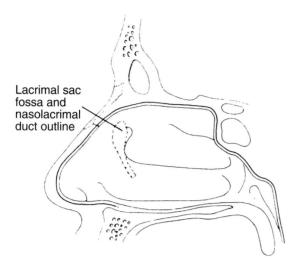

FIG. 4. Relationship of the lacrimal drainage system to the lateral wall of the nose.

turbinate relative to the lacrimal fossa can present additional difficulties at the time of surgery. Excision of the middle turbinate is frequently required to adequately complete a thorough DCR and to allow the creation of sufficient nasal and lacrimal flaps (Fig. 4).

LACRIMAL EXCRETORY PASSAGES

Structure

Ongoing investigation of the anatomy of the lacrimal excretory system continues to contribute valuable information to the understanding of this system and helps to explain phenomena seen clinically, such as the nonregurgitating mucocele.

The three-dimensional configuration of the excretory system reveals a great deal of variability that is often experienced at the time of probing of the nasolacrimal duct. Specifically, variation is known to exist in the width, length, and angulation of the nasolacrimal canal. Angulation differences in osteology and differences that may exist between male and female anatomy explain much of what is seen clinically by the ophthalmologist. Recent communication by Linberg and colleagues demonstrates the presence of acute angulation at the level of the canaliculi and the entrance of the common canaliculus into the lacrimal sac. Their studies using rigid anatomic casts of the lacrimal outflow system demonstrate that at the junction of the upper and lower canaliculus, the common canaliculus angles anteriorly at a mean angle of approximately 118°. As a result, the common canaliculus enters the lacrimal sac at a mean angulation of approximately 58° (2). This acute angulation of the common canaliculus as it enters the lacrimal sac potentially explains the nonregurgitating lacrimal sac mucocele and acute dacryocystic retention. The upper and lower cana-

liculi have an angle of approximately 50° as they enter the common canaliculus (9) (Fig. 5).

Variation is also found in the angulation of the lacrimal sac and canal. Generally, the lacrimal sac and canal assume a 15° posterior inclination with a great deal of variability seen in the lateral angulation. This angulation varies from 0 to 30° depending on the anatomy and location of the canthi, and the osteology of the individual (6). Individuals with wider noses or with narrower intercanthal distances generally are seen to have a greater angulation of the nasolacrimal canal. An understanding of these variations and a respect for them is critical, particularly when undertaking probing of the nasolacrimal excretory system.

Puncta and Canaliculi

The lacrimal puncta represent the most proximal portion of the lacrimal excretory system. The normal puncta are patent superiorly and inferiorly and are positioned in such a way that they point posteriorly into the lacrimal lake lateral to the caruncle. They are slightly elevated above the normal level of the lid margin, resting on what is termed the "lacrimal papilla." The upper puncta is generally located approximately 8 mm from the tear sac

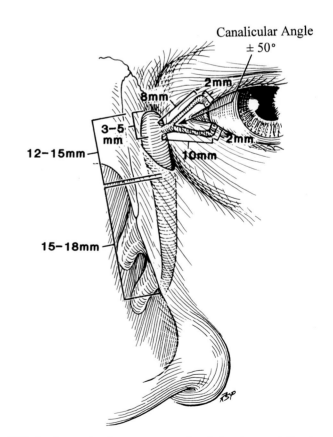

FIG. 5. Approximate measurements of structures relating to the lacrimal drainage pathways. (Courtesy of Richard Pennell, Lexington, KY.)

and the lower approximately 10 mm from the tear sac (10). It is not uncommon to see additional nonpatent supernumery puncta. The normal puncta lie lateral to the caruncle and plica semilunaris. Figure 4 demonstrates the generally accepted lengths of each portion of the canaliculi, but these may vary significantly from individual to individual. The initial portion of the canaliculi underneath the puncta is vertical and 2 mm in length. This vertical portion of the canaliculi terminates in the ampulla. The ampulla is a saccular dilatation surrounded by Horner's muscle. It can expand and contract with blinking and may therefore exhibit variations in intraluminal pressure, which may be important in the drainage of tears through the canaliculi. The horizontal segments of the canaliculi differ in length, being approximately 8 mm in the upper eyelid and 10 mm in the lower eyelid. The canaliculi are not entirely horizontal but meet to form the common canaliculus in virtually all individuals. This fact can be confirmed on dacryocystography. False passaging though the canaliculi into the lacrimal sac at the time of DCR surgery may give the false perception that the canaliculi enter the sac separately. The average length of the common canaliculus is 1.2 mm, but its length may reach 3 to 5 mm (2). Some have termed this region the "sinus of Maier" (Fig. 5).

Histologic examination of a cross section of the eyelid demonstrates a fibrous ring that contributes to the formation of the lacrimal papilla. In most individuals the canaliculi lie deep in the eyelid surrounded by orbicularis muscle. On occasion, the canaliculus can be seen to lie on the superficial aspect of the eyelid just underneath the epithelial and subepithelial tissues of the eyelid. The fibrous ring beginning at the papilla surrounds the canaliculus and extends to develop into the lacrimal fascia surrounding the lacrimal sac. The vertical and horizontal portions of the canaliculi comprise a stratified squamous epithelium. A gradual transition occurs at the common canaliculus developing into the columnar epithelium of the nasolacrimal sac and duct (11). Superficial to the mucosal lining of the canaliculi is the elastic and fibrous tissue noted above. The lacrimal canaliculi parallel the course of the eyelids, frequently joining to form a common canaliculus subsequently penetrating the lacrimal fascia described by Jones (12), passing behind the medial canthal tendon and entering the lacrimal sac. The lacrimal fascia surrounds the lateral and superficial aspect of the lacrimal sac in the lacrimal fossa. Horner's muscle divides into posterior fibers that originate from the pretarsal orbicularis muscle and anterior fibers that originate from preseptal orbicularis muscle. Superiorly, the anterior fibers of Horner's muscle insert onto the lacrimal fascia. The inferior lacrimal fascia receives a similar contribution from the deep head of the medial canthal tendon below the level of Horner's muscle. These fibers also attach onto the lacrimal fascia. These deep fibers of the medial canthal tendon insert finally on the posterior

lacrimal crest (13). Anteriorly and posteriorly, the lacrimal fascia attaches to the lacrimal fossa crests (Fig. 3). Thus, the medial canthal tendon and Horner's muscle each have attachments on the lacrimal fascia with the medial canthal tendon passing both anteriorly and posteriorly to the fascia, inserting on the lacrimal crests, and being surrounded superiorly, inferiorly, and posteriorly by Horner's muscle (10) (Fig. 1).

Nasolacrimal Sac and Duct

The nasolacrimal sac varies in size and configuration, with a larger and more vertical sac being present frequently in the male. Generally, the sac measures 12 to 15 mm vertically, 4 to 8 mm anteroposteriorly, and 3 to 5 mm in width (5,10,12). Approximately one third of the lacrimal sac lies above the level of the medial canthal tendon. The amount of lacrimal sac covered by the bone varies significantly as noted above under "Osteology." A significant amount of variability is encountered in the relationship between the lacrimal sac and fossa to the ethmoids and cribriform plate. The cribriform plate and floor of the anterior cranial fossa varies considerably in location, with 21% of individuals having a medial canthal tendon that is 3 mm or less in distance from the floor of the anterior cranial fossa. This distance can extend to as great as 30 mm above the level of the medial canthal tendon (14). The superior aspect of the lacrimal sac most frequently terminates at a level lateral and slightly inferior to the cribriform plate. Creation of a rhinostomy extending to the superior aspect of the nasolacrimal sac can put the surgeon in close proximity to the cribriform plate. Vigorous twisting or manipulation of the bone in this region can result in a fracture of the cribriform plate and potential cerebrospinal fluid leak. Variation in the inferior extent of the cribriform plate will therefore place some patients more at risk for this complication. The ethmoidal sinuses display far greater variability than the location and position of the cribriform plate. Most individuals demonstrate ethmoidal air cells that may be encountered at the time of DCR. Creation of the normal rhinostomy incorporates portions of the lacrimal, maxillary, and nasal bones. A small number of individuals will display pneumatization of the lacrimal bone with the anterior positioning of the ethmoidal air cells. Removal of the anterior aspect of the lacrimal bone and nasal bone will therefore result in entrance into the ethmoidal air cells medial and posterior to this rhinostomy. Frequently these air cells will need to be removed to expose nasal mucosa. The nasolacrimal duct passes through the maxillary bone aligned just medial to the wall of the antrum until its point of exit beneath the inferior nasal turbinate (Fig. 6).

The lacrimal sac and nasolacrimal duct are distinct and separate entities, although anatomically contiguous.

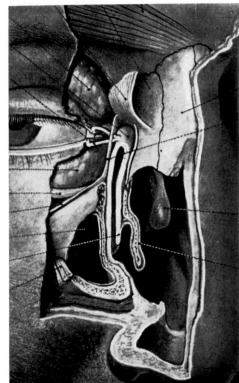

Medial palpebral ligament (turned up)

Frontal process

Corrugator supercilii

Orbital fat

Lacrimal sac

Inf. canaliculus

Orbital fat

Inf. oblique

Periorbita

Maxillary sinus

"Valve" of Hasner

Infraorbital artery and nerve

Nasal bone

Lacrimal fascia

Middle concha

Inf. concha

FIG. 6. Relationship of the lacrimal drainage system to mid-facial structures. (Courtesy of R.J. Last, ref. 16.)

Many authors feel that a narrowing occurs, particularly in females, at the transition from the nasolacrimal sac to the nasolacrimal duct within the confines of the nasolacrimal canal. Some have labeled this narrowing the "valve of Krause" (Fig. 7). The length and extent of the nasolacrimal duct varies, ranging from 22 mm in the infant to approximately 35 mm in the adult. The nasolacrimal sac and duct are lined by a columnar epithelium and surrounded by the fibrous tissue of the lacrimal fascia, which continues inferiorly to envelop the nasolacrimal duct. Numerous investigations have described the diverticulae and valves of the nasolacrimal duct, as demonstrated in Fig. 5 (15). The most critical of these is the valve of Hasner lying underneath the inferior turbinate. The location of the valve of Hasner and its patency varies significantly. The sac lies anterior to the anterior tip of the middle turbinate (Fig. 6). The duct at its inferior aspect runs into the inferior meatus. The angulation anteroposteriorly as well as laterally will determine the actual point of exit of the nasolacrimal duct underneath the inferior turbinate. Extension of the nasolacrimal duct to the nasal floor will produce an imperforate duct that may not respond to probing, as demonstrated by Jones and

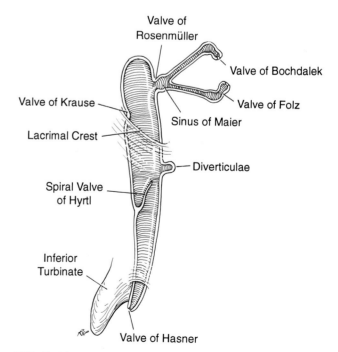

Valve of Rosenmüller

Valve of Bochdalek

Valve of Krause

Valve of Folz

Sinus of Maier

Lacrimal Crest

Diverticulae

Spiral Valve of Hyrtl

Inferior Turbinate

Valve of Hasner

FIG. 7. Valves and sinuses of the lacrimal excretory passages. (Courtesy of Richard Pennell, Lexington, KY.)

Wobig (12). Hasner's valve (Fig. 7) is the terminal soft tissue component of the lacrimal excretory passages. An imperforate valve will result in the pediatric patient with epiphora and signs of congenital nasolacrimal duct obstruction. The relationship between the distal opening of the nasolacrimal duct and the inferior turbinate is highly variable. A narrow inferior meatus or abnormally positioned valve of Hasner will be more prone to obstruction and the treatment often requires outfracture of the inferior turbinate, combined with dilation and probing of the patient with congenital nasolacrimal duct obstruction.

REFERENCES

1. Horner WE. Description of a small muscle at the internal commissure of the eyelids. *Phila J Med Phys Sci* 1824;8:70.
2. Linberg JV, Tucker SM, Tucker NA. Anatomy of the common canaliculus. *Paper presentation at the 25th Annual Scientific Symposium*. American Society of Ophthalmic Plastic and Reconstructive Surgery: San Francisco, October 1994.
3. Farkas LG, Posnick JC, Hreczko TM. Growth patterns in the orbital region: a morphometric study. *Cleft Palate–Craniofac J* 1992;29:315–318.
4. Jones JT. An anatomical approach to problems of the eyelids and lacrimal apparatus. *Arch Ophthalmol* 1961;66:111.
5. Bailey JH. Surgical anatomy of the lacrimal sac. *Am J Ophthalmol* 1923;6:665.
6. Lemke BN. Anatomy of the ocular adnexa and orbit. In: Smith BC, et al., eds. *Ophthalmic plastic and reconstructive surgery*, vol 1. 1987;1–47.
7. Patton JM. Regional anatomy of the tear sac. *Ann Otol Rhinol Laryngol* 1923;32:58.
8. Whitnall SE. The relations of the lacrimal fossa to the ethmoidal cells. *Ophthalmol Rev* 1911;30:321.
9. Corin S, Hurwitz JJ, Jaffer N, Botta EP. The true canalicular angle, a mathematical model. *Ophthalmic Plastic Reconstr Surg* 1990;6:42–45.
10. Lemke BN. The lacrimal anatomy. In: Bosniak SL, Smith BC, eds. *Advances in ophthalmic plastic and reconstructive surgery*. 1984:3;11–23.
11. Cowen DE, Nianiaris N, Howarth D, Hurwitz JJ. Lacrimal sac histopathology and lacrimal sac stone formation: new insights. In: *VIIIth International Symposium on the Lacrimal System*, June 1994; Toronto, Canada.
12. Jones LT, Wobig JL. *Surgery of the eyelids and lacrimal system*. Birmingham, AL: Aesculapius Publishers; 1976.
13. Ahl, NC, Hill JD. Horner's muscle and the lacrimal system. *Arch Ophthalmol* 1982;100:448.
14. Kurihashi K, Yamashita A. Anatomical considerations for dacryocystorhinostomy. *Ophthalmologica* 1991;203:1.
15. Aubaret E. The valves of the lacrymo-nasal passages. *Ophthalmascope* 1908;6:900–903.
16. Last RJ, *Wolff's anatomy of the eye and orbit, 6th ed.* H.K. Lewis and Company, 1968.

CHAPTER 4

Physiology of the Lacrimal Drainage System

Jeffrey Jay Hurwitz

The lacrimal drainage pathway must function as a conduit to remove those tears secreted into the palpebral aperture to cover the cornea, and prevent tears from pooling over the eye and from running down onto the cheek. The mechanism is extremely complicated; despite the fact that a tremendous number of research papers have been published over the last few decades, the exact mechanism is still conjectural. However, enough is known so that one can postulate a mechanism of tear flow in normal and abnormal states.

TEAR SECRETION

It would seem that tears are secreted at the rate of 1.2 μl/min with a total 24-hour secretory volume of approximately 10 ml (1). The average total volume of the fluid in the conjunctival sac at any point in time is approximately 7 mm^3 (2). It would seem that the fornix of the conjunctiva fills up first and can hold approximately 3 to 4 μl. The act of blinking carries the fluid upward to establish the precorneal tear film. Once the fornices are filled, any extra fluid goes into the marginal tear strips on the upper and lower lids. These tear strips can together hold approximately 2 to 3 μl of tears. If more fluid than this is present in the marginal tear strips, the level will rise above the punctal opening and will pass through the puncta and down through the canalicular system. The rate of tear flow through the nasolacrimal duct is probably slower than 0.06 mm^3/min, which would suggest that much of the fluid is absorbed by the nasolacrimal system or is lost through evaporation. This is even more obvious when one considers that lacrimal fluid can be seen to be running into the puncta at approximately 0.6 mm^3/min (3).

J. J. Hurwitz: Oculoplastics Program, Mount Sinai Hospital; and Department of Ophthalmology, University of Toronto Faculty of Medicine, Toronto, Ontario M5S 1A8, Canada.

TEAR ELIMINATION

Movement of Tears from the Superolateral Fornix to the Lacrimal Lake

With blinking, as the orbicularis contracts, the palpebral aperture closes initially in the lateral commissure, and closure occurs from lateral to medial. This has the effect of propelling tears medially toward the lacrimal lake. Also, the attachments of the medial canthal tendon to the anterior lacrimal crest, with slips going to the lacrimal diaphragm on the lateral wall of the sac, on contraction, will cause an increase in the potential size of the lacrimal lake. This may cause a relative negative pressure in the lacrimal lake that will cause suctioning from the tear menisci into the lake.

The tears pass from the superolateral aspect of the palpebral aperture along the marginal tear strips of the upper and lower lids. The tears probably do not bathe the surface of the cornea initially. With a blink, the tears from the adjacent upper and lower tear menisci will coalesce, and then on separating the newly secreted tears will cover the cornea. Thus, it may be suggested that the menisci may act as a reservoir of tears, with the newly secreted ones covering the cornea. It has been postulated that there is a negative pressure in the tear film meniscus and this tends to suction tears from the adjacent tear film, thereby covering the cornea (4).

Passage of Tears from the Lacrimal Lake Through the Puncta (Fig. 1)

The puncta are two mounds that sit on the upper and lower lids just lateral to the tear lake. The upper punctum lies slightly medial to the lower punctum. As blinking begins, the puncta move toward each other. In fact, the puncta strike each opposing eyelid and are occluded by contact of the lid margin when the eyelids are approxi-

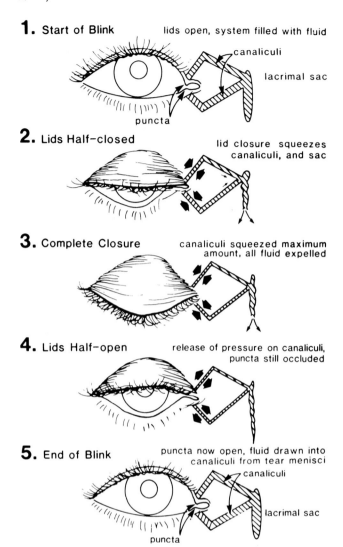

1. Start of Blink   lids open, system filled with fluid

canaliculi

lacrimal sac

puncta

2. Lids Half-closed   lid closure squeezes canaliculi, and sac

3. Complete Closure   canaliculi squeezed maximum amount, all fluid expelled

4. Lids Half-open   release of pressure on canaliculi, puncta still occluded

5. End of Blink   puncta now open, fluid drawn into canaliculi from tear menisci

canaliculi

lacrimal sac

puncta

FIG. 1. The blink-driven tear drainage process. (From Doane, ref. 18, with permission.)

mately one third closed. Further closure squeezes the tears already through the puncta into the canaliculi. On opening the eye, as the lids are approximately one third open, the puncta are still occluded, but there is a release of pressure on the canaliculi. As the lids are approximately two thirds open, the force of lid opening pops the puncta apart and tear fluid can enter the puncta. The tears enter the puncta for three reasons:

1. a negative pressure would develop just inside the punctum to suck in tears
2. the act of capillarity that would suction tears through the small capillary tube
3. the Krehbiel effect.

The Krehbiel effect suggests that there is always a flow of tears from the lacrimal lake through the puncta regardless of blinking (5). The compressive action of one lid against the other is mandatory in the drainage of tears

through either canaliculus. If the lower punctum is everted, tears will not flow through the punctum, but tears probably will also not flow through the punctum because some of these forces (mainly the difference in pressure effect) may not occur. However, there may be some drainage through the upper canaliculus because of capillarity and because of the Krehbiel effect. It would seem that a slit canaliculus functions because the puncta are pressed against the globe by the orbicularis muscle (3). In addition to the pumping action of the orbicularis, the effect of gravity might have something to do with the tears draining into the lacrimal lake and through the puncta—the lateral canthus is usually slightly higher than the medial canthus and this might conceivably help tears flow "downhill" to the medial canthus and through the lower punctum. It would seem that whereas each punctum is important for the drainage of tears, the lower punctum is probably more important than the upper punctum (6).

The diameter of the punctum enlarges as one approaches the canaliculus. Because of this, there would be a tendency for more pressure variation within the distal punctum than within the proximal punctum. For this reason, and because of the fact that the muscular sphincter around the most proximal aspect of the punctum is of a smaller diameter than the sphincter at the most distal aspect of the punctum, there is little reflux of tears from the canaliculus into the lacrimal lake. Despite the fact that the Krehbiel flow is mainly from the lacrimal lake to the canaliculus, there may be some retrograde flow to a small degree.

Flow Through the Canaliculi

The tensor tarsi (Horner's) muscle originates on the posterior lacrimal crest and passes laterally and forward, and divides to surround the canaliculi. It then becomes continuous with the pretarsal portions of the orbicularis muscle. This is important for the movement of the eye margin nasally when the eyelids are closed. The lacrimal pump mechanism, as proposed by Jones (7), suggests that the canaliculi are important in propelling tears into the tear sac. When one closes the eyes, the canaliculi shorten and move nasally. The tears within the canaliculi are propelled toward the lacrimal sac. It has been shown that upon lid closure, the pressure within the canaliculi increases, and when the lids are open, as the canaliculi elongate, the pressure decreases (8).

The vertical and horizontal limbs of the canaliculi are joined at the ampulla, which is a saccular dilatation surrounded by muscles. There is probably a change of pressure with blinking within the ampulla that has a greater variation than within the vertical and horizontal limbs of the canaliculi. This suctioning effect may play a role in transporting tears through the puncta into the ampulla, along the vertical limb of the canaliculus. The changes in pressure may have a role in transporting tears with orbicularis contraction along the horizontal limb of the canaliculus. The Bernoulli principle may come into effect here because as there is movement over a low pressure area, a suctional effect exists. This probably not only exists in the ampulla, but is also probably present where the upper and lower canaliculi join with the common canaliculus. The common canaliculus is a larger structure and probably has more of a fluctuation of pressure within it (9). The flow along the canaliculi toward the common canaliculus probably is also due to the Venturi tube effect (9).

The Venturi tube effect suggests that when a conduit narrows, the speed of movement of the conducted liquid is forced to increase. The canaliculi narrow close to the common canaliculus, thereby increasing the speed of flow from lateral to medial. The reason the canaliculus does not collapse totally at its junction with the common canaliculus is because of the encasing structure of the medial canthal tendon tissues. Therefore, flow through one canaliculus may augment flow through the other and, in fact, occluding one canaliculus may increase the flow through the other uninvolved canaliculus (10).

Flow from the Canaliculi into the Sac

The canaliculi come together and join the common canaliculus, which is a definite structure that can be seen on dacryocystography (11) and can also be shown anatomically. Because the common canaliculus is larger in diameter than the individual canaliculi, there is more of a change in positive and negative pressure during blinking. Because of this and because of the suctioning effect, tears flow quickly from the canaliculi through into the sac. Because of this, it is difficult to image tracer in the common canaliculus when one is performing a nuclear lacrimal scan (12).

Traditionally, one has postulated that there is a valve at the junction of the common canaliculus and the sac at the level of the common internal punctum that prevents back flow of tears from the sac into the canaliculi. Linberg's group has suggested that the common canaliculus angles anteriorly at approximately 118° and enters the lacrimal sac at a mean angle of 58°. They propose that this angulation may account for the one-way valve effect noted clinically at the site of the common canaliculus. They feel that perhaps because the common canaliculus enters the lateral lacrimal sac at an acute angle of 58°, when the sac expands with fluid, the distal canaliculi would collapse and perhaps this is why reflux of fluid is prevented (13). Also, the angle at which the upper and lower canaliculi join the common canaliculus has been

shown to be approximately 50° to 55°—an acute angle that may also, on increased sac pressure and lateral expansion, cause the distal canaliculi to collapse, thereby preventing reflux of tears (14).

The common internal punctum has sphincteric muscle around its opening, a fact that also may prevent reflux of tears from the sac into the common canaliculus. The "canalicular pump" is probably more important than the "sac pump" because, following the dacryocystorhinostomy (DCR), when the sac ceases to exist, tears are still drained through the canaliculi into the nose. In the post-DCR patient, if there is a facial paralysis and the orbicularis is not functioning, even though there may be a patent opening, tears will not drain into the nose because the orbicularis cannot operate the canalicular pump (17).

Flow from the Lacrimal Sac to the Nose

The orbicularis muscle attaches to the lacrimal diaphragm, which is present along the lateral wall of the sac. With blinking, the sac may distend and contract. There are different theories as to whether the sac expands with closure of the eyes or with opening of the eyes, and vice versa, for opening of the eyes. However, what one might surmise is that there is indeed an active peristaltic mechanism that flows from the superior aspect of the sac down to the lower aspect of the duct. This can be seen radiographically with cine-photography.

Tears enter the sac through the common internal punctum via a pumping mechanism, but also perhaps because of the principle of Bernoulli (9). The flow of tears from the sac down through the duct has been postulated to be a siphoning effect and a gravitational effect (15). Tears will flow through the lacrimal system when one is lying down, or even when one is standing on his head, but at a decreased rate (16). Some of the tears may be absorbed through the lining of the nasolacrimal duct, especially in the distal duct where microciliation is present. The sac probably passively fills up with fluid, and when it reaches a critical pressure, tears are probably impelled down through the duct. On each blink, both the canaliculi and the sac expel the little fluid that they have accumulated, and it is felt that the system is virtually empty all the time. The fluid that does go through the nasolacrimal duct probably is absorbed by the lining of the duct before it reaches the nose. The canaliculi have a capacity of pumping approximately 100 mm³/min, and any tearing above this would not be able to be passed through the canaliculi into the sac, and would spill out onto the cheek (2).

The effect of respiration probably has some value in drainage of tears from the duct into the nose. Here Bernoulli's principle must have a role to play. However, because the duct narrows as one reaches the valve of Hasner, the effect is probably minimal. It has been shown, however, when a DCR has been performed and the common canaliculus drains directly into the nose, that the effect of respiration has more of a role to play than it would in the unoperated patient (17). In this situation, the sac ceases to exist as a structure and the Bernoulli principle probably has more of a role.

Blinking is the main factor in draining tears through the sac and duct. When the eyelids are closed, the canaliculi are squeezed and fluid is pushed into the sac. When the eyes are opened, the canaliculi relax and the fluid can squirt down into the duct (18).

FACTORS IN TEAR FLOW

The Pumping Action of the Orbicularis Muscles

Certainly in a facial palsy, tears will not be pumped through the lacrimal system. Even with a Jones tube in place, if the orbicularis function is not normal, there will be a decrease in tear flow (17). The orbicularis muscle is important in pumping of tears in a number of regions in the system:

1. The palpebral aperture. The orbicularis contracts from lateral to medial and propels the tears nasally and to a certain extent in a downwards direction.
2. The Horner's muscle around the canaliculi pumps tears from the punctum through to the sac.
3. The orbicularis attaching to the lacrimal diaphragm will cause changes in pressure in the lacrimal sac. On closing of the eyes, the canaliculus shortens and tears are expressed into the sac, which fills up with fluid as the lacrimal diaphragm is pulled laterally. On opening the eyes, the tension on the lacrimal diaphragm is released, the sac collapses, and the sac expels fluid down through the nasolacrimal duct (Fig. 2).

The maximum closing velocity of the eyelids is 18.7 cm/sec, and the maximum opening velocity is 9.7 cm/sec (19). This would suggest that there is probably more action in closing than in opening, and this would be in keeping with Jones's theory (7).

Bernoulli's Principle

Bernoulli's principle suggests that as gases or fluids pass over an orifice in a conduit, a low pressure area occurs and there is a suctional effect. This probably takes place in the lacrimal system at the nasal cavity sucking tears from the valve of Hasner area into the nose, in the ampulla, and just distal to the common internal punc-

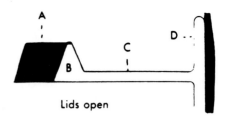

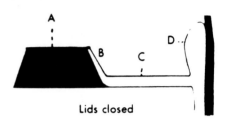

FIG. 2. Schematic drawing of the lacrimal pump. (From Jones, ref. 23, with permission.)

tum (9). This would also tend to decrease back flow through the system.

Capillarity

The small canaliculi may act as capillary tubes. Both the canaliculi and nasolacrimal duct narrow as one proceeds more distally in each structure. Capillarity tends to occur more strongly in narrow bore tubes than in wider ones and, therefore, capillarity probably does exist in these two areas. However, capillarity is not the only factor in drawing tears through the punctum, because a slit canaliculus where capillarity has been destroyed usually functions well for other reasons.

Venturi Tube Effect

The Venturi tube effect suggests that when a conduit narrows, the speed of movement of the conducted liquid increases. This probably plays a role at the distal canaliculus, as mentioned above (9).

Krehbiel Effect

Krehbiel suggested that even in the resting phase of the blink cycle, tears pass from the punctum through into the canaliculus. This may be due to changes of pressure within the lacrimal sac. However, if a DCR is performed, this effect may not be seen and, therefore, it is probably not the intracanalicular suction that is causing this effect, but sac suction (20).

Gravity

Gravity may be significant because the nasolacrimal duct is lower than the sac. This effect definitely has a role to play because of the fact that even on lying down, or standing on one's head, tears will still be seen to flow through the system but at a lower rate (16). Murube feels that gravity causes a negative pressure in the sac as opposed to the lower nasolacrimal canal, and is responsible for sucking tears through the canaliculi and into the sac (15).

Respiration

The effects of respiration have a small role to play in draining tears through the system, especially from the lower nasolacrimal duct through the valve of Hasner and into the nose. The Bernoulli principle probably has a role to play here. The effect of respiration on the drainage of tears through the system is much increased in a post-DCR situation as compared to an unoperated system (17).

Reabsorption

Microciliation has been demonstrated at the lower end of the nasolacrimal duct as it approaches the nose, but also in the lacrimal sac (21). This would suggest that reabsorption does occur within not only the lacrimal duct, but also the sac. This would explain why there is much less flow of tears through the nasolacrimal sac than one sees entering the puncta through the lacrimal lake. In the resting state, probably any tears going down through the nasolacrimal system are absorbed through the mucosa of the sac and duct so that the system is, generally speaking, empty most of the time.

Evaporation

Schirmer felt that approximately half the secreted tears were lost by evaporation (22). In situations of low humidity, cold, and wind, the evaporation will increase, thereby further decreasing the amount of tears that flow down through the nasolacrimal passageways.

Valves

Valves have been described at many areas of the nasolacrimal drainage pathway, but most of these are mucosal folds that play a role in decreasing retrograde flow of tears from the nose toward the palpebral aperture. The most important valve is probably the valve of Hasner at the lower end of the nasolacrimal duct. This valve prevents air currents from within the nose being drawn up into the lacrimal duct. The valve at the common internal punctum, the valve of Rosenmuller, has been said to prevent back flow from the sac into the canaliculi. However, this valve probably has the "valve-like" effect because of the anatomic angulation of the canaliculi and common canaliculus (13,14), as well as the punctum at the common internal opening. Other valves have been described at the punctum, the ampulla, and at the junction of the nasolacrimal sac and duct. However, these are probably related to mucosal folds and probably do not have much of a function. The valve of Rosenmuller is probably important in preventing back flow of tears from the sac into the canaliculi, especially after a DCR. The fact that a DCR functions with little back flow, even though one may be able to blow air from the nose back to the canaliculi into the palpebral aperture, suggest that the valve may be "a one-way valve."

CONCLUSION

The drainage of tears is multifactorial, dependent on the unique anatomic configuration of the nasolacrimal passages, and the effects of muscle function, physical effects, capillarity, gravity, respiration, reabsorption, and evaporation. The action of the orbicularis is probably the main factor. Without proper orbicularis pumping, the patient usually experiences epiphora even though the drainage pathways are completely open.

REFERENCES

1. Norn MS. Tear secretion in normal eyes. *Acta Ophthalmol* 1965;43:567.
2. Mishima S, Gasset A, Klyce S, Baum J. Determination of tear volume and tear flow. *Invest Ophthalmol* 1965;5:264.
3. Maurice DM. The dynamics drainage of tears. *Int Ophthalmol Clin* 1973;13:103.
4. McDonald JE. Surface phenomena of tear films. *Trans Am Soc Ophthalmol* 1968;66:905.
5. Krehbiel J. Uberdiemuskulatur der die muskulatur der Traneswege und der Augenlider. *Diss. en Jahresbericht d. Ophth. Jes.* In Munchen Page 31. 1878.
6. Rabinovitch J, Hurwitz JJ, Chin-Sang A. Quantitative evaluation of canalicular flow using lacrimal scintillography. *Orbit* 1985;3:263.
7. Jones LT. Epiphora II. Its relation to the anatomic structure and surgery of the medial canthal region. *Am J Ophthalmol* 1957;43:203.
8. Hill JC, Bethell W, Smirmaul HJ. Lacrimal drainage—a dynamic evaluation. Part I Mechanics of tear transport. *Can J Ophthalmol* 1974;9:411.
9. Sisler HA. Lacrimal drainage. *Adv Ophthalmol Plastic Reconstruct Surg* 1984;3:25.
10. Daubert J, Nik N, Chandeyssoun PA, El-Choufi L. Tear flow analysis through the upper and lower systems. *Ophthal Plastic Reconstruct Surg* 1990;6:193.
11. Hurwitz JJ, Welham RAN, Lloyd GAS. The role of intubation macrodacryocystography in management of problems of the lacrimal system. *Can J Ophthalmol* 1975;10:361.
12. Chavis RM, Welham RAN, Maisey MN. Quantitative lacrimal scintillography. *Arch Ophthalmol* 1978;96:2066.

13. Linberg JV, Tucker SM, Tucker NA. Anatomy of the common canaliculus. Proceedings of the American Society of Ophthalmic Plastic and Reconstructive Surgery. San Francisco; 1994.

14. Corin S, Hurwitz JJ, Jaffer N, Botta EP. The true canalicular angle: a mathematical analysis. *Ophthal Plastic Reconstruct Surg* 1990;6: 42.

15. Murube del Castillo J. On the gravity as one of the impelling forces of lacrimal flow. *Asahi Evening News* 1978:51.

16. Hurwitz JJ, Maisey MN, Welham RAN. Quantitative lacrimal scintillography. I method and physiological application. *Br J Ophthalmol* 1975;59:308.

17. Nik NA, Hurwitz JJ, Chin Sang H. The mechanism of tear flow after DCR and Jones' tube surgery. *Arch Ophthalmol* 1984;102: 1643.

18. Doane MG. Blinking and tear drainage. *Adv Ophthal Plastic Reconstruct Surg* 1984;3:39.

19. Doane MG. Interaction of eyelids and tears in corneal wetting and the dynamics of the normal human eye blink. *Am J Ophthalmol* 1980;89:507.

20. Frieberg P. Uber die Mechanik der Tranenebelitung met bescndere Hinsicht ung die Ergebnisse ver neureren Tranen sack operatienen. *Z Augenheilkd* 1917;37:42.

21. Radnot M. Scanning electron microscopy of the lacrimal sac. *Asahi Evening News* 1978:35.

22. Schirmer O. Studien zur Physiologie und Pathologie der Tranenebsonderung und Tranenabfuhr. *Arch Ophthalmol* 1903;56:197.

23. Jones LT. The cure of epiphora due to canalicular disorders, trauma, and surgical failures on the lacrimal passages. *Trans Am Acad Ophthalmol Otolaryngol* 1962;66:506.

CHAPTER 5

Embryology of the Nose and Sinuses

Ian J. Witterick and Jeffrey Jay Hurwitz

NASAL CAVITIES

In the human embryo at the end of the fourth week of gestation, bilateral nasal placodes develop on each side of the lower part of the frontonasal prominence (Fig. 1). Each nasal placode consists of an oval-shaped thickening of surface ectoderm that becomes surrounded by mesenchyme at the margins, forming horseshoe-shaped elevations called the medial and lateral nasal prominences (elevations). As the face develops, the nasal placodes become depressed, forming nasal pits that deepen to form primitive nasal sacs. The sacs are initially separated from the oral cavity by the oronasal membrane, but this ruptures, bringing the nasal and oral cavities into communication and forming the primitive choanae. The lateral palatine processes fuse with each other and the nasal septum, separating the oral and nasal cavities again. After the secondary palate and septum develops, the choanae are located at the junction of the nasal cavity and pharynx. Elevations on the lateral wall of each nasal cavity form superior, middle, and inferior turbinates, and ectodermal epithelium in the roof of each nasal cavity becomes specialized as the olfactory epithelium.

SINUSES

The sinuses form from the walls of the nasal cavities as diverticula but not all develop during fetal life. The newborn infant has maxillary sinuses that are approximately 3 to 4 mm in diameter and several smaller anterior and posterior ethmoidal air cells. There are no frontal or sphenoidal sinuses at birth. The maxillary sinuses grow slowly until puberty, but they are not fully devel-

I. J. Witterick: Department of Otolaryngology, Mount Sinai Hospital, University of Toronto Faculty of Medicine, Toronto, Ontario M5S 1A8, Canada.

J. J. Hurwitz: Oculoplastics Program, Mount Sinai Hospital; Department of Ophthalmology, and University of Toronto Faculty of Medicine, Toronto, Ontario M5S 1A8, Canada.

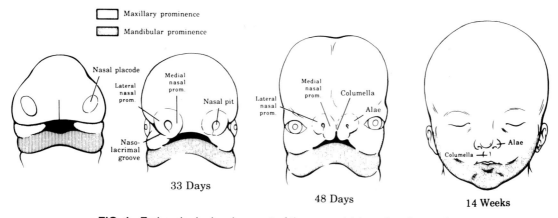

FIG. 1. Embryologic development of the nose at 14 weeks of gestation.

oped until all the permanent teeth have erupted. The ethmoid sinuses do not begin to grow until age 2 years, but it is not until age 6 to 8 years that they begin to grow rapidly. The frontal sinuses are formed by the growth of the two most anterior ethmoidal air cells into the frontal bone at approximately age 2 years. The frontal sinuses are not visible on x-rays until age 7 years. There is great variety in the pneumatization of the frontal bone; the midline septum dividing the two frontal sinuses is rarely in the midline. In a similar fashion, the sphenoid sinuses are formed from the two most posterior ethmoid air cells growing into the sphenoid bone, also resulting in great variation in the size and shape of the sphenoid sinuses.

SUGGESTED READING

Mann I. *Developmental abnormalities of the eye.* Philadelphia: JB Lippincott; 1957.

CHAPTER 6

Anatomy of the Nose and Sinuses

Ian J. Witterick and Jeffrey Jay Hurwitz

A thorough knowledge of the anatomy of the nose is important for the surgeon diagnosing lacrimal dysfunction and planning drainage surgery into the nose.

EXTERNAL NOSE

The external nasal skeleton is made up of bone and cartilage. The nasal bones make up the upper one third and the lower two thirds is formed by cartilage. There is tremendous variation in the size and shape of the nose largely because of differences in the cartilage. The two nasal bones vary in size and join each other in the midline. They articulate with the frontal bone superiorly and with the frontonasal processes of the maxillary bones laterally. The cartilaginous portion of the nose is formed by the upper and lower lateral cartilages. The upper lateral cartilages occupy the middle one third of the nose between the nasal bones superiorly and the lower lateral cartilages inferiorly. The lower lateral cartilages give shape to the nostrils and are made up of medial and lateral crura. The nasal septum forms part of the dorsum or bridge of the nose as it extends between the two upper lateral cartilages. The columella is the caudal supporting structure of the nose dividing the two nostrils and is made up of the caudal margin of the septum, the two medial crura, and the overlying soft tissues.

INTERNAL NOSE

The nares, or nostrils, are the two openings into the nasal cavities. The vestibule of the nose is the anterior, skin-lined portion containing nasal hairs (vibrissae). The junction of the skin and nasal mucous membrane occurs at a variable distance inside the nose and is usually clearly discernible by the differing colors between skin and mucosa. The choanae are the posterior limits of the nasal cavities dividing the nose from the nasopharynx. The nasal septum divides the nose into right and left nasal cavities. The septum comprises cartilage anteriorly (quadrilateral/septal cartilage) and bone posteriorly (perpendicular plate of the ethmoid bone posterosuperiorly, vomer bone posteroinferiorly, and the crest of the maxilla inferiorly).

The lateral wall of the nose is an important but complex structure. There are three to four paired nasal turbinates (inferior, middle, superior, and sometimes supreme turbinates) with a corresponding meatus under each turbinate (Fig. 1). The inferior turbinate is the largest turbinate and is a separate bone, whereas the other turbinates are part of the ethmoid bone. The middle turbinate is smaller than the inferior turbinate but may contain an air cell (concha bullosa) that can enlarge and block the sinuses draining under the middle meatus. The superior and supreme turbinate (if present) are usually small and insignificant in size compared with the other two turbinates.

The size of the meatus under each turbinate may be large or small, corresponding to the size of the bone making up the turbinate and varying with the state of mucosal and vascular engorgement of the overlying epithelium. These anatomic and mucosal factors can dramatically influence the structures draining into each meatus. The nasolacrimal duct is the only structure draining into the inferior meatus and this opens toward the anterior end of the meatus. The middle meatus is critical for drainage of the maxillary, frontal, and anterior ethmoid sinuses. The air cells forming the posterior ethmoid sinus drain into the superior meatus and the sphenoid sinus drains into the sphenoethmoidal recess above the superior and supreme turbinates. The delinea-

---

I. J. Witterick: Department of Otolaryngology, Mount Sinai Hospital, University of Toronto Faculty of Medicine, Toronto, Ontario M5S 1A8, Canada.

J. J. Hurwitz: Oculoplastics Program, Mount Sinai Hospital; and Department of Ophthalmology, University of Toronto Faculty of Medicine, Toronto, Ontario M5S 1A8, Canada.

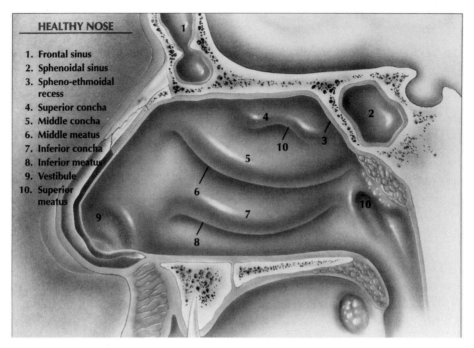

FIG. 1. A ''healthy nose.'' (From *Medical Management,* illustrated by Witterick and Hawke, with permission.)

tion between anterior and posterior ethmoid air cells is the attachment of the middle turbinate to the lateral wall of the nose. This separation has been given various names including "ground" lamella, "grand" lamella, and "basal" lamella. The ostia of the sinuses are rarely seen clinically because most are covered by other structures (with the exception of the sphenoid sinus), thus preventing easy examination.

The lateral wall of the nose in the region of the middle turbinate and middle meatus is complicated (Figs. 2 and 3). Located just anterior to the middle turbinate is the lacrimal bone. Posterior to the lacrimal bone is the unci-

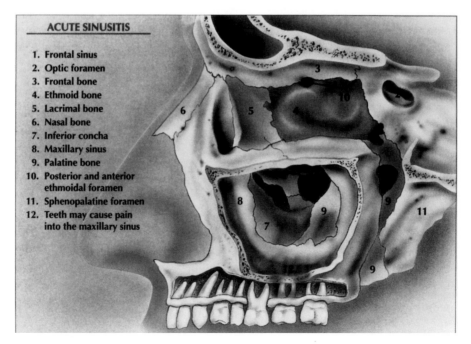

FIG. 2. ''Acute sinusitis.'' (From *Medical Management,* illustrated by Witterick and Hawke, with permission.)

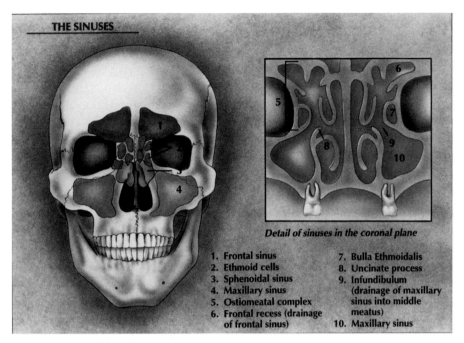

FIG. 3. "The sinuses," showing sinuses and ostiomeatal complex. (From *Medical Management,* illustrated by Witterick and Hawke, with permission.)

nate process, a thin, sickle-shaped bone covering the area where the sinuses drain. Posterior to the uncinate process and approximately midway along the meatus, the ethmoidal bulla (the largest anterior ethmoid air cell) bulges from the lateral wall. There is a sickle-shaped opening between the uncinate process and the ethmoidal bulla called the hiatus semilunaris. The hiatus semilunaris is the doorway to a three-dimensional space called the infundibulum. The frontal sinus drains into the anterosuperior end of the infundibulum through the nasofrontal duct, which is also referred to as the frontal recess. The anterior ethmoid cells drain along with the frontal sinus, anteriorly and superiorly. The maxillary sinus drains into the posteroinferior portion of the infundibulum inferior to the ethmoidal bulla. The agger nasi is an anatomic variation from pneumatization of the frontal recess that appears as an elevation of the lateral wall of the nose just anterior to the attachment of the middle turbinate. Agger nasi cells become clinically significant if they enlarge and mechanically constrict the frontal recess.

BLOOD SUPPLY OF THE NOSE

Arterial Blood Supply

Branches of the external carotid artery supply the majority of blood to the internal and external nose, but there are important contributions from the internal carotid artery (1).

External Carotid Artery Supply

The most important branch of the external carotid artery supplying the nasal lining is the maxillary artery, followed by the facial artery. The maxillary artery is still frequently referred to as the "internal maxillary artery," but current anatomic nomenclature has designated it as the "maxillary artery" (2). Similarly, the "external maxillary artery" is now known as the "facial artery."

The maxillary artery is a terminal branch of the external carotid artery that has been arbitrarily divided into three divisions by anatomists as it travels through the infratemporal and pterygopalatine fossae. The first division lies between the mandibular ramus and sphenomandibular ligament and the second division is that portion that travels over the lateral pterygoid muscle. The third division is the terminal portion of the maxillary artery that enters the pterygopalatine fissure and divides into several branches in the pterygopalatine fossa. The pterygopalatine fossa is located posterior to the maxillary sinus and lateral to the posterior aspects of the nasal cavity.

Two important branches of the third division of the maxillary artery are the sphenopalatine and greater palatine arteries (Fig. 4). The sphenopalatine artery enters the nasal cavity through its foramen near the posterior end of the middle turbinate. It divides into a medial nasoseptal branch and one or two lateral branches. The medial branch travels over the rostrum of the sphenoid bone to the posterior edge of the nasal septum to become the

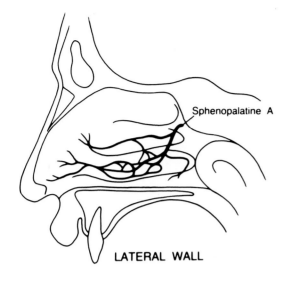

LATERAL WALL

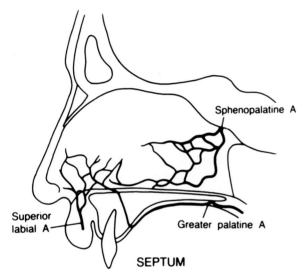

SEPTUM

FIG. 4. External carotid artery blood supply to the septum and lateral nasal wall. (From Hengerer, ref. 5, with permission.)

branch to the anterior septum and an alar branch to the nasal ala.

Internal Carotid Arterial Supply

The internal carotid artery does not have any branches in the neck before it enters the petrous temporal bone (petrous portion) at the skull base. It courses through the cavernous sinus (cavernous portion) and pierces the dura near the anterior clinoid process. The first major branch of the intracranial portion of the internal carotid artery is the ophthalmic artery, which again becomes extracranial after passing through the superior orbital fissure to the orbit. The ophthalmic artery gives off several branches including the central retinal artery and two branches (anterior and posterior ethmoidal arteries) to the nose.

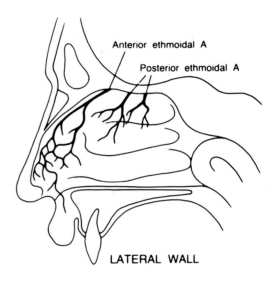

LATERAL WALL

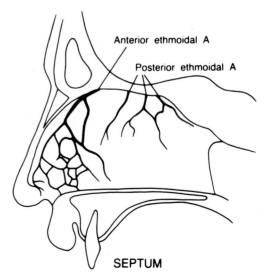

SEPTUM

FIG. 5. Internal carotid artery blood supply to the septum and lateral nasal wall (From Hengerer, ref. 5, with permission.)

posterior septal artery that travels anteriorly along the septum. The lateral branch(es) of the sphenopalatine artery supply the inferior and middle turbinates and occasionally the superior turbinate.

The greater palatine artery branch of the maxillary artery travels inferiorly to the palate through the greater palatine canal. It then travels along the alveolar ridge to the incisive foramen, where it turns superiorly through this foramen to supply the anterior/inferior nasal septum.

The other important arterial contribution from the external carotid artery is the facial artery. After the facial artery courses diagonally over the mandible and lower face it gives off a superior labial branch to the upper lip. The superior labial artery in turn gives off a septal

The anterior ethmoidal artery is the more constant and larger nasal branch. Both anterior and posterior ethmoidal arteries leave the orbit through their respective canals and travel through the ethmoid sinuses and then briefly again through the intracranial cavity before descending into the nose through the cribriform plate. The anterior third of the septum and lateral nasal wall are predominantly supplied by the anterior ethmoidal artery (Fig. 5). The posterior ethmoidal artery supplies the superior turbinate and a corresponding portion of the superior septum.

Important Arterial Anastomoses

The most important anastomosis of arteries is the region of the anterior nasal septum called Kiesselbach's plexus or Little's area. Approximately 80% of epistaxis arises from this anastomosis and is the region where branches of the external carotid artery (posterior septal artery, greater palatine artery, and superior labial arteries) anastomose with a branch of the internal carotid artery (anterior ethmoidal artery). Another potentially important anastomosis responsible for persistent bleeding exists between the ophthalmic artery and the middle meningeal and maxillary arteries (3). This anastomosis allows persistent bleeding from branches of the maxillary artery to the ethmoid artery or vice versa following single-vessel ligation of one vessel.

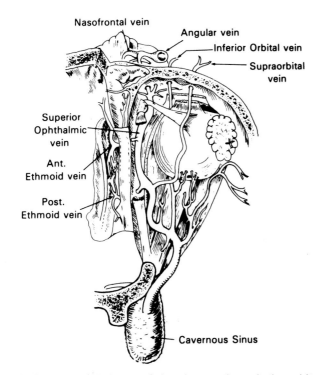

FIG. 6. Venous drainage of the sinuses through the orbit. (From Goodwin and Godley, ref. 6, with permission.)

Venous Drainage

The venous drainage of the nasal cavities follows the basic arterial pattern. The anterior portion of the nasal cavity drains inferiorly through the facial veins. The posterior nasal cavity drains via the sphenopalatine vessels into the pterygoid venous plexus within the infratemporal fossa. Veins in the roof of the nasal cavities drain through the ethmoidal veins to the ophthalmic veins in the orbit (Fig. 6). Angular veins from the external nose also drain to the inferior ophthalmic vein. The ophthalmic veins in turn course posteriorly into the cavernous sinuses and become part of the drainage pattern of the dural venous sinuses. These connections can have life-threatening consequences in the presence of infectious diseases in the nose and paranasal sinuses.

NERVE SUPPLY OF THE NOSE

The muscles of the external nose are supplied by the facial nerve and the skin receives sensory supply from the trigeminal nerve through its first division (nasociliary, external nasal, and infratrochlear nerves) and second divisions (intraorbital nerve). The general sensory nerve supply to the internal nose also comes from the first (ophthalmic) and second (maxillary) divisions of the trigeminal nerve. The anterior ethmoidal/nasociliary nerve is a branch of the ophthalmic division and supplies the superior and anterior part of the septum and lateral nasal wall. Maxillary division branches arising from the sphenopalatine ganglion (lateral posterior superior or "short sphenopalatine," medial posterior superior or "septal," nasopalatine or "long sphenopalatine" and greater palatine nerves) supply most of the posterior part of the nose.

The sphenopalatine ganglion is a parasympathetic ganglion and the sensory nerves pass through it without synapsing. Preganglionic parasympathetic fibers come from the greater petrosal nerve, a branch of the facial nerve. Postganglionic parasympathetic fibers are distributed in the branches of the sphenopalatine ganglion to the nasal septum and lateral nasal wall and ultimately to the glandular epithelium. The sphenopalatine ganglion also supplies the lacrimal gland and palate mucosal glands with parasympathetic fibers.

Sympathetic fibers leave the spinal cord through spinal nerves T1-T3 and reach the sympathetic trunk by white rami communicantes. The fibers travel up the cervical sympathetic trunk and synapse in the superior cervical ganglion. Postsynaptic fibers travel along the sympathetic plexus of the internal carotid artery. Some of these fibers condense to form the deep petrosal nerve. The deep petrosal nerve (postganglionic sympathetic) joins the greater petrosal nerve (preganglionic parasympathetic) to form the Vidian nerve, also called the nerve of the pterygoid canal. The Vidian nerve connects to the sphenopalatine ganglion and the preganglionic parasympathetic fibers synapse in the ganglion and the postganglionic parasympathetic fibers exit the ganglion along with postganglionic sympathetic fibers to be distributed by nasal and greater palatine branches to glands and microvasculature of the nasal mucosa.

Sympathetic and parasympathetic stimulation of the nasal mucosa generally produce opposite effects. Parasympathetic stimulation promotes serous and mucinous secretion and dilates the blood vessels. Tonic sympathetic innervation maintains blood vessel tone and stimulation promotes vasoconstriction that decreases turbinate engorgement and hence nasal resistance.

The specialized olfactory epithelium is located in a narrow crevice in the roof of the nose along the cribriform plate and adjacent superior nasal septum and lateral nasal wall. The cell bodies are located in the mucous membrane and send fibers upward through the cribriform plate to the olfactory bulb and on to the olfactory nerves.

LYMPHATICS OF THE NOSE

Lymphatic drainage of the nose is extensive and parallels the venous drainage. The lymphatics of the external nose and nasal vestibule drain laterally along the course of the facial vein into the submandibular lymph nodes. The posterior nasal cavity and sinuses generally drain posteriorly into the retropharyngeal nodes and eventually to the deep cervical lymph nodes. These regional lymphatic chains are important in the dissemination of malignant neoplasms and infections of the nose and sinuses.

THE PARANASAL SINUSES

There are four paired sinuses filled with air and lined by mucous membrane: the maxillary sinus, ethmoid sinus, frontal sinus, and sphenoid sinus.

Maxillary Sinus

The maxillary sinus (antrum of Highmore) is the largest of the sinuses, with a volume of approximately 15 mL. It lies in the body of the maxillary bone and has a pyramidal shape with the base directed toward the nasal cavity and the apex toward the zygomatic process. In adults, the floor is 3 to 5 mm inferior to the level of the nasal cavity. In children, the floor is at or above the level of the nasal floor. The medial wall is thin and corresponds to the lateral wall of the nose. The medial wall is in close proximity to the nasolacrimal canal, and is separated by thin bone. The anterior wall is thicker and

forms the outline of the "cheek." The superior wall or roof of the sinus serves as the floor of the orbit. The infraorbital nerve traverses the roof of the sinus and is usually covered in a bony canal but it may be covered only by mucous membrane. The posterior wall overlies the pterygopalatine and infratemporal fossae that contain branches of the maxillary artery and sphenopalatine ganglion.

Ethmoid Sinus

The ethmoid sinuses are located between the middle turbinate and the medial orbital wall (lamina papyracea). The roof is formed by the superior plate of the ethmoid bone and the sinus opens inferiorly to the middle meatus. There are a variable number of air cells (7–15 per side) in each ethmoid sinus with a total volume of approximately 14 mL. The lamina papyracea may contain natural dehiscences that can potentially be a direct route of spread for ethmoid infection to the orbit. Posterior ethmoid cells may be in close proximity or directly adjacent to the optic nerve (cells of Onodi). The roof of the ethmoid sinus can vary from an almost horizontal to almost vertical orientation. The cribriform plate is not part of the ethmoid sinus but is located medial to the attachment of the middle turbinate and separates the nose from the anterior cranial fossa. The two cribriform plates are separated from each other by the crista galli and both plates lie posterior to the posterior table of the frontal sinus. Each cribriform plate measures approximately 2 cm from anterior to posterior and 0.5 cm from medial to lateral. Olfactory nerve endings traverse small openings in each cribriform plate to reach the olfactory bulb (first cranial nerve). The cribriform plate is 4 to 7 mm inferior to the ethmoidal roof in 70% of patients but lies 12 to 16 mm below the ethmoidal roof in 18% of patients (4). In these patients, the medial aspect of the ethmoidal roof is formed by the lateral lamellae of the cribriform plate.

Frontal Sinus

The frontal sinuses are located in the frontal bone superiorly and posterior to the superior orbital ridge. The frontal sinuses form an irregular pyramid with the apex directed superiorly. They are usually of unequal size and variable depth, with a midline septum rarely in the midline. The ostia of the frontal sinus vary from 2 to 10 mm in diameter and are located in the anteromedial aspect of the sinus floor. The anterior table of the frontal bone is thicker than the posterior table that separates the sinus from the frontal lobe of the brain. These tables may contain marrow that can become infected from sinusitis and disseminate the infection through the vascular channels found in the marrow.

Sphenoid Sinus

The sphenoid sinuses are located within the body of the sphenoid bone and vary greatly in size and shape. They are commonly deep in their anteroposterior dimensions. Laterally they may extend into various parts of the sphenoid bone including the greater and lesser wings, pterygoid processes, and lateral pterygoid plates. The midline septum usually divides the two sinuses unequally. The sphenoid ostia are superior and medial on the anterior wall and drain into the sphenoethmoidal recess.

The anterior portion of the sphenoid sinus abuts against the posterior ethmoid air cells. There are several important relationships with surrounding structures. The brain stem (pons, basilar artery) lies posterior to the sphenoid sinus. The optic chiasm and pituitary gland lie superior to the sinus and the pituitary gland commonly bulges into the superior wall. The optic nerves, carotid artery, and cavernous sinus are important lateral relationships. The nasopharynx is inferior to the sphenoid sinus.

REFERENCES

1. Lander MI, Terry O. The posterior ethmoid artery in severe epistaxis. *Otolaryngol Head Neck Surg* 1992:106;101–103.
2. International Congress of Anatomists. *Nomina Anatomica,* 6th ed. New York: Churchill Livingstone; 1989:A54.
3. Pearson BW, MacKenzie RG, Goodman WS. The anatomic basis of transantral ligation of the maxillary artery in severe epistaxis. *Laryngoscope* 1969;79:969–984.
4. Keros P. Uber die praktische Bedeutung der Niveau-Unterschiede der Lamina cribrosa des Ethmoids. In: Naumann HH, ed. *Head and neck surgery, vol 1, face and facial skull.* Philadelphia: WB Saunders; 1980:392.
5. Hengerer AS. Epistaxis. In: Lee KJ, ed. *Textbook of otolaryngology and head and neck surgery.* Norwalk, CT: Appleton & Lange; 1989.
6. Goodwin WJ Jr, Godley F. Developmental anatomy and physiology of the nose and paranasal sinuses. In: Lee KJ, ed. *Textbook of otolaryngology and head and neck surgery.* Norwalk, CT: Appleton & Lange; 1989.

CHAPTER 7

Physiology of the Nose and Sinuses

Ian J. Witterick and Jeffrey Jay Hurwitz

The functioning of the nose plays an important role in the etiology of tearing problems and in the results of lacrimal surgery.

EPITHELIUM AND MUCOUS BLANKET

The first 1 to 2 cm of the nasal cavity is composed of keratinized, stratified squamous epithelium containing hair follicles. The nose posterior to the vestibule and the paranasal sinuses is lined by ciliated, pseudostratified, columnar (respiratory) epithelium. The submucosa contains nerves, blood vessels, mucous-producing glands, and inflammatory cells (e.g., lymphocytes, plasma cells) capable of a rapid inflammatory response to potential invaders.

The epithelium is protected by a mucous blanket composed of an outer viscous layer called the gel phase and an inner thin serous layer called the sol phase. The cilia beat in the sol phase, which in turn moves the gel phase. The balance between the sol and gel phases is critically important for the maintenance of normal mucociliary clearance. The viscous layer is produced by goblet cells interspersed between the epithelium and the thinner fluid is produced by serous glands within the lamina propria deep to the mucous membrane. The predominant component of nasal mucous is water (96%), but other substances found include inorganic salts, sulphated mucoproteins and mucopolysaccharides, antibodies (primarily IgA), fibrinolytic enzymes, glucose, and lysozyme. Approximately 1 L of seromucinous fluid is produced by the nasal and sinus mucosa each day (1). The nasal mucous traps particulates, removes potentially toxic substances, and is important in water retention, humidification, and heat exchange.

The mucous blanket is propelled by the cilia on the surface of the respiratory epithelium. The cilia in the sinuses are oriented to move the mucous to the natural ostia, where it is emptied into the nose. The mucous from the sinuses and the nasal mucosa is propelled posteriorly to the nasopharynx, where it is either swallowed or expectorated. The coordinated ciliary action is capable of moving the nasal and sinus mucous blanket at approximately 5 to 10 mm/min. Mucociliary clearance is an important nasal physiologic function that can be impaired by extremes of temperature, dryness, smoke, pollution, viral infections, and inadequate nasal secretions. Congenital ciliary dysfunction (e.g., Kartagener's syndrome) is rare.

NASAL MICROVASCULATURE

The nasal microvasculature consists of arterioles, venules, submucosal periglandular capillary beds, and an extensive sinusoidal network of large capacitance vessels. Important concentrations of vascular tissue include the inferior turbinates and anterior septum, where large capacitance vessels form areas of "erectile tissue." Autonomic nerves and chemical mediators are important in controlling the flow of blood through the nasal vascular beds. When the net outflow of blood is less than inflow, the mucosa expands and functionally increases the net surface area. As the surface area increases, so too does the nasal resistance, thereby slowing the nasal airflow and enhancing the conditioning and filtering properties of the nose. In addition, there are multiple arteriovenous anastomoses that serve an important temperature-regulating function by increasing nasal blood flow and

I. J. Witterick: Department of Otolaryngology, Mount Sinai Hospital, University of Toronto Faculty of Medicine, Toronto, Ontario M5S 1A8, Canada.

J. J. Hurwitz: Oculoplastics Program, Mount Sinai Hospital; and Department of Ophthalmology, University of Toronto Faculty of Medicine, Toronto, Ontario M5S 1A8, Canada.

heat exchange without creating changes in nasal blood volume.

Nasal blood flow is primarily regulated by neuropeptides released by autonomic nerves. Sympathetic stimulation causes emptying of the venous sinusoids, thus reducing nasal blood flow and mucosal congestion. Parasympathetic stimulation causes vasodilatation and glandular secretion, resulting in nasal congestion and a watery nasal discharge. Continuous sympathetic discharge produces a certain level of ongoing vasoconstriction. The resting tone oscillates between nasal cavities causing the vasculature of one side to constrict while the other side becomes congested. This naturally occurring "nasal cycle" is present in approximately 80% of the population and the cycle length varies widely between 30 minutes and 6 hours (2,3).

Blood flow can be affected by a variety of local and systemic factors. Local factors include temperature, humidity, trauma, exercise, infection, and vasoactive drugs. Systemic factors include thyroid hormone imbalance (hyper- or hypothyroidism) and elevated estrogen levels (e.g., during menstruation and pregnancy). Emotional stress may cause either vasoconstriction or vasodilatation. In addition, postural changes may affect the erectile tissue of the nasal cavity. Recumbency congestion is common when lying supine or with one nasal cavity dependent. The mucosa of the dependent nasal cavity becomes congested as blood pools in the venous sinusoids, leading to the symptoms of nasal obstruction and congestion on that side (4).

FUNCTIONS OF THE NOSE

The nose has a large internal surface area (100–200 cm^2) in relation to its external size, which helps in the filtration, warming, and humidification of inspired air. In an average day, the adult nose conditions 10,000 to 20,000 L of inspired air (5). The anterior nose, in a region called the nasal valve, is responsible for approximately 50% of the total resistance to airflow from the atmosphere to the alveoli. The increased resistance in this region slows the air so it can interact more effectively with the nasal mucosa, particularly the turbinates. In addi-

tion, some turbulence in the nasal airflow increases contact with the mucosal surface.

Filtration of inspired air is important because of the billions of infectious, allergenic, irritative, and toxic materials found in it. Filtration is accomplished by several mechanisms. Large particles are filtered by the nasal vestibular hairs (vibrissae) and smaller particles (>4 μm in diameter) are trapped in the mucous blanket (6). The mucous blanket in health is constantly replenished and moves trapped substances to the nasopharynx for expectoration or swallowing and inactivation by gastric acid. In addition, the sneezing reflex may help to remove foreign substances from the nasal cavities.

Inhaled air is warmed from ambient temperatures to 31°C or higher in the pharynx and 35°C in the trachea. Air reaching the nasopharynx has a constant relative humidity of 75% to 80%. The actual amount of fluid lost varies with the relative humidity of the inspired air. For example, if the relative humidity is high, little (if any) fluid is lost from the mucous membrane. The water is replenished from the submucosal glands. The nose is so efficient at warming and humidifying that even extremely cold and dry air is almost instantaneously warmed to body temperature and completely humidified during nasal transit.

Another important function of the nose is olfaction, which is important for taste perception and warnings against detectable toxic gases and foods. In addition, the nasal and sinus cavities contribute to the resonant properties of speech.

REFERENCES

1. Assessing and treating rhinitis—a practical guide for Canadian physicians. *Can Med Assoc J* 1994:151(4)(suppl); 1–27.
2. Stoksted P. The physiologic cycle of the nose under normal and pathological conditions. *Acta Otolaryngol* 1952:42; 175–179.
3. Arbour P, Kern EB. Paradoxical nasal obstruction. *Can J Otolaryngol* 1975:4; 333–338.
4. Cole P. *The respirology role of the upper airways: a selective clinical and pathophysiological review.* St. Louis: Mosby Year Book; 1993.
5. Bridger GP. Physiology of the nasal valve. *Arch Otolaryngol* 1970: 92; 543–553.
6. Brain JD, Valberg PA. Deposition of aerosol in the respiratory tract. *Am Rev Respir Dis* 1979:120; 1325–1373.

CHAPTER 8

Lacrimal Secretion

Raymond Stein and Jeffrey Jay Hurwitz

Dry eye conditions can be subdivided into five principle categories:

1. aqueous deficiency
2. mucin deficiency
3. lipid abnormalities
4. lid-surfacing problems
5. epitheliopathy.

There are a variety of methods to diagnose a dry eye condition. The clinician goes through the process of a detailed history, biomicroscopic examination, and specific tests to detect abnormalities of the tear film.

HISTORY

A patient with a dry eye may not necessarily complain of specific dryness. A significant proportion of patients report irritation, burning, itching, eyestrain, and other irritative symptoms. It is not uncommon for patients with a dry eye to complain of intermittent blurred vision when reading, watching television, or working at a computer terminal. This is usually secondary to staring and poor tear flow over the ocular surface. Symptoms are usually worse as the day progresses. A history of intolerance to drafts, wind, smoke, and air conditioning are indicative of dry eye symptoms. These symptoms are most common in the elderly, whose tear secretion is diminished from age-related atrophy of the lacrimal gland and who have a reduced outflow of tears. When outdoors, the patient may have tearing (reflex-stimulated tear secretion exceeds the reduced outflow of tears), and indoors

R. Stein: Cornea and External Disease Program, Mount Sinai Hospital, Toronto, Ontario M5G 1X5, Canada.

J. J. Hurwitz: Oculoplastics Program, Mount Sinai Hospital; and Department of Ophthalmology, University of Toronto Faculty of Medicine, Toronto, Ontario M5S 1A8, Canada.

the nonstimulated tear secretion is so minimal that the condition may be characterized as that of a dry eye.

A history of contact lens intolerance may indicate a dry eye. A patient who is asymptomatic with a marginal tear film may become symptomatic when wearing contact lenses.

The cause of the patient's dry eye must be determined. With the specific diagnosis, the ophthalmologist can recommend specific therapeutic interventions. Several causes of dry eye may be present in the same patient. For instance, keratitis sicca and blepharitis often are found together and both must be treated to resolve the patient's symptoms. To determine whether a patient has keratitis sicca, a careful and thorough history and clinical examination should be performed and supplemented by clinical and laboratory tests and treatment trials.

The patients with keratitis sicca have often a multitude of symptoms including foreign body sensation, burning, and photophobia. Tearing or epiphora often are attributed to keratitis sicca, but other causes such as blepharitis, exposure keratopathy, and nasolacrimal duct obstruction must be ruled out. However, tearing (with or without grittyness) may be the predominant symptom. Ocular irritaton stimulates V1 afferents, and via a reflex arc back to the lacrimal gland, increased reflex tears are secreted.

The patients can be asked whether they produce increased tears from irritant phenomena or as an emotional response. Increased tear production when peeling onions or when crying suggests a certain level of function from the lacrimal glands. A negative response suggests an inability of the lacrimal glands to secrete tear fluid in response to any stimuli. The ability to generate irritant tears is lost before the ability to produce emotional tears in keratitis sicca.

The time course of these dry eye symptoms is important. How long have the symptoms been present? Are they related to the menstrual cycle, menopause, hysterectomy, or oophorectomy? Are there fluctuations in the symptoms that occur on an hourly, day to day, or month to month cycle? For patients with keratitis sicca, the symptoms are usually less significant on awakening and worsen during the course of the day. Patients with blepharitis are highly symptomatic on awakening, usually better within an hour, and often worse later in the day. Is there a seasonal component? What effect does the patient's environment have on his or her symptoms? Patients with dry eyes are worse in dry environments and under conditions of increased evaporation. Air conditioners and car heaters often worsen symptoms.

A detailed history of past ocular treatments should be documented. A list of topical lubricants and medications should be obtained. Are the artificial tears or ointment preserved or unpreserved? How long has the patient used the medication and how often? The severity of keratitis sicca can often be determined from how frequently the topical lubricants are used.

The clinician should ask whether or not temporary collagen plugs or reversible silicone plugs have been tried. If so, note whether there was an improvement in symptoms and whether epiphora occurred. Ask whether permanent occlusion with laser or cautery has been performed. Systemic medication should be documented. Many systemic medications affect tear secretion such as antihistamines, antidepressants, anticholinergics, and diuretics. Any associated systemic symptoms or diseases should be determined. Does the patient have a history of dry mouth (xerostomia). The patients should be questioned as to whether they have ever been told they have Sjogren's syndrome, systemic lupus erythematosus, rheumatoid arthritis, scleroderma, thyroid disease, lymphoma, or acquired immunodeficiency syndrome. A family history should be obtained with inquiry as to whether there is a relative with keratitis sicca,

Sjogren's syndrome, collagen vascular disease, or other eye diseases.

CLINICAL EXAMINATION

Nonocular Examination

A limited physical examination is helpful to rule out conditions that may be responsible for patient's dry eye. The facial skin is examined to rule out the possibility of acne rosacea and the malar rash of systemic lupus erythematosus. The scalp is examined for evidence of dandruff suggestive of seborrheic dermatitis. Palpation of the thyroid gland is performed to rule out enlargement and nodules. Hypothyroidism is commonly seen in patients with dry eyes. Hyperthyroidism may be seen in patients with superior limbic keratoconjunctivitis. Proptosis and diminished blinking, which may occur in Graves' disease, can cause symptoms of a dry eye (Fig. 1). The tongue may be examined for evidence of dryness. The hands may be assessed for joint inflammation, indicative of rheumatoid arthritis and scleroderma.

Ocular Examination

Before the slit lamp examination, the patient's eyelids should be evaluated. The completeness of the blink, the blink rate, and the function of the eyelids should be assessed. Is there lagophthalmos? Is there a forced eyelid closure? Laxity of the upper lid should be evaluated to determine the presence of the floppy lid syndrome.

Slit lamp examination should be done to evaluate the marginal tear strip, the lid margin and lashes, the puncta, the palpebral and bulbar conjunctiva, and the cornea.

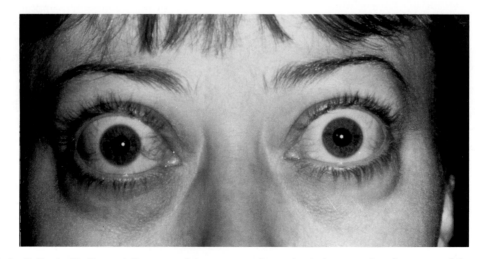

FIG. 1. Patient with Graves' disease and dry eye symptoms due to increased surface area of the palpebral aperture, and relative tear film instability.

The examination of the fornices should be done to rule out shortening and symblepharon formation.

The marginal tear strip in a normal eye has a height of 0.2 to 0.5 mm. In a dry eye patient the meniscus height is usually 0.1 mm or less. The preocular tear film is evaluated for the presence of debris and mucin. In a normal eye, the tear film is clear. Are the eyelids in proper position? Is ectropion or entropion present? Are all the puncta present or are they occluded? Are the puncta in normal position or are they everted? Misdirected puncta can result in epiphora.

Chronic blepharitis should be ruled out based on thickening of the lid margins, erythema, scales on the lashes, and misdirection of the cilia. The health of the meibomian gland should be assessed. Plugged or missing meibomian gland orifices or the presence of an oily or a foamy tear film suggest meibomian gland dysfunction. Inflammation of the posterior eyelid margins suggests a diagnosis of meibomianitis.

The conjunctiva is evaluated for the presence of follicles, papillae, shortening of the fornices, symblepharon, and injection. A papillary reaction involving the inferior conjunctiva is a nonspecific finding and not uncommonly seen in Sjogren's syndrome. The causes of inflammation of the upper eyelid are usually restricted to atopic eye disease, vernal, giant papillary conjunctivitis, superior limbic keratoconjunctivitis, floppy eyelid syndrome, and trachoma. In keratitis sicca the conjunctiva and cornea may appear dry and lusterless.

In more advanced cases of keratitis sicca, a filamentary keratitis may be seen. The filaments in a severe dry eye patient usually form inferiorly where the incomplete blink stops. The presence of a punctate epithelial keratopathy, epithelial erosions, or corneal irregularity should be noted. A keratopathy is usually seen in more severe dry eye patients or secondary to toxicity from a preservative in a lubricating drop.

MEASUREMENT OF TEAR SECRETION

In 1903, Otto Schirmer introduced his tear production test with tear paper absorbing tears from the conjunctival sac. The length of the moistened paper outside the conjunctiva is measured in millimeters. A standardized filter paper (Whatman's #41) is used. The paper strips are delivered in a precut size enclosed in polythene envelopes, with two strips in each individually closed envelope. Each filter paper has an indentation. The proximal part is rounded, 5 mm long, and prepared for insertion into the conjunctival sac. The distal part below the indentation is 35 mm long. The two strips are folded at the sites of the indentations. The patient is informed about the purpose of the test and is told that the procedure will take approximately 5 minutes. The patient is instructed to look upward; the clinician folds the lower lid and inserts the short rounded end of the filter paper inside the lateral one third of the lower lid with as little manipulation as possible (Fig. 2). The 5-mm long proximal section of the filter paper is thus contained in the conjunctival sac, and the 35-mm long section distal to the indentation hangs down before the cheek. Generally both eyes are subjected to the test simultaneously.

The filter paper must sit correctly and not touch the cornea. The patient should sit with both eyes closed and remain quiet. After exactly 5 minutes, the filter strips are removed. These are both read after having been placed on the enclosed millimeter scale. The distance from the fold to the site of transition from moist to non–tear-stained paper is measured. The filter paper should be read immediately after its removal from the eye because the fluid extends further over the paper with time.

As originally described, Schirmer's test I is performed on an opened eye. Schirmer's test II measures reflex-stimulated tear secretion that is precipitated by homolateral nostril irritation. Schirmer's test III measures reflex-stimulated tear secretion provoked by letting the patient look in the direction of the sun. Schirmer's test I with an opened eye gives a higher value with an anesthetized opened eye than with an anesthetized closed eye (1). Schirmer's test with local anesthesia gives a lower value than a test without anesthesia, which represents the basal tear secretion.

An abnormal Schirmer's test reveals less than 10 mm of wetting for a test period of 5 minutes (Fig. 3). Schirmer himself took 15 mm as the cutoff but he tested with an opened eye. Van Bijsterveld tested 550 normal subjects in 43 patients with keratitis sicca and found 5.5 mm to be the best cutoff point (2). Zappia has suggested the following age-related values in 5 minutes: 11–20 years, 19 mm; 21–30 years, 20 mm; 31–40 years, 18 mm; 41–50 years, 13 mm; 51–59 years, 13 mm; and 60 years or above, 9 mm (3).

Schirmer's test is a course test and it is therefore tempting to express the result in relation to "gray zone" of 5 to 15 mm in 5 minutes. A test result above 15 mm is regarded as normal and one below 5 mm is pathologic. A result following in the gray zone is inconclusive. If a cutoff value of 3 mm of wetting in 5 minutes is used it is extremely specific (100%). Many patients with dry eyes are missed because of the insensitivity of the test (10%).

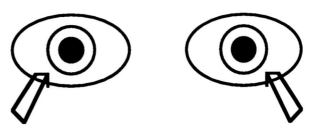

FIG. 2. Schirmer's test is performed with filter strips and measures tear production.

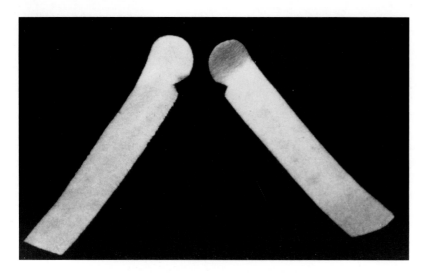

FIG. 3. Schirmer's strips showing decreased secretion (less than 5 mm from notch) in patient with keratitis sicca.

MEASUREMENT OF TEAR FILM INTEGRITY

Rose bengal staining is probably the most useful clinical test in the work-up of a suspected dry eye patient. This dye stains devitalized epithelial cells, filaments, and mucus in the tear film. Rose bengal in a 1% solution is preferable to the impregnated strips. A small amount of rose bengal dye (5 μl) is placed on the eye. The patient is asked to blink several times and the amount of staining is recorded after 1 minute. In dry eyes there is characteristic staining of interpalpebral conjunctiva and cornea. The conjunctiva tends to stain earlier than cornea and the nasal conjunctiva earlier than the temporal conjunctiva.

The red-free (green) filter on slit lamp is used for an examination of the conjunctiva and cornea. The amount of staining is recorded for both the nasal and temporal conjunctiva and cornea. Interpalpebral bulbar conjunctiva and corneal staining is consistent with keratitis sicca. Inferior corneal staining may be seen in blepharitis, ophthalmos, toxic keratopathy, and in factitious causes. Superior corneal and limbal staining may be seen in superior limbic keratoconjunctivitis and secondary to a retained foreign body beneath the upper lid. Staining of the entire cornea may be seen in advanced cases of kera-

titis sicca and ocular inflammatory diseases such as cicatricial pemphigoid and Stevens-Johnson syndrome (Fig. 4).

MEASUREMENT OF EPITHELIAL INTEGRITY

Sterile fluoroscein-impregnated strips or a 2% solution can be used to determine epithelial cell loss. Fluoroscein is applied to the inferior marginal tear strip. After the patient has blinked several times, the amount of conjunctival and corneal staining can be graded as done with rose bengal testing. As with rose bengal dye, the conjunctiva stains in mild to moderate keratitis sicca and corneal staining in advanced dry eyes.

TEAR FILM BREAK-UP TIME

The tear break-up time (BUT) is a measurement of time as it elapses from the blink to the appearance of corneal dry spots after the application of topical fluorescein to the tear film. This is a measurement of tear film stability and is usually abnormal in patients with moderate to severe keratitis sicca. Normal values are greater

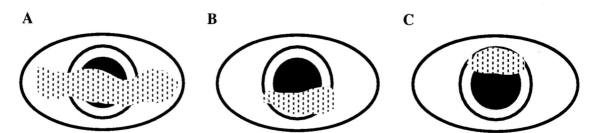

FIG. 4. A: Interpalpebral staining with rose bengal dye is characteristic of keratitis sicca. **B:** Inferior staining is suggestive of blepharitis or exposure keratopathy. **C:** Superior staining is seen in superior limbic keratoconjunctivitis (often in Graves' disease), floppy lid syndrome, or foreign body in the upper tarsal conjunctiva.

than 10 seconds. The test should be repeated three times and results averaged. Tear break-up time is decreased with topical anesthestics, drug preservatives, ocular ointments, and during the estrogen phase of the menstrual cycle (4). It is increased by the use of artificial tears.

LABORATORY TESTS

Tear Film Osmolality. The osmolality of the tear film is increased in patients with diminished tear film secretion, increased evaporation, and increased ocular exposure.

A commercially available osmometer has the ability to measure osmolality on tear samples from freezing-point depression (5). Tear film osmolality is normally between 303 and 305 mosm/L. In patients with a dry eye, this is greater than 312 mosm/L (84% specific, 76% sensitive).

Electrolyte Composition. Potassium and sodium concentrations can be measured by absorption spectrometry in tears. The electrolyte composition in keratitis sicca may be abnormal (6).

Protein Composition. The technique of electrophoresis can be used to separate the various proteins in tears. There are qualitative differences in the electrophoretic pattern of tears from normal subjects in patients with keratitis sicca (7).

Lysozyme. Tear film lysozyme levels account for 20% to 40% of the total tear protein. Tear lysozyme levels of less than 1 mg/mL are consistent with the diagnosis of keratitis sicca. The levels of lysozyme can be measured by a variety of biochemical techniques including enzyme-linked immunosorbent assay, radioimmunodiffusion, electroimmunodiffusion, and turbidimetric assays.

Lactoferrin. Lactoferrin levels are often reduced by 50% in patients with keratitis sicca. A commercially available radioimmunodiffusion assay is available for measuring lactoferrin levels.

CONJUNCTIVAL CYTOLOGY

In keratitis sicca, the bulbar conjunctival surface may undergo squamous metaplasia, which results in keratinization of the epithelial cells and loss of goblet cells. Conjunctival impression cytology removes the superficial layers of the conjunctival epithelium and goblet cells. Discs or strips of acetate filter material are applied to the conjunctival surface for a few seconds. Specimens are then removed, fixed, and stained using periodic acid-Schiff stain. These specimens are then dried and covered. The specimens are graded in terms of the number of goblet cells present and the degree of epithelial cell abnormality. In keratitis sicca, the bulbar conjunctival surface is abnormal, whereas the inferior palpebral conjunctival surface is normal. In addition to squamous metaplasia in keratis sicca, other changes include a decrease in goblet cell density, an increase in epithelial cell size, a decrease in epithelial cell cohesion, and a decrease in the size of the nucleus.

REFERENCES

1. Rieger G. Schirmer's test with topical anesthesia with opened or closed eyes? *Fortschr Ophthalmol* 1986;83:179–180.
2. Van Bijsterveld OP. A diagnostic test in sicca syndrome. *Arch Ophthalmol* 1969;82:10–14.
3. Zappia RJ. Fluorescein dye disappearance test. *Am J Ophthalmol* 1972;74:160–162.
4. Lemp MA, Hamill JR. Factors affecting tear break-up in normal eyes. *Arch Ophthalmol* 1973;89:103–105.
5. Farris RL, Stuchell RN, Mandel ID. Basal and reflex human tear analysis I physical measurements: osmolality, basal volumes, and reflex flow rate. *Ophthalmology* 1981;88:852–857.
6. Gilbard JP, Rossi SR. An electrolyte-base solution that increases corneal glycogen and conjunctival goblet-cell density in a rabbit model for keratoconjunctivitis sicca. *Ophthalmology* 1992;99:600–604.
7. Boukes RJ, Boonstra A, Breebaart AC. Analysis of human tear protein profiles using high performance liquid chromatography. *Doc Ophthalmol* 1987;67:105–113.

CHAPTER 9

Epiphora

Jeffrey Jay Hurwitz

HISTORY

Tearing

It must be ascertained whether the tearing is unilateral or bilateral. If the tearing is unilateral, it is more suggestive of a local condition such as an obstruction of the tear duct or a local irritative phenomenon such as a foreign body. If the tearing is bilateral, it is more suggestive of an oversecretion problem such as allergy, or keratoconjunctivitis. However, tearing may certainly be bilateral and this occurs, in our experience, in 40% of cases. If the tearing is bilateral, it should be ascertained as to whether the eyes tear equally or whether one eye tears more than the other because this is important when one is contemplating surgery. Other symptoms associated with tearing are important:

1. *Pain.* If the eye is painful as well it suggests causes other than lacrimal obstructions such as foreign bodies, keratitis (Fig. 1), iritis, or glaucoma. Pain and tearing that is worse in the morning suggests a recurrent erosion.
2. *Itchiness.* Itchiness in conjunction with tearing is suggestive of an allergic problem. This would be often associated with a response in the conjunctiva.
3. *Grittiness and burning of the eyes.* Grittiness and burning associated with tearing is suggestive of a problem with the tear film, such as one sees in keratitis sicca.

One should also consider psychological stress, seasonal factors (allergy), and environmental factors. In a woman, a history of eye make-up should be obtained because it is now recognized that there may be an associa-

tion between elements in the make-up and lacrimal obstruction (1).

A history of eye medications is important. Medications such as epinephrine, pilocarpine, phospholine iodide, and idoxuridine can all cause lacrimal obstruction. A history of any previous chemotherapy and radiotherapy is important as these may also cause canalicular obstruction.

Any surgery in the nose or the sinus region should be elucidated as there may be secondary iatrogenic causes of lacrimal obstruction due to the initial surgery.

Previous Lacrimal History

It should be ascertained whether the patient has had previous probings or previous lacrimal surgery. It may be often impossible to see a scar from a previous dacrocystorhinostomy (DCR). As well, tearing may be due to eyelid abnormalities related to cosmetic eyelid surgery and questions related to this should be asked. History of intracranial surgery or parotid surgery that may have led to a seventh nerve dysfunction is important.

One should also invesitgate whether the tearing is associated with eating because "crocodile tearing" gets worse with chewing and is often associated with aberrant regeneration of the seventh nerve.

A history of previous conjunctivitis is important because it may be the inciting factor in obstruction. As well, the conjunctivitis may be secondary to a blockage. It should be ascertained whether the discharge is clear, purulent (which suggests bacterial infection), mucoid (which suggests viral or allergic etiology), or bloody (which suggests a tumor).

The intermittency and the duration of tearing is important. One must ascertain how much of a problem the tearing is to the patient when one decides whether surgical management, if appropriate, is indicated. We feel that the patient must have lived with the tearing for a

J. J. Hurwitz: Oculoplastics Program, Mount Sinai Hospital; and Department of Ophthalmology, University of Toronto Faculty of Medicine, Toronto, Ontario M5S 1A8, Canada.

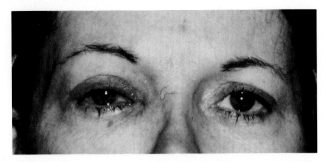

FIG. 1. Patient with herpes zoster keratitis and secondary tearing due to increased secretion of tears.

long enough period of time to appreciate the relative nuisance value of the tearing in order to contemplate surgery and be satisfied with the results.

PHYSICAL EXAMINATION

Examination of the Face and Periorbital Structures

Involuntary closing of the eye while trying to open the mouth suggests aberrant regeneration of the facial nerve, a potential etiology of tearing. So does a brow droop and, in younger people, lid retraction secondary to an orbicularis dysfunction.

Redness and inflammation in the orbital area should be ascertained. Redness, pain, and tenderness in the lacrimal sac area suggest a dacryocystitis. Masses around the lacrimal sac with a dacryocystitis suggest granuloma formation secondary to a pericystitis. Palpation by pressing on the lacrimal sac will reveal whether there is regurgitation through the punctum and canaliculus. It must be noted whether there is reflux through one canaliculus or both. Reflux through both canaliculi suggest that both canaliculi are open and the obstruction is in the lacrimal sac or duct. The nature of the reflux should be ascertained as to whether it is clear, purulent, or bloody. If there is no regurgitation, the lesion may still be a swollen lacrimal sac, and the fluctuant nature of the mass should be ascertained to confirm that it is indeed a swollen lacrimal sac (Fig. 2). A firm, hard, nonfluctuant mass may indeed be a tumor. A mass that moves within the sac may be a large lacrimal stone. Masses in the lacrimal sac area may also be due to foreign bodies that lodge in the lacrimal sac (2).

The facial symmetry should be ascertained, and evidence of trauma assessed. Hypertelorism would suggest previous facial trauma. One should look for scars around the face, specifically on the side of the nose related to a previous DCR, on the lids if a previous blepharoplasty has been performed, or in the conjunctival cul-de-sac if other surgeries have been undertaken.

The relationship of the eyelids to the lacrimal lake should be assessed. Occasionally in people with large

noses and prominent anterior limbs of the medial canthal tendon the punctum may be pulled anterior to the lacrimal lake in the lower lid (centurion syndrome).

When one examines a mass at the medial canthus, a mass above the medial canthal tendon suggests a lesion emanating from the ethmoids, and a mass below the medial canthal tendon suggests a lacrimal sac etiology. However, we have certainly seen swellings above the medial canthal tendon that are of lacrimal sac etiology, and swellings below the medial canthal tendons that are of ethmoidal etiology. One should also look for evidence of a fistula. A fistula emanating from a lacrimal sac or canaliculus etiology is located usually inferolaterally to the lacrimal sac and, on pressure, fluid may be seen to come from the fistula. A fistula of the ethmoidal sinuses has constant drainage and pressure in the area does not seem to increase the amount of the drainage through it.

Examination of the Eyelids

One should look for ptosis whereby the lid may obstruct the lacrimal punctum or possibly cause change in the dynamics of the relationship of one punctum to the other punctum (Fig. 3). As well, one should look for lid retraction, which may be due to a facial palsy but more commonly due to previous surgery or, especially, thyroid eye disease. One should ask the patient to open and close the eye to see if there is any lagophthalmos or evidence of orbicularis dysfunction (Fig. 4). On opening and closing the eyelids, one should be able to determine a change in the position between the upper lid and lower lid such as one sees in a floppy eyelid or eyelid imbrication syndrome. If one holds the eyebrow against the bone and

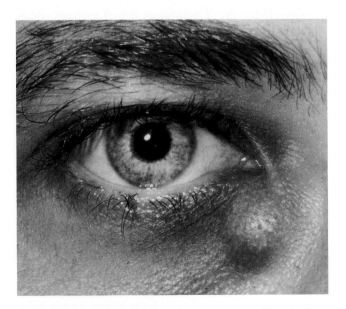

FIG. 2. Patient with mass in lacrimal sac area. Mass is fluctuant—lacrimal sac mucocele.

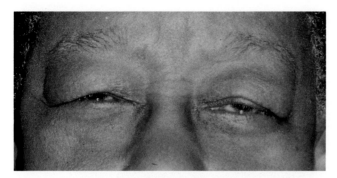

FIG. 3. Patient with severe ptosis changing relationship of the punctum of the upper lid to that of the lower lid. The upper punctum overhangs the lower punctum and, therefore, tears cannot get into the canaliculi, which causes symptoms of tearing.

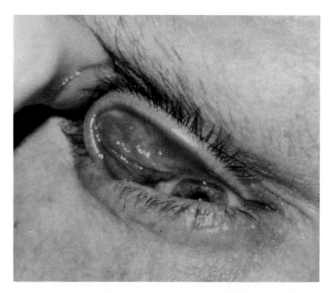

FIG. 5. Patient with extreme upper lid laxity producing floppy eyelid syndrome.

asks the patient to look down, in a floppy eyelid syndrome the upper lid will be seen to evert and there may be some follicular reaction on the conjunctiva (Fig. 5).

The resiliency and laxity of the lower lid should be ascertained. A distraction test in which the lower lid is pulled away from the globe should be performed (Fig. 6). The lid should not be able to be pulled away from the globe more than approximately 8 mm (3). The resiliency of the lid can be ascertained with the "snap back" test. When the patient looks up the lower lid can be pulled inferiorly and then released. The eyelid should be seen, when released, to snap back against the globe. Decreased "snap back" suggests eyelid laxity. which may be the cause of the tearing (Fig. 7). The eyelid margin should be examined on slit lamp and evidence of trichiasis or distichiasis noted. Certainly, lashes irritating the cornea might cause increased tearing.

The position of the puncta should be noted. One should not be able to see the back wall of the lower punc-

tum on examination with the patient looking straight ahead (Fig. 8). With the patient opening and closing the eyes, the lower punctum should be seen to hit against the upper lid and the upper punctum to hit against the lower lid. The upper punctum is located 1 to 2 mm medial to the upper lid. The lower punctum should rest just lateral to the plica, and the upper punctum tends to rest just medial to the lateral edge of the plica close to the lateral aspect of the caruncle.

On forced opening and closing of the eye one should ascertain whether an entropion is present. This is cer-

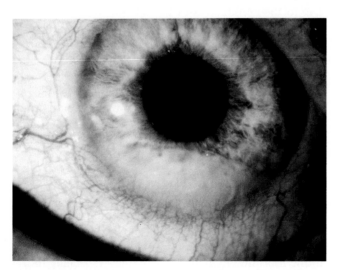

FIG. 4. Patient with nocturnal lagophthalmos with superficial punctate keratopathy and tearing.

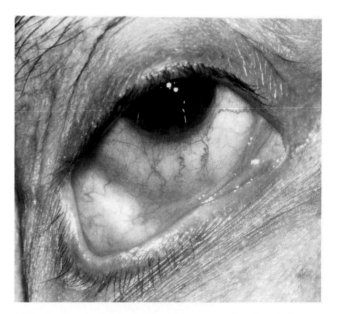

FIG. 6. Distraction test. The lid is grasped and pulled away from the globe. More than 8 mm of distraction between the lid and the cornea is suggestive of laxity.

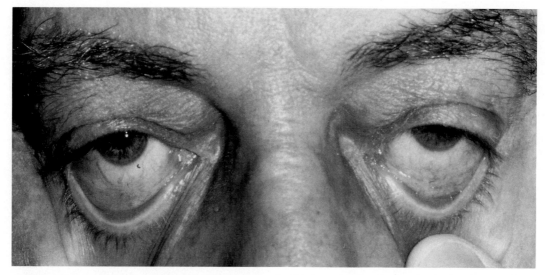

FIG. 7. The resiliency or ''snap back'' test. Pulling the lid downward and releasing it should allow for an immediate ''snap back'' against the globe. If the lid does not snap back, one can theorize a lacrimal pump dysfunction.

tainly one of the causes of intermittent tearing and irritation. The relation of the lower lid to the inferior limbus should be examined. If there is scleral show this may cause a lacrimal pump problem and tears may not be pumped adequately into the lacrimal lake and through the punctum. The presence of blepharitis should be ascertained because scaling, discharge, and meibomian gland hypertrophy may cause secondary tearing because of scales falling into the palpebral aperture and irritating the eye to cause secondary oversecretion of tears (Fig. 9).

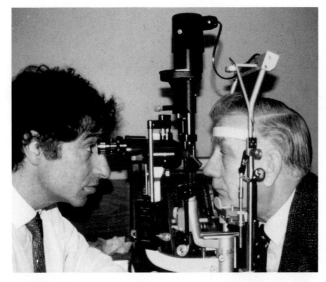

FIG. 8. Slit lamp examination is essential to determine the position of the upper punctum relative to the lower punctum on blinking.

Examination of the Conjunctiva

One may observe on gross examination symblepharon formation when one everts and pulls down the lower lid. Subepithelial fibrosis may be seen on the slit lamp as may symblepharon (Fig. 10). Symblepharon formation is suggestive when one pulls the lower lid downward and the globe moves downward at the same time. This will happen only if there is symblepharon formation, which suggests an etiology such as ocular pemphigoid, Stevens-Johnson syndrome, or burns. One should evert the upper lid to see whether there is any scarring or evidence of trachoma such as an Arlt's line. Certainly any patient with trichiasis of the upper lid should be checked for an etiology of trachoma. The position of the punctum relative to the conjunctiva of the lid should be examined. Redundant conjunctiva may fold over the punctum, thus preventing tears from getting into the lower punctum, and also interfere with apposition of the lid and the globe. This has been called ''conjunctivochalasis'' (4). Hypertrophy of the plica may also interfere with the position of the punctum and may push the punctum out of the lacrimal lake and prevent tears from getting into the punctum.

Examination of the Cornea

Evidence of corneal scarring or staining with fluorescein and/or rose bengal should be looked for (Fig. 11). If there has been a recurrent erosion, this may be seen only in the morning. Evidence of fine lines, especially in the superior aspect of the cornea vertically, may suggest a

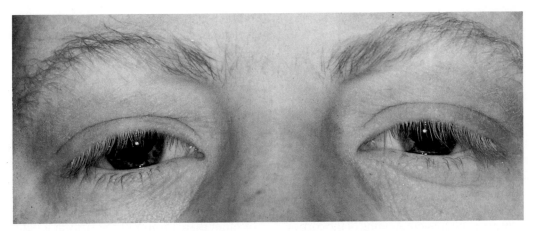

FIG. 9. Blepharitis. The crusts and scales may irritate the eye to cause an increased secretion of tears.

conjunctival foreign body under the upper lid and this should be looked for. If trichiasis is suspected, one should determine whether there are any corneal changes from the aberrant lashes.

Examination of the Vision

Tearing may cause visual problems especially in patients with lax lids in whom the increased tear lake pools in front of the cornea. Also, if one has a dacryocystitis, the vision should be checked carefully. Any signs of visual compromise, especially color vision and/or visual field deficit, would suggest a posterior tracking of pathogens. In fact, severe visual loss may occur from dacryocystitis with posterior cellulitis (5,6).

Examination of the Caruncle

Lesions of the caruncle may cause secondary obstruction of the puncta, interfere with the relative position of the puncta to each other and to the lacrimal lake, and may directly extend from the caruncle posteriorly to involve the common canaliculus. The distance between the posterior aspect of the caruncle and the common canaliculus is short (7): only 2 to 3 mm. Lesions of the caruncle may be inflammatory or neoplastic. The neoplastic lesions may be benign or malignant with the common lesions being nevi, cysts, and papillomas (8). Approximately only 5% of the lesions of the caruncle are malignant.

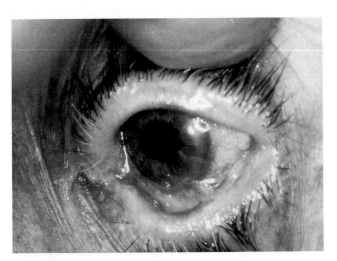

FIG. 10. Symblepharon. Patient with ocular pemphigoid and secondary canalicular obliteration producing epiphora.

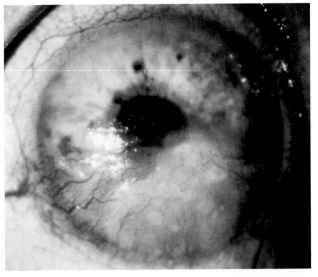

FIG. 11. Patient with corneal superficial punctate keratopathy causing secondary oversecretion of tears.

CLINICAL TESTS IN PATIENTS WITH TEARING (TABLE 1)

Secretory Tests

Fluorescein Test

A drop of fluorescein may be placed at the external canthus on the lower lid. One may observe, using the slit lamp, how the fluorescein travels from lateral to medial across the eyelid. There should be a 1-mm marginal tear strip along the upper lid and the lower lid. The absence of any tear strip is suggestive of a dry eye syndrome. One can assess if there is any fluorescein staining of the cornea as the fluorescein passes from the lateral canthus to the medial lacrimal lake. One can then evert the lids medially to see if fluorescein got into each punctum. We find it useful at this point to, with a cotton swab, milk the canaliculus from the lacrimal sac toward the punctum and see if fluorescein passes out of the punctum.

One can then perform, with the fluorescein, a fluorescein dye disappearance test. One can wait 5 minutes and then determine how much fluorescein remains in the conjunctival cul-de-sac. The amount of fluorescein can then be graded on a scale from 0 to 4, where 0 represents no dye remaining and 4 represents all the dye remaining and thereby a lacrimal dysfunction (9). As the fluorescein passes across the cornea one should also determine, with the patient blinking, whether holes develop in the tear film. This test, called the "tear break-up time," will suggest problems with the components of the tear film due to a mucous deficiency, or perhaps a reflex hypersecretion of the aqueous component of the tears. The normal break-up time should be approximately 15 to 30 seconds. A break-up time of less than 10 seconds indicates a deficiency. We have found in patients with a severe deficiency that the break-up time is almost instantaneous. We have not found it as useful to quantitate the time for the film to break up because, in our hands, there seems to be a gray area between a normal and abnormal break-up time.

The fluorescein may then be looked for in the nose. One may do this in an adult by having the patient blow the nose and see if there is any fluorescein on the tissue.

In the pediatric age group, it is often difficult to get the patient to blow the nose. One may look with an otoscope in the nose and see if there is any fluorescence in the area of the inferior meatus (10).

Schirmer's Test

A strip of Whatman filter paper measuring 35×5 mm may be placed at the junction of the medial two thirds and lateral one third of the lower eyelid with the 5-mm end folded around the lid. The patient, without any eyedrops in the eyes, and in a semidarkened room, is asked to sit quietly and blink normally for 5 minutes. A wetting of more than 15 mm of the strip in a patient under 40 years of age should be expected. If the patient is over 40 years of age one should expect a wetting of at least 10 mm. Decreased wetting suggests a decreased "reflex" aqueous tear secretion. This test is called Schirmer's I test.

If a dry eye syndrome is suspected, and the Schirmer's I is normal, one may then perform a "Schirmer with anesthetic." A drop of anesthetic eye drop is placed on the conjunctiva and wiped out after a few minutes. The Schirmer's test is then repeated and the amount of wetting ascertained. Normally there should be 10 mm of wetting in a patient under 40 years of age and 5 mm of wetting in a patient over 40 years of age. Decreased wetting on the Schirmer's with anesthetic test suggests a deficiency of the accessory lacrimal glands and the secretors. We have found these tests to be useful in patients in whom we suspect a lacrimal gland inflammatory dysfunction such as one sees with Sjogren's syndrome, sarcoidosis of the lacrimal gland, and acute and chronic dacryoadenitis (11).

The Schirmer's II test determines whether there is a reflex block of lacrimal secretion. If there is a chronic dry eye and there is no oversecretion of tears, one stimulates the first division of the trigeminal nerve afferent in the nose with a cotton tip applicator. This sensory irritation may cause a secondary oversecretion of tears in the lacrimal gland that is no longer being stimulated through the reflex arc of the afferent coming from the conjunctiva and cornea. We have not clinically found this test to be useful.

TABLE 1. *Tearing*

Lacrimation Tests of secretion	Epiphora	
	Anatomical tests	Physiologic tests
Fluorescein and rose bengal	Palpation of the lacrimal sac	Saccharin test
Schirmer's test	Irrigation and diagnostic probing	Jones dye test
	Dacryocystography	
Tear film breakup	(computerized tomography-dacryocystography)	Lacrimal nuclear scan (scintillography)
Tear lysozyme	Magnetic resonance imaging	Fluorescein dye disappearance
	Ultrasonography	
	Nasal examination	

For all the Schirmer's tests, one may wait 1 minute only, and multiply the results by three and this will approximate the results after 5 minutes (12).

Tear Lysozyme Measurement

Lysozyme is an enzyme in the tear film that may be measured by using a filter paper disk 6 mm in diameter and placing it in the conjunctiva to absorb the tears. The amount of lysozyme activity and concentration is measured by inhibition of the growth of the bacterium *Micrococcus lysodikticus.* If there is an oversecretion of tears, the lysozyme concentration is diluted. In hyposecretion states as well, such as Sjogren's disease, the lysozyme activity may also be low (13). We have not found it necessary to use this test.

Excretory Tests

Saccharin test

The saccharin test as described initially by Lipsius (14) has been popularized by Hornblass (15). A drop of saccharin is placed into the conjunctival cul-de-sac after the eye is anesthetized. A 0.4 ml of a 2% drop is used. The average time from ocular instillation to the time that the patient tastes saccharin is 3.5 minutes. It must be ascertained whether the patients have any problem with tasting before this test is done. The test is useful in determining whether the system is patent. Hornblass found that 90% of patients had a positive response in 15 minutes. We have not found, in our practice, a need to perform this test because it is not an anatomical test. However, if it cannot be determined whether a patient has tearing due to an increased secretion of tears or a decreased drainage of tears, this test might be useful.

Lacrimal Syringing

Syringing of the lacrimal drainage system is an anatomical test to determine if an obstruction exists within the system. Before performing a syringing, the patient should be informed as to what to look for and what to report to the physician. The patient should be told that this is a test and not meant to be treatment. The physician should tell the patient that the test will be performed on the eyelid and that if the system is open the patient will feel some water going to the nose and throat. One may apply a drop of topical anesthetic such as Ophthaine to the conjunctival sac. We have done a doubleblind study using Ophthaine on one side and saline on the other, and the patients cannot report much of a difference as far as the discomfort during the syringing. The lower punctum or upper punctum may be used, but we prefer to use the lower punctum because it is more accessible and does not cause as much discomfort as does syringing of the upper punctum. The lower punctum is dilated with a small dilator large enough to insert the end of a #23 lacrimal cannula. A 3-cc syringe is used (Fig. 12). During the procedure, the lower lid is put on the stretch by pulling the lid with a finger laterally. This straightens out the canaliculus and decreases the chance of false passaging through the ampulla. We prefer to do the dilatation with the patient fixated in the head rest of the slit lamp. This allows for easy access to the punctum and dilatation. After the punctum is dilated widely enough to accept the end of the cannula, we sit the patient back against the head rest and then insert the cannula. In patients with tiny puncta, we prefer to use the small double-tapered lacrimal dilator (Pilley). In those cases in which even the smallest dilator cannot be passed, or when the punctum is virtually obstructed, at the slit lamp, one may insert a #25 needle vertically into the punctum and vertical canaliculus and then move the end of the #25 needle in a medial direction. This, in fact, is a small "one snip" procedure. This allows the dilator to be passed. The end of the cannula is inserted approximately 4 mm inside the lower punctum and then the fluid is irrigated. One need not use saline—regular tap water may be used. One of three results may be found on syringing:

1. fluid passes through into the nose and throat
2. fluid regurgitates through the canaliculus, common canaliculus, and sac and comes out the upper punctum
3. fluid comes directly back through the lower canaliculus.

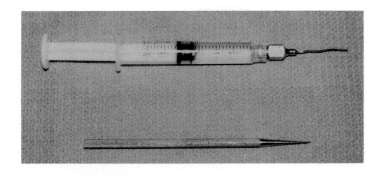

FIG. 12. A small Nettleship lacrimal dilator is used to dilate the punctum large enough to insert the end of a #23 lacrimal cannula for syringing.

Of course, there may be a combination of any two or three of these findings.

If the fluid passes through to the throat, this means the system is patent, but does not mean that the system is normal. If fluid regurgitates around the common canaliculus and comes out the upper canaliculus, the obstruction may be located in the duct, sac, or common canaliculus. At this point it is convenient to pass the cannula toward the medial aspect of the sac so that it hits on the bone of the lacrimal fossa. If there is a "hard stop" (i.e., on bone), it suggests that the cannula has passed into the sac. Therefore, the obstruction is in the sac or duct. If one feels a "soft stop" and cannot pass the cannula to a "hard stop," the obstruction is probably within the common canaliculus. It is convenient to look at the inner canthus while one is advancing the cannula toward the hard stop. If the obstruction is indeed in the sac, then the inner canthus should not shift. However, if there is a medial shift of the inner canthus while one is advancing the cannula toward the bone of the lacrimal fossa, it indicates that the cannula must be dragging the common canaliculus medially toward the bone, and that even if a soft stop (i.e., not reaching bone but appearing to stop on soft tissues) is not palpated, the obstruction is probably within the common canaliculus. This is a significant differentiation because the treatment of an obstruction in the sac or duct versus the common canaliculus is different.

If on syringing of the lower canaliculus there is regurgitation back through the lower punctum, one should insert a probe and advance it until a stop is obtained. Then, a small artery forceps can be placed against the punctum on the probe and the probe withdrawn. The distance from the end of the artery forceps to the end of the probe can be measured, and this will indicate the distance from the punctum that obstruction is present. If the lower canaliculus is obstructed, it is mandatory that the upper also be irrigated. If the upper canaliculus is also blocked, then there will be reflux of fluid back along the upper canaliculus and in a similar fashion the distance from the punctum to the obstruction should be measured. It may be found that the upper punctum is patent with syringing through to the nose. If there is an obstruction within the sac and the lower canaliculus is blocked, one would see the sac filling up when irrigated. If this happens, one should press on the sac to see if indeed there is reflux of fluid down into the nose or back through the upper canaliculus and punctum. One may also find that there is an obstruction within the common canaliculus on irrigation of the upper canaliculus. As one passes the cannula one would find a dragging of the medial canthus medially, indicating a soft stop and a common canalicular blockage.

There is one other situation that one may encounter: one may syringe into the sac and there seems to be no obstruction, and the patient cannot feel fluid going into the nose and throat. This suggests that there is a communication through into the maxillary antrum. If the patient quickly tips the head forward, the fluid may drain out of the antrum through its opening into the middle meatus and run out the nose. The usual cause of this is trauma or following sinus surgery.

Patency to syringing does not mean a normal system because there may be some stenosis within the system that causes the tearing. If some of the fluid passes through to the nose and some refluxes, the examiner might attempt to determine what percentage of the fluid passes through to the nose and what percentage of the fluid passes back through either punctum. On the other hand, if the system is completely obstructed it does not necessarily mean that by doing an operation on the tear duct to open up the tear duct that this will get rid of the tearing. In older patients, a lax lid must be looked for as well, and also a tear film instability (dry eye) should also be assessed because these may coexist with a blocked tear duct, especially in older patients, and be the main cause of the tearing.

We have not found it necessary to use a tiny lacrimal probe, which has a sharp tip on the end, to serve as a dilator. We are concerned that when we are doing our diagnostic probing, the sharp tip may damage some of the canalicular mucosa (16).

It is useful to draw a diagram of the lacrimal system on the patient's chart and indicate the findings (Fig. 13).

Jones Dye Test (17)

The Jones dye test (Table 2) is a physiologic test to determine whether the lacrimal system, which is patent to syringing, has a drainage defect at the lower end of the system (sac-duct). If this is the case, one would do a DCR; if the blockage is at the upper end of the system, one would insert a bypass tube (Jones). The primary dye test is meant to determine whether the system is "normal" or not. It is mandatory that one understands that the Jones tests are of no value if the system is blocked

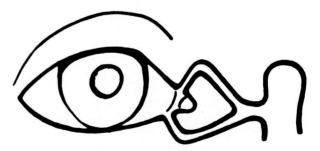

FIG. 13. Diagram of lacrimal system that can be put on a patient's chart to indicate findings of syringing and diagnostic probing.

TABLE 2. *Jones test*

Jones I	Jones II	Location of abnormality	Suggested surgery
Positive (dye in nose)	Positive (dye on irrigant)	Normal	
Negative (no dye in nose) →	Positive (dye on irrigant)	Lower system block	DCR
↘	Negative (no dye on irrigant)	Upper system block	?Jones tube ?Lid surgery

DCR, dacrocystorhinostomy.

to syringing. The system should be irrigated first before performing a Jones test. If the system is blocked, a Jones test has no value. In a system that is patent to syringing, one may perform a primary Jones dye test. The nose is cocainized with 4% cocaine spray. A topical anesthetic should not be used. A drop of fluorescein is placed into the palpebral cul-de-sac and then 5 minutes later a cotton swab is placed in the inferior meatus of the nose and is examined to see if the dye is retrieved. There is a 22% false-negative rate for this test, meaning that 22% of patients with no problems will not have retrievable dye in the nose (18). The less the tear secretion (based on Schirmer's test), the less the chance of retrieving dye in the nose in a normal patient. Also, gravity and the fluorescein volume affect the passage of fluorescein through to the nose (19). One may look for fluorescein within the nose or the oropharynx using an ultraviolet light; the positive yield of this increases to 90% (20).

The yield of retrieving fluorescein in the nose is increased if one uses a flexible endoscope (21). It would also seem that the more experienced the examiner, the greater the chance of a positive yield (22).

In practice we do not use the Jones dye test. We find that it is not helpful from an anatomical point of view in diagnosing a complete obstruction. In those situations in which an incomplete obstruction exists, a negative Jones 1 and a positive Jones 2 would indeed suggest that one could perform a DCR. However, in those cases, we prefer to get anatomical lacrimal imaging to determine whether indeed a DCR would give a reasonable hope of curing the patient. If the Jones 1 and Jones 2 are negative, it would suggest an upper system block, that is, in the common canaliculus, canaliculus, or punctum. There are a number of different treatment options and one certainly requires more information than is obtainable with a Jones test before one determines what the appropriate line of action should be surgically. As well, the Jones test does not differentiate whether the treatment should be based on a lid laxity problem or an obstruction. This situation may be even more confusing in an elderly patient with an obstruction or incomplete obstruction, and one certainly must get more information before a definitive lacrimal procedure is performed.

A difficult situation also exists in a patient who has had an enucleation, wearing an artificial eye, that has a lacrimal obstruction and presents with epiphora. Many patients with a longstanding enucleation and artificial eye have decreased sensation of the socket and, therefore, the feedback to increase the tearing through the V1 afferents in the conjunctiva would be decreased and, therefore, decrease tear secretion. Even though the tear duct might be blocked, the appropriate treatment may not necessarily be lacrimal surgery in these patients. In fact, many patients with anophthalmic sockets may have obstructed tear ducts and have no symptoms of tearing whatsoever (23).

We do use a modification of the Jones test after DCR surgery or Jones tube surgery. This can be referred to as the "Jones 3" test. Fluorescein can be placed in the conjunctival cul-de-sac and the cotton swab passed into the *middle* meatus, where the DCR or the Jones tube would drain. There should be, within seconds, appearance of fluorescein through to the cotton swab. The rate of drainage will depend on the lacrimal pump. If there is a normal orbicularis function, then the appearance of the fluorescein on the cotton swab should be almost instantaneous. However, if there is a problem with eyelid closure and lacrimal pumping, the appearance may be delayed (24).

We agree with Tucker and Codere that if one places many drops of fluorescein in the conjunctiva, the transit time to the nose of retreivable fluorescein will decrease (25). This allows for fewer false negatives.

REFERENCES

1. Heathcote G, Eplett C, Holmyard D, Hurwitz JJ. Makeup fragments in lacrimal disease. Presented at Annual Research Day, University of Toronto; 1990.
2. Felt DP, Frueh BR. Exogenus ball valve in the lacrimal sac. *Ophthal Plast Reconstruct Surg* 1985;1:115.
3. Hill JC. Analysis of senile changes in the palpebral fissure. *Trans Ophthal Soc UK* 1975;95:49.
4. Bosniak SL, Smith DC. *Advances of ophthalmic plastic reconstructive surgery*, vol 3. Pergamon Press; 1984.
5. Molgat YM, Hurwitz JJ. Orbital abscess due to acute dacryocystitis. *Can J Ophthalmol* 1993;28:181.
6. Nunery WR, Martin RT. Visual loss secondary to nasolacrimal duct obstruction. Proceedings of the American Society of Ophthalmic Plastic and Reconstructive Surgeons; 1989.
7. Kathuria S, Hurwitz JJ, Howarth D. Anatomy of the caruncle.

Proceedings of the Ophthalmology Research Day, University of Toronto; 1994.

8. Santos A, Gomez-Leal A. Lesions of the lacrimal caruncle clinical pathologic features. *Ophthalmology* 1994;101:943.
9. Zappia RJ, Milder B. Lacrimal drainage function. 2. The fluorescein dye disappearance test. *Am J Ophthalmol* 1972;74:160.
10. Jacobson ME, Pashby RC, Crawford JS. A new diagnostic method of lacrimal assessment. Poster. *Am Soc Pediatr Ophthalmol Strabismus* 1987.
11. Weiss RA, Hurwitz JJ. Lacrimal gland infections and inflammations. In: Hornblass A, ed. *Oculoplastic orbital and reconstructive surgery*, vol 2. Baltimore, Hong Kong, London and Sydney: Williams & Wilkins; 1990:1507.
12. Jones LT. The lacrimal secretory system and its treatment. *Am J Ophthalmol* 1966;62:47.
13. Hornblass A, Hershorn BJ. Lacrimal diagnosis. In: Smith BC, Della Rocca RC, Nesi FA, Lisman RD, eds. *Ophthalmic plastic and reconstructive surgery*, vol 2. St. Louis: CV Mosby; 1967:914.
14. Lipsius EI. Sodium saccharin for testing the patency of the lacrimal passages. *Am J Ophthalmol* 1956;41:320.
15. Hornblass A. A simple taste test for lacrimal obstruction. *Arch Ophthalmol* 1973;90:435.
16. Khan JA. Combination of punctal dilator and lacrimal probe. *Ophthal Plast Reconstruct Surg* 1991;7:69.
17. Jones LT. An anatomical approach to problems of the eyelids and lacrimal apparatus. *Arch Ophthalmol* 1961;66:111.
18. Zappia RJ, Milder B. Lacrimal drainage function. 1. The Jones fluorescein test. *Am J Ophthalmol* 1972;74:154.
19. Chavis RM, Welham RAN, Maisey MN. Quantitative lacrimal scintillography. *Arch Ophthalmol* 1978;96:2066.
20. Flach A. The fluorescein appearance test for lacrimal obstruction. *Ann Ophthalmol* 1979;11:237.
21. Becker BB. Flexible endoscopy in primary dye testing of the lacrimal system. *Ophthal Surg* 1990;21:577.
22. Wright MM, Bersani TA, Frueh BR, Musch DC. Application of the primary dye test. *Ophthalmology* 1989;96:481.
23. Larned DC. Lacrimal mechanics in the enucleated state. *Ophthal Plast Reconstruct Surg* 1992;8:202.
24. White WL, Glover AT, Buckner AB. Effect of blinking on tear elimination as evaluated by dacryoscintillography. *Ophthalmology* 1991;98:367.
25. Tucker MA, Codere F. The effect of fluorescein volume on lacrimal outflow transit time. *Ophthal Plast Reconstruct Surg* 1994;10:256.

CHAPTER 10

The Nose and Sinuses

Per Gunnar Liavaag, Jeremy L. Freeman, and Jeffrey Jay Hurwitz

EXTERIOR OF THE NOSE

The external nose is examined by inspection and palpation. The skin is inspected for any cutaneous abnormalities. Inspection is also made for structural problems, including displacement or deformity of the bony or cartilaginous skeleton of the nose.

INTERIOR OF THE NOSE

The interior of the nose is examined with the nasal speculum and head mirror using indirect lighting or head light using direct lighting (anterior rhinoscopy) (Fig. 1). The posterior choanae (the posterior opening of the nasal cavities facing the nasopharynx) can be visualized by a mirror placed through the oral cavity and carefully positioned behind the edge of the soft palate (posterior rhinoscopy). An excellent view of the whole of the nasal cavities including the nasopharynx is afforded by the fiberoptic nasopharyngoscope or by rigid endoscopes (Fig. 2).

Nasal Vestibule

The vestibule is the hair-bearing (vibrissae) skin-lined anterior aspect of the internal nose. It is pear-shaped in adults, with a narrow upper angle. The skin is inspected either by direct visualization and manual manipulation

P. G. Liavaag: Department of Otolaryngology, Mount Sinai Hospital, Toronto, Ontario M5G 1X5, Canada.

J. L. Freeman: Head and Neck Program, Mount Sinai Hospital, and Department of Otolaryngology, University of Toronto Faculty of Medicine, Toronto, Ontario M5S 1A8, Canada.

J. J. Hurwitz: Department of Ophthalmology, Oculoplastics Program, Mount Sinai Hospital; and University of Toronto Faculty of Medicine, Toronto, Ontario M5S 1A8, Canada.

or by using a short-bladed speculum, placed just within the nares.

Septum

The septum is composed of bone (perpendicular plate of the ethmoid, vomer, and maxillary crest) and cartilage covered by mucosa; it separates the nasal cavities into its two chambers. Using the nasal speculum or fiberoptic telescopes, one inspects for structural or other disorders such as tumors, ulcerations, or perforations.

Lateral Wall, Roof, and Floor

These areas are best inspected with the speculum or the fiberoptic telescope—the application of topical anesthesia and vasoconstrictors may obviate this. Direct examination is the mainstay of diagnosis of nasal disorders in this site.

OTHER METHODS IN THE EVALUATION OF THE NASAL CAVITIES

Other ancillary modalities are helpful in the management of nasal problems. These include imaging in the form of plain films, computed tomography (CT) and magnetic resonance imaging (MRI). The patency of the nose may be measured by rhinomanometry or nasal Doppler. Biopsy of any suspicious masses can be performed either directly through a speculum or using the nasal endoscope as a guide.

Sinuses

Physical examination of the sinuses is performed in the course of nasal examination. By the use of the specu-

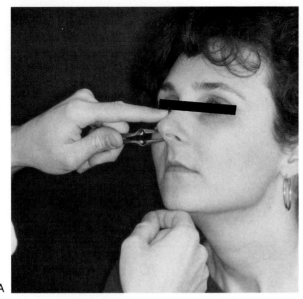 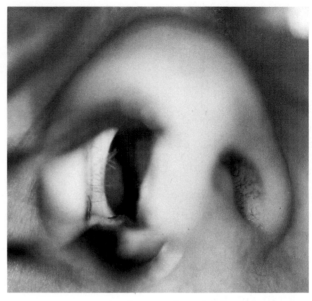

FIG. 1. A: The performance of anterior rhinoscopy is done by the use of indirect or direct lighting (from a headlight) with the nasal speculum. **B:** View obtained by anterior rhinoscopy. Visualization is limited to the anterior aspect of the nasal cavity unless a decongestant is applied. The septum, lateral wall, and floor of the nose is seen.

lum or endoscope the borders of the sinuses as they abut on the nasal cavity can be appreciated (see Chapter 17) (Fig. 2, and see Colorplate 1 after page 142). Better visualization of the areas of the ostia may be effected with sinus endoscopes. The presence of purulent material and tumors that have transgressed the sinus into the nose may be detected.

Transillumination of the frontal and maxillary sinuses is an unreliable maneuver—a sinus that fails to "glow" red in a darkened room has been purported to harbor "disease," but this is not necessarily the case.

The anterior wall of the maxillary sinus and the zygomaticomaxillary complex can be examined by palpation of these on the face. In acute maxillary and frontal

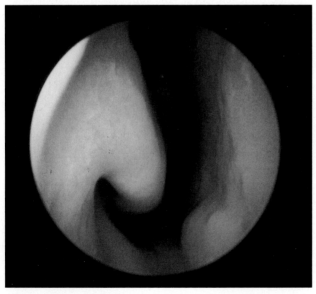

FIG. 2. Endoscopic view of the normal nasal anatomy in the middle meatus. (Courtesy of Dr. Michael Hawke, Toronto.)

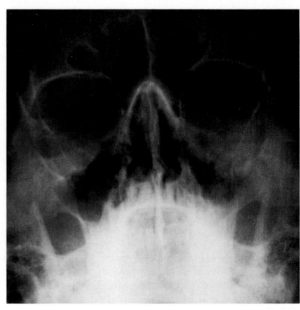

FIG. 3. Plain film demonstrating nasal and sinus anatomy.

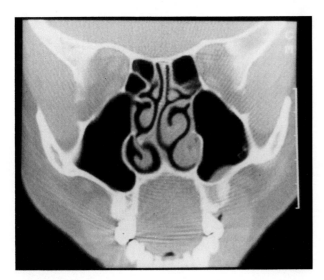

FIG. 4. Coronal CT of the nose and paranasal sinuses.

sinusitis palpation of the sinus wall may elicit some tenderness.

Palpation of the facial skeleton is important in trauma to diagnose or exclude fractures. Antral tumors can grow through the anterior wall of the sinus as well as through the palate and present as a palpable mass.

Radiologic Examination

Plain x-ray examination is still the most common imaging method of the sinuses. The anteroposterior and Waters views give the best image of the frontal and maxillary sinuses, and the lateral view best depicts the sphenoid sinus (Fig. 3).

CT is the modality of choice in the evaluation of the sinuses, both in inflammatory and neoplastic disease. This is also an excellent method of delineating abnormalities of bone, such as erosion (Fig. 4).

The use of MRI is useful in the evaluation of sinus disease, especially the soft tissue component, and is complementary to CT.

SUGGESTED READINGS

1. Ballantyne J, Groves J. *Diseases of the ear, nose and throat,* vol 3, 4th ed. London: Butterworths; 1979.
2. Cummings CW, Fredrickson JM, Harker LA, Krause CJ, Schuller DE. *Otolaryngology—head and neck surgery,* vol 1. St. Louis: CV Mosby; 1986.
3. McCaffrey TV, Kern EB. Rhinomanometry. In: English GM, ed. *Otolaryngology,* rev ed. Philadelphia: JB Lippincott; 1986.
4. Noyek AM, Zizmor J. Radiology of the nose and paranasal sinuses. In: English GM, ed. *Otolaryngology,* rev ed. Philadelphia: JB Lippincott; 1980.
5. Stammberger H, Hawke M. *Essentials of functional endoscopic sinus surgery.* St. Louis: CV Mosby; 1993.

CHAPTER 11

Examination of the Pediatric Lacrimal Patient

Robert Pashby and Jeffrey Jay Hurwitz

The causes of epiphora in the pediatric age group are numerous (1–3). They include nasolacrimal obstruction, punctal occlusion or agenesis, conjunctivitis, foreign body, keratitis, lid abnormalities such as epiblepharon, entropion, ectropion, distichiasis, trichiasis, glaucoma, iritis, and seventh nerve palsy. Elimination of the causes other than nasolacrimal obstructive or nasolacrimal abnormalities is mandatory before one proceeds with the frequently performed procedure of nasolacrimal probing.

CLINICAL EVALUATION

Palpation over the sac will determine whether a mucocele is present. Regurgitation of mucus through the puncta confirms a nasolacrimal obstruction.

The puncta should be assessed and the size of the openings determined. If the punctum is stenotic, one must determine if there is a membrane covering a normal punctum, or whether the whole of the punctum (including the papilla) has not developed. Accessory puncta should be noted, as should the presence and location of fistulas.

Any other nasal and facial abnormalities should be noted, such as cleft lip, nasal malformation, facial asymmetry, etc.

R. Pashby: Department of Ophthalmology, Oculoplastic Program, Mount Sinai Hospital, Hospital for Sick Children, and Department of Ophthalmology, University of Toronto Faculty of Medicine, Toronto, Ontario M5S 1A8, Canada.

J. J. Hurwitz: Oculoplastics Program, Mount Sinai Hospital and Hospital for Sick Children; and Department of Ophthalmology, University of Toronto Faculty of Medicine, Toronto, Ontario M5S 1A8, Canada.

LACRIMAL EVALUATION

Secretory Tests

Schirmer's test is divided into the Schirmer I and Schirmer II test. Schirmer's I test consists of the use of a Schirmer tear test strip, which is inserted into the inferior fornix and is used to measure tear production. The 5-minute reading is usually between 10 and 30 mm; however; the 1-minute reading multiplied times three is an adequate assessment. Schirmer's II test is rarely used in the pediatric age group. In this test the Schirmer tear strip paper is inserted as in test I and the nasal mucosa in the middle turbinate is irrigated and the amount of tears measured.

Irrigation of the lacrimal system in the office is impractical in infants, but can be done in an older child. This will give the definite assessment of patency. If accessory puncta or a fistula exists, and if irrigation is possible, one should irrigate through all of the openings to determine patency.

Excretory Tests

The Jones 1 and Jones 2 tests, which are mentioned in standard texts, are rarely used in the authors' experience. One test that has been practical (4) is the use of a fluorescein drop into the conjunctival sac. A modified otoscope with a cobalt blue filter is then used to look into the appropriate naris after 5 minutes to see whether there has been a passage of the fluorescein through the nasolacrimal apparatus to exit under the inferior turbinate into the inferior meatus. During the 5-minute period it is required to keep the child in a vertical position with normal blinking.

Dacryocystography, often used in the study of nasolacrimal problems in the adult (5), is rarely used in the infantile and pediatric age groups. A general anesthetic is required and, unless a significant mass lesion is suspected, the use is minimal. Microscintillography with Technetium 99 can measure the rate of lacrimal excretion but it is seldom used in children, in particular the infantile age group, as a cooperative child with the head in the vertical position and a normal blinking pattern is required. In a sedated or anesthetized child in the supine position without the normal blink, the results cannot be properly interpreted.

NASAL EXAMINATION

Nasal examination is often difficult to perform in the infant. A large inferior turbinate may make it difficult to examine the middle meatus. If possible, the inferior meatus should be assessed for congenital abnormalities. A nasal endoscope may help in assessment.

REFERENCES

1. Isenberg J, ed. *The eye in infancy.* Chicago: Yearbook Medical Publishers; 1989:209–215.
2. Welham RAN. In: Collin RJO, ed. *A manual of systematic eye lid surgery.* New York: Churchill Livingstone; 1982.
3. Morin, Crawford, eds. *The eye in childhood.* New York: Grune & Stratton; 1983:183.
4. Jacobson ME, Pashby RC, Crawford JS. A new diagnostic method of assessing lacrimal function. Presented at American Association for Paediatric Ophthalmology and Strabismus; April 1987.
5. Hurwitz JJ, Welham RAN. The role of dacryocystography in the management of congenital nasolacrimal duct obstruction. *Can J Ophthalmol* 1975; 10:346.

CHAPTER 12

Dacryocystography

Jeffrey Jay Hurwitz and Edward Kassel

Contrast dacryocystography, first described in 1909, remains the most common and definitive test for assessing the anatomy of the nasolacrimal drainage system (1). Dacryocystography (DCG) is performed by the cannulation of the superior or inferior puncta allowing direct introduction of radiopaque contrast media into the drainage system. This test is therefore an anatomic rather than a physiologic display of the drainage system (Fig. 1).

DCG is performed with the patient in the supine position on a radiographic table. A short-acting topical ophthalmic anesthetic solution may be instilled into the conjunctival sac. The punctum is dilated with a lacrimal dilator with the selected lid slightly everted and minimal traction laterally to help stabilize the punctum. The lacrimal sac is palpated to detect any mass lesion or to express any fluid present from the sac through the punctum or into the nose. A lacrimal cannula connected to a tubing filled with contrast media free of air bubbles is then placed into the selected (usually inferior) punctum. Various cannulas may be used, ranging from blunted 27 gauge lymphangiogram needles, to commercially available dacryocystogram catheters with fine metallic cannulas, to finely tapered Teflon tubing catheters. Using a variety of techniques, the contrast medium is introduced and followed radiographically. Most commonly used techniques now are intubation macrodacryocystography (2) and digital subtraction DCG (3). Intubation macrodacryocystography utilizes a magnification technique combined with distention techniques, i.e., radiographs

obtained during the injection of a contrast medium rather than following the injection of the contrast medium. Tomographic DCG using complex motion tomography may help assess fine detail of the nasolacrimal apparatus. More recently, digital subtraction DCG combines the techniques of DCG with digital subtraction fluoroscopic capabilities of modern medical imaging departments. Such equipment has high resolution digital imaging capabilities such that the image quality is superb and the overlying facial skeleton is immediately digitally subtracted, avoiding the time-consuming commitment for the previous conventional photographic subtraction techniques. Radiation dose to the lens is significantly less with digital subtraction DCG compared to conventional DCG. Digital subtraction DCG allows for real-time imaging during the introduction of contrast media. Images are usually taken at a rate of approximately one image every 1 to 2 seconds. Images are collected until patency or obstruction of the drainage system is defined. Digital subtraction DCG is also superior in demonstrating the upper drainage system, especially the common canaliculus, before reflux into the conjunctival sac obscures information regarding canalicular patency. The increased contrast sensitivity of digital imaging also allows greater flexibility of contrast agents.

Philosophy and personal preference determine whether DCG studies are routinely done unilaterally or bilaterally. An advantage of bilateral injections (simultaneous injection using a Y connector) allows for further information regarding comparative flow through the nasolacrimal drainage system. The patient is advised that he may experience a taste during the injection because the contrast medium enters the nasal cavity and subsequently the naso-oropharynx. We seldom require a lateral projection; however, such images may be useful in isolated circumstances.

Many options for contrast media now exist. The pre-

J. J. Hurwitz: Department of Ophthalmology, Oculoplastics Program, Mount Sinai Hospital; and University of Toronto Faculty of Medicine, Toronto, Ontario M5S 1A8, Canada.

E. Kassel: Department of Medical Imaging, Mount Sinai Hospital, and Department of Medical Imaging, University of Toronto Faculty of Medicine, Toronto, Ontario M5S 1A8, Canada.

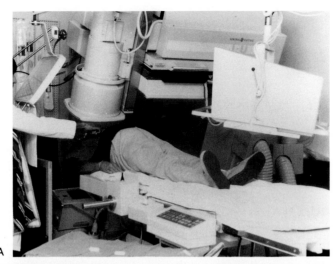

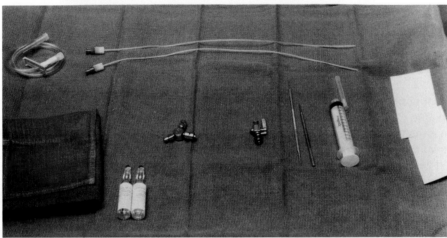

FIG. 1. A: DCG set-up. Patient lying on bed. Injection of contrast material given by examiner. **B:** Materials for DCG (digital subtraction): pediatric sialography catheters, Y-connector with one syringe, dilators, and low viscosity water-soluble contrast medium.

vious widespread use of oil-based contrast medium is being replaced by water-soluble contrast media. Oil-based contrast media such as iodized oil (Lipiodol) or ethiodized oil (Ethiodol) are less miscible with tears and may fail to display the nasolacrimal system to full advantage. If extravasated, they may remain in the soft tissues for many years, creating a granulomatous inflammatory lesion. Such oil-based solutions are more viscous and often require heating to reduce the viscosity before injecting.

Sinografin, a more physiologic ionic aqueous nonirritating contrast medium solution, miscible with tears and having a viscocity and pH similar to tears, has been replaced by a variety of nonionic aqueous-based contrast media. These new nonionic or lower osmolarity agents allow a great variety of options in iodine concentration as well as viscosity. Such variation allows both personal preference and adaptation of contrast media to DCG

performed using either conventional modalities or digital subtraction fluoroscopic control. The increased contrast sensitivity of the digital subtraction units allows for contrast media of lower volumes and lower iodine concentration. All aqueous solutions, however, have an unpleasant taste in contrast to the oil-based products, which are either tasteless or more agreeable in taste.

Approximately 1 to 2 cc of radiopaque contrast medium is injected. The lower viscosity and greater miscibility with tear fluid allow greater ease of injection and faster flow of the contrast medium through the nasolacrimal drainage system, features that are better followed with a digital DCG technique.

The concentration of iodine solutions can vary from 200 gm/L to 370 g/L. The inherent risk of granuloma formation from tissue extravasation of oil-based contrast media is obviated by the use of water-soluble contrast.

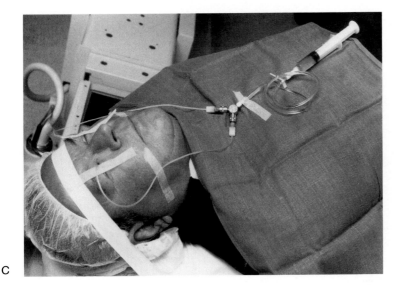

C

FIG. 1. (*Continued*.) **C:** Catheters inserted just inside the puncta and held in place with tape on cheek. Simultaneous injection possible through Y-connector.

INDICATIONS FOR DCG (FIGS. 2 AND 3)

1. *Complete obstructions.* When it is difficult to determine whether there is a "hard stop" or "soft stop," a dacryocystogram will determine if the obstruction lies in the sac or the common canaliculus. The size of the sac may be determined, and one may visualize the exact location of the obstruction (Figs. 4–8).

In patients who have had trauma to the midface and/or reconstructive surgery, if a lacrimal drainage proce-

dure is to be performed, it is useful to determine the anatomy of the lacrimal system and to view the pathology of the surrounding structures (Figs. 9 and 10).

Following failed lacrimal surgery, it is useful to determine the state of the remaining lacrimal passages (Figs. 11–15). In canalicular obstruction where canaliculitis is suspected, a DCG will show enlarged canaliculi if canaliculitis is present (Fig. 16).

2. *Incomplete obstructions.* If a patient is patent to syringing and has tearing, regardless of whether the system

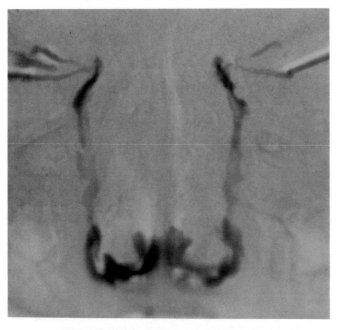

A

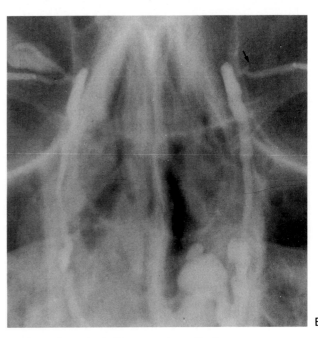

B

FIG. 2. A: Normal dacryocystogram (intubation macrography, subtraction). The normal canaliculi, common canaliculi, and the rest of the system can be seen. **B:** Normal dacryocystogram showing a lack of reflux through the superior canaliculus on the left side (this is probably a normal variant in older patients). (From Hurwitz et al., ref. 8, with permission.)

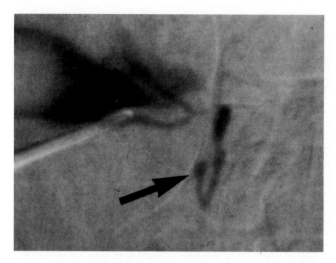

FIG. 3. Diverticulum of the lacrimal sac (*arrow*). This is a normal finding in approximately 5% of dacryocystograms. (From Hurwitz et al., ref. 8, with permission.)

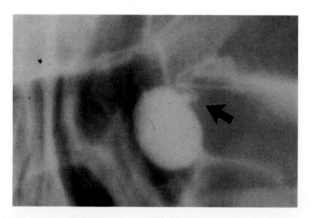

FIG. 4. Dacryocystogram demonstrating obstruction at the junction of the sac and the duct; large sac. The common canaliculus is kinked (*arrow*), preventing reflux of the mucocele on pressure. (From Rosenstock and Hurwitz, ref. 9, with permission.)

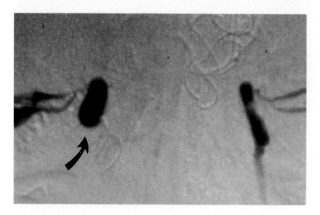

FIG. 5. Digital subtraction DCG showing one side normal system and the other with obstruction (*arrow*). (From Hurwitz et al., ref. 8, with permission.)

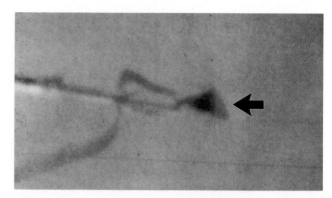

FIG. 6. Dacryocystogram demonstrating sac obstruction; small sac. (From Hurwitz et al., ref. 8, with permission.)

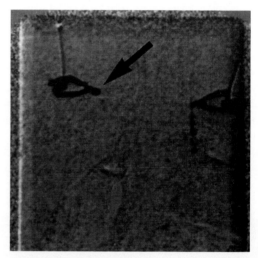

FIG. 7. Dacryocystogram demonstrating normal left system and completely obstructed right common canaliculus at its medial end (junction of sac). (From Hurwitz and Molgat, ref. 12, with permission.)

is fully or partially patent, a DCG will accurately outline if a stenosis exists within the system, and will locate the stenosis exactly (Figs. 17–21). Patients harboring stones are best sorted out using DCG (Figs. 22–25). This includes a previously performed DCR in which there is patency to syringing, and the patient still has epiphora (see above).

3. *Patients with suggested sac tumors* are assessed with DCG (Fig. 26).

4. *Adnexal problems.* Previous surgery to the nose, sinuses, or orbits may cause lacrimal dysfunction and it is useful to perform a DCG to help with the diagnosis. We now prefer to perform a DCG with a computed tomographic (CT) scan in those patients (see below).

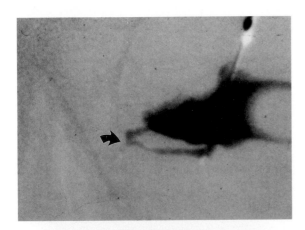

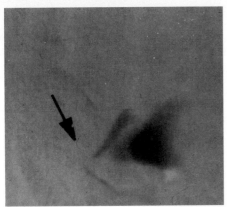

FIG. 8. Dacryocystograms demonstrating complete obstruction of the upper and lower canaliculi at the junction of the common canaliculus. (From Hurwitz et al., ref. 8, with permission.)

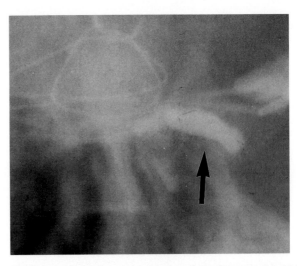

FIG. 10. Dacryocystogram of patient following motor vehicle accident and reconstruction. The left lacrimal sac is displaced superiorly and laterally (*arrow*), well out of the lacrimal fossa. This is important when one is contemplating DCR surgery. (From Hurwitz et al., ref. 8, with permission.)

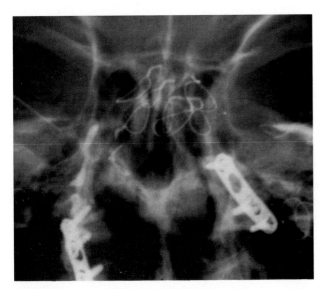

FIG. 9. Dacryocystogram of patient with severe trauma demonstrating plates and screws in the area of the nasolacrimal ducts. The location of the hardware is important when one is contemplating DCR surgery. (From Hurwitz et al., ref. 8, with permission.)

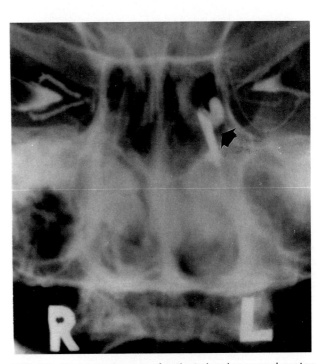

FIG. 11. Dacryocystogram of patient showing normal postoperative appearance of left DCR (*arrow*) and obstructed right lacrimal sac. (From Hurwitz et al., ref. 10, with permission.)

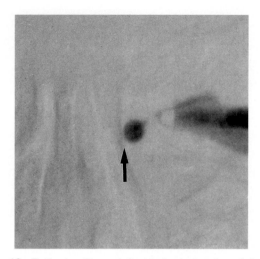

FIG. 12. Patient with a left-sided obstruction following DCR—a tiny sac is visualized. This patient is probably best reconstructed using a canaliculo-dacryocystorhinostomy rather than a reoperation at the site of the previous anastomosis.

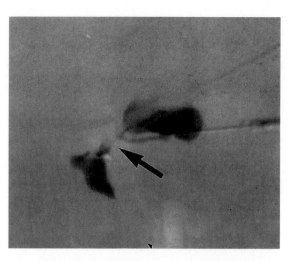

FIG. 14. Patient with tearing following a DCR in which the system is patent. A stenosis of the common canaliculus is obvious, and the patient was cured with a canaliculo-dacryo-cystorhinostomy. (From Hurwitz et al., ref. 8, with permission.)

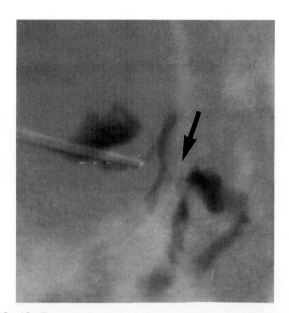

FIG. 13. Dacryocystogram showing right-sided incomplete obstruction of a dacryocystorhinostomy. The patient is tearing in spite of patency of the DCR, because of a stenosis that was cured with reoperation and fabricating a larger anastomosis. (From Hurwitz et al., ref. 10, with permission.)

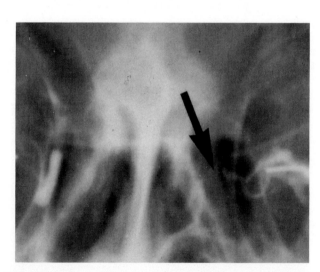

FIG. 15. Dacryocystogram using a cannula demonstrates a complete obstruction at the medial end of the common canaliculus on the left side following a previous dacryocystectomy. The patient was cured with a common canaliculorhinostomy. (From Hurwitz et al., ref. 8, with permission.)

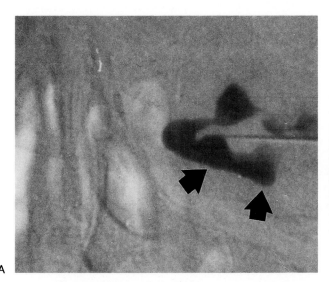
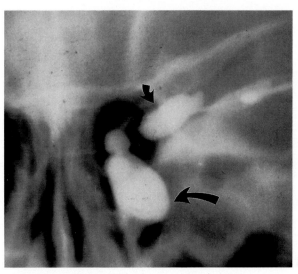

A

B

FIG. 16. A: Canaliculitis patient with canaliculitis demonstrating tremendous saccular dilatations (*arrow*) of the canaliculi, especially on the left side. Because the patient was 85 years of age, she was not having symptoms of tearing, but only chronic discharge. She was cured of the discharge with a canaliculotomy. **B:** Dacryocystogram of a 20-year-old patient with upper canaliculitis (*small arrow*) and a dilated sac (*large arrow*), both structures full of stones. The patient was cured with a canaliculotomy, dacryocystorhinostomy, and removal of the stones. (From Demant and Hurwitz, ref. 11, with permission.)

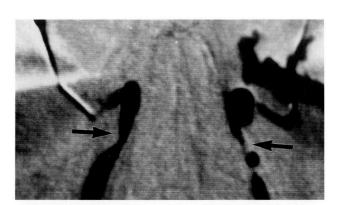

FIG. 17. Patient with bilaterally stenosed sacs at the sac-duct junction, treated with a bilateral DCR. (From Hurwitz and Molgat, ref. 12, with permission.)

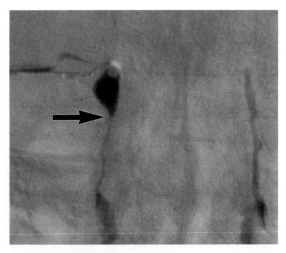

FIG. 18. Patient with a prestenotic dilatation of the sac and a filling defect within the sac. There was an incomplete obstruction within the sac. No stone was found at DCR surgery. (From Rosenstock and Hurwitz, ref. 9, with permission.)

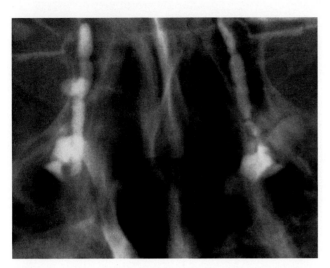

FIG. 19. Patient with bilaterally patent systems but there is drainage into the maxillary antrum. This patient had sustained previous facial fractures from a motor vehicle accident. The epiphora was relieved with a bilateral DCR draining the sacs into the middle meatus. (From Rosenstock and Hurwitz, ref. 9, with permission.)

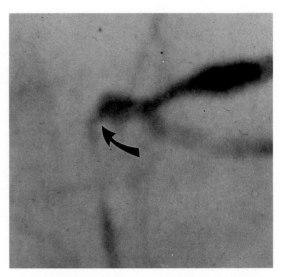

FIG. 21. Patient with tearing in spite of a patent system. There is an incomplete obstruction within the common canaliculus at its junction with the sac. Treatment is a DCR and common internal punctoplasty with insertion of a temporary tube. (From Hurwitz et al., ref. 10, with permission.)

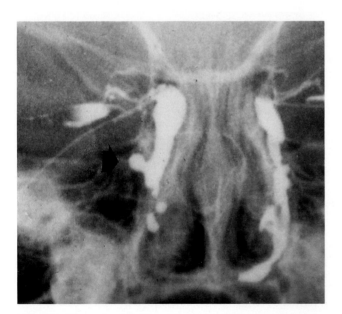

FIG. 20. Stenosis of right sac in 2-year-old (incidental diverticulum is noted).

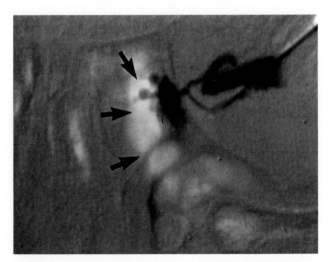

FIG. 22. Patient with left-sided tearing and patency to syringing. The dacryocystogram shows a filling defect within the sac and a large stone was found. A dacryocystorhinostomy was performed. (From Rosenstock and Hurwitz, ref. 9, with permission.)

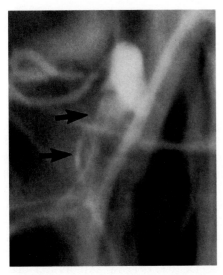

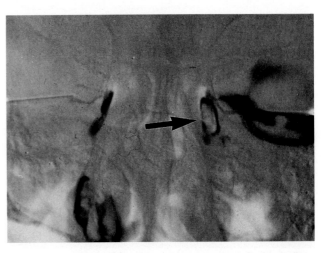

FIG. 23. A 20-year-old patient with patency to syringing on the right side. A filling defect indicative of a stone was found and this was confirmed at DCR surgery. (From Rosenstock and Hurwitz, ref. 9, with permission.)

FIG. 24. A patient with a filling defect on the left side indicative of a stone. This was confirmed at DCR surgery. There is also a filling defect on the right side, but symptoms were minimal and, therefore, surgery was performed only on the left side.

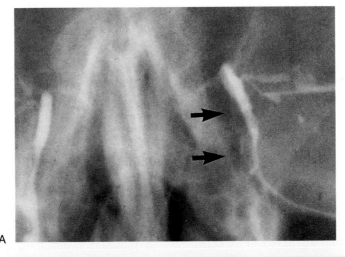

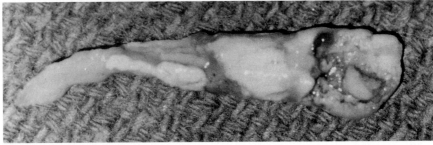

FIG. 25. A: Patient with left-sided tearing and patency to syringing. The ribbon of contrast is deflected laterally because of a filling defect within the sac. At the time of dacryocystorhinostomy surgery, a huge stone was found taking up the whole of the sac and part of the nasolacrimal canal. **B:** Stone taken from lacrimal sac. (From Herzig and Hurwitz, ref. 13, with permission.)

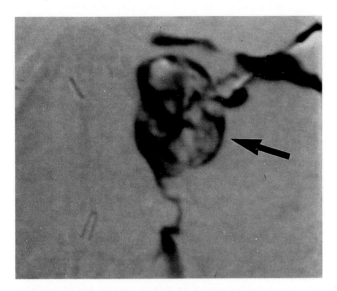

FIG. 26. Patient with tearing, mass in the lacrimal sac region, and patent system. The dacryocystogram highlights an enlarged sac with a diffuse filling defect pattern indicative of a lacrimal sac tumor. (From Hurwitz and Molgat, ref. 12, with permission.)

OUR PRACTICE REGARDING DCG

In practice, approximately 1,500 patients a year are seen in our oculoplastic clinic with complaints of tearing. Approximately 450 lacrimal drainage pathways operations are performed, and more than 250 patients undergo surgery to their eyelids for physiologic dysfunction in the lacrimal drainage. The remainder have minor office procedures such as punctal surgery, or are treated nonsurgically. Of the patients presenting with tearing, approximately 150 to 200 dacryocystograms are performed per year. Of the 450 lacrimal drainage surgeries, approximately 90 of these will have had previous dacryocystograms. Of these, approximately half will have been done for incomplete obstructions to help diagnose the significance of the stenosis and the need for lacrimal drainage surgery. The other half will have had DCG performed when complete obstructions existed, either in a post-traumatic situation, after previously failed lacrimal surgery, or to give better anatomical localization that could not be obtained by an office syringing and probing.

All our DCGs are now performed using digital subtraction rather than conventional DCG with bone subtraction. This seems to give better resolution (4). As well, digital substraction gives a lower radiation dose to the lens of the eye as compared to conventional DCG (5). Migliorati and Montanara state that in the examinations with direct magnification (macrodacryocystography), the dose to the lens is 0.17 mGy per film (6). They also state that a water-soluble contrast material gives less possibility of producing a short-term keratitis than does ultrafluid Lipiodol. In fact, they feel that it is important to protect the cornea with a solution such as methylcellulose. In our experience, we have not had anyone complaining of keratitis. Since we have been using water-soluble contrast material for our digital subtraction dacryocystography, we do not use any methylcellulose on the cornea.

More recently, DCG has been used to help determine which patients should not be treated with a laser-assisted endoscopic DCR (7). These authors feel that a DCR should be attempted by laser only if there is a large sac and if one can rule out the possibility of stones and/or tumors.

REFERENCES

1. Ewing AE. Ronetgen ray demonstration of the lacrimal abscess cavity. *Am J Ophthalmol* 1909;26:1.
2. Lloyd GAS, Welham RAN. Subtraction macrodacryocystography. *Br J Radiol* 1974;47:379.
3. Galloway JE, Kavic TA, Raflo GT. Digital subtraction macrodacryocystography. *Ophthalmology* 1984;91:956.
4. Steinkogler FJ, Karnel S, Canigiani G. Digital dacryocystography. *Klin Mbl Augenahilk* 1987;191:55.
5. Gmelin E, Bastian GO, Rinast E. Digital subtraction dacryocystography. *Klin Mbl Augenahilk* 1987;191:484.
6. Migliorati G, Montanara A. Short term keratitis after macrodacryocystography. In: Van Bijsterveld OP, Lemp MA, Spinelli D, eds. *The lacrimal system symposium on the lacrimal system.* Amsterdam Berklin, Milano: Kugler and Ghedini Publications; 1991.
7. Mannor GE, Millman AI. The prognostic value of preoperative dacryocystography in endoscopic intranasal dacryocystorhinostomy. *Am J Ophthalmol* 1992;113:134.
8. Hurwitz JJ, Welham RAN, Lloyd GAS. The role of intubation macrodacryocystography in the management of problems of the lacrimal system. *Can J Ophthalmol* 1975;10:361.
9. Rosenstock T, Hurwitz JJ. "Functional obstruction" of the lacrimal drainage pathways. *Can J Ophthalmol* 1982;17:249.
10. Hurwitz JJ, Welham RAN, Maisey MN. Intubation macrodacryocystography and quantitative scintillography—the "complete lacrimal assessment." *Trans Am Acad Ophthalmol Otolaryngol* 1976;81:575.
11. Demant E, Hurwitz JJ. Canaliculitis—review of twelve cases. *Can J Ophthalmol* 1980;15:73.
12. Hurwitz JJ, Molgat Y. Nasolacrimal drainage system evaluation. *Ophthalmol Clin North Am* 1994;7:393.
13. Herzig S, Hurwitz JJ. Lacrimal sac calculi. Can J Ophthalmol 1979;14:17.

CHAPTER 13

Nuclear Lacrimal Scanning

Jeffrey Jay Hurwitz and Joel Kirsch

Nuclear lacrimal scanning is a simple, noninvasive physiologic test to evaluate patency of the lacrimal system. Fine anatomic detail is not available as it is with contrast dacryocystography (DCG), but physiologic assessment is more accurate because no instrumentation is necessary. Furthermore, the scintigraphic images are usually acquired on a computer so that, in addition to simple image enhancement, quantitative assessment of rate of drainage and percent clearance can be obtained from each palpebral aperture. Less sophisticated physiological tests have been utilized in the past.

One may instill drops of ultrafluid Lipodol (a low viscosity oil) or Angiographin (a water-soluble contrast material) into the palpebral aperture and follow the passage of the material through the lacrimal system radiographically (1). Although this test is more physiologic than a DCG because there is no instrumentation, anatomical information is lacking. As well, there is not enough resolution of the contrast material to give an accurate assessment of lacrimal function. The nuclear lacrimal scan gives far superior information and with much less radiation.

The *nuclear lacrimal scan* was first described in 1972 in which a drop of technetium was placed in the conjunctival cul-de-sac and followed through the system using a pinhole collimator gamma camera (2) (Figs. 1–4). Computer interfacing to the system allowed one to determine the outflow of tracer from the palpebral aperture and from the lacrimal sac in a quantitative fashion (3) (Figs. 5 and 6).

J. J. Hurwitz: Department of Ophthalmology, Oculoplastics Program, Mount Sinai Hospital; and University of Toronto Faculty of Medicine, Toronto, Ontario M5S 1A8, Canada.

J. Kirsch: Division for Nuclear Medicine Program, Mount Sinai Hospital, and Department of Medical Imaging, University of Toronto Faculty of Medicine, Toronto, Ontario M5S 1A8, Canada.

PROCEDURE

Materials

1. gamma camera equipped with a micropinhole collimator ($\frac{1}{16}$ inch) and interfaced to a nuclear medicine computer
2. a 10-μL drop of technetium 99 m pertechnetate (Eppendorf pipette); this contains 5 to 10 MBq of radioactivity
3. a headrest specially designed for this test.

Method

1. Set up the computer for 20 minutes of acquisition. These are 64×64 frames at 10 sec/frame and results in about 3 K counts per frame.
2. Drop the activity in each conjunctival sac and position at a distance so that both eyes are in the field of view. Patient may blink as needed.
3. Delayed images may be obtained.
4. Have patient wash out the eyes after procedure is completed.

The images may then be formatted on film or viewed in line mode on the computer monitor. One can assess transit times, symmetry, and alterations of flow patterns.

INDICATIONS FOR NUCLEAR LACRIMAL SCANNING

1. *Interpretation of anatomical tests such as syringing or dacryocystogram.* The nuclear lacrimal scan is helpful if one cannot determine accurately with syringing whether the system is fully patent or not. If a dacryocystogram demonstrates what is a questionable minor ste-

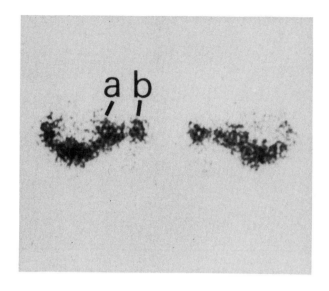

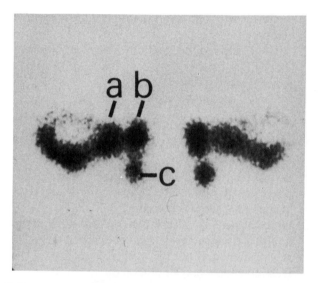

FIG. 1. Nuclear lacrimal scan. *Upper image* demonstrates tracer after 10 seconds. "a" indicates the inner canthus pool of tracer and "b" the sac pool of tracer. The second image shows, after collection of tracer at 1 minute, that activity is present down in the nasolacrimal duct ("c"). (From Hurwitz et al., ref. 9, with permission.)

nosis, the nuclear lacrimal scan may be useful in determining if indeed the stenosis is significant or not. If the stenosis is significant, tracer will be seen to halt in its flow at the level of the stenosis. If the stenosis is not significant, there will be good flow of tracer beyond the area of question (Figs. 7–9).

2. *Patients with completely normal lacrimal systems with questionable lid laxity* (Fig. 10). One can usually determine if a lid is lax enough to be the cause of a lacri-

mal pump dysfunction and epiphora. If the clinical examination is not conclusive, a nuclear lacrimal scan will be helpful because there may be seen, in a lax lid with a lacrimal pump dysfunction, to be pooling of the tracer in the lid and slow flow from the palpebral aperture into the lacrimal sac.

3. *A questionable punctal stenosis* (Fig. 11). One can usually determine at the slit lamp if a punctum is obstructed or not. However, a relative stenosis may occasionally be difficult to be sure of clinically. A nuclear lacrimal scan will be helpful because if the stenosis is significant there will be flow along the lid to the stenosis quite rapidly, and then a slow flow through the punctum into the lacrimal sac.

4. *To determine whether a system is normal or abnormal.* The lacrimal scan is the best method for measuring the dynamics of tear drainage (4). If the nuclear lacrimal scan is normal, then it is extremely unlikely that the tearing is due to a problem related to drainage of tears.

5. *Questionable pediatric obstructions.* In a baby in whom one may not be able to perform a syringing in the office, lacrimal scanning may be useful in determining whether the system is patent or not (5). However, we have not performed lacrimal scanning in babies because there is some radiation (although very low) and one may adequately determine the status of the lacrimal system by putting fluorescein into the conjunctiva and looking in the nose with an otoscope (6).

6. *Facial nerve palsy.* Patients with a seventh nerve palsy may have tearing for a variety of reasons. A lacrimal scan will help determine whether it is on the basis of a lacrimal pump dysfunction (7) (Fig. 12). One may use color coding images to get some degree of quantitation as to where the concentration of the tracer is the "hottest" (see Colorplates 2 and 3 after page 142).

7. *Thyroid eye disease.* If one studies patients with thyroid eye disease complaining of epiphora with lacrimal scanning, one may find a holdup of tracer in the palpebral aperture. As well, the sac may be flattened because of the increased orbital pressure. The lacrimal scan may be useful in determining whether a thyroid patient with tearing has a drainage problem or a hypersecretion of tears (8).

8. *Assessment of punctal occlusion.* When permanent punctal occlusion is performed surgically, or temporary punctal occlusion is performed with the insertion of punctal plugs, a lacrimal scan will determine the efficacy of occlusion. If the puncta are inadequately occluded, one may be able to see tracer flow through the canaliculi and into the sac (8).

PRACTICAL ASPECTS OF DCG AND NUCLEAR SCANNING

In practice, we do not perform lacrimal scanning routinely because in our practice it seems that for patients

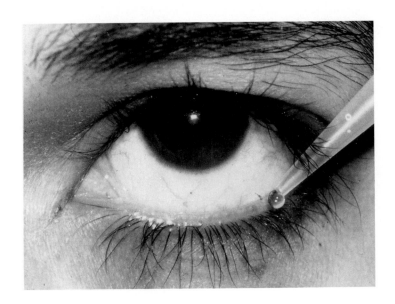

FIG. 2. Delivery of technetium sulfur colloid: 0.10–0.13 μL is dropped onto the marginal tear strip. (From Hurwitz et al., ref. 3, with permission.)

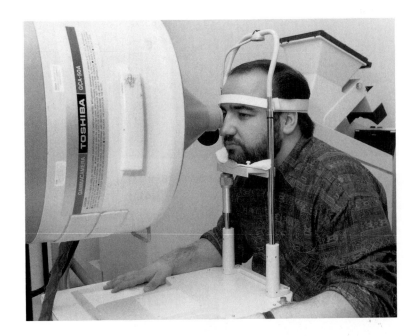

FIG. 3. Set-up for nuclear lacrimal scan. The patient sits upright with the head fixed in a head rest of a slit lamp head holder in front of the pinhole collimator of a gamma camera. Serial images are taken as the tracer passes through the system.

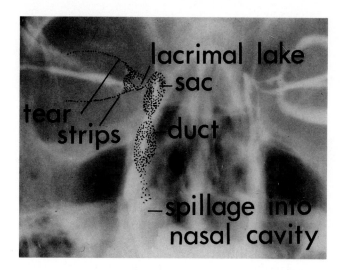

FIG. 4. Superimposition of scan images on a dacrocysto-gram. One can see the tear strips, the lacrimal lake, the lacrimal sac, the duct, and spillage into the nasal cavity. (From Hurwitz et al., ref. 9, with permission.)

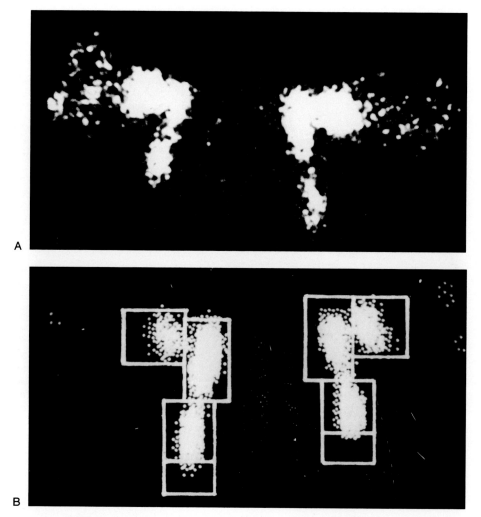

FIG. 5. A: A normal lacrimal scan image taken from an asymptomatic patient—1-min scan. **B:** On the images areas of interest can be outlined and time-activity curves can be constructed on the computer. (From Hurwitz et al., ref. 9, with permission.)

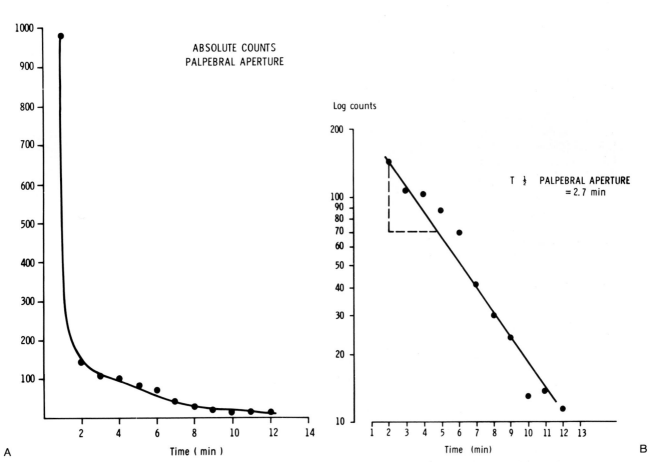

FIG. 6. A: Diagrammatic representation of a time-activity curve of drainage of tracer from the palpebral aperture. **B:** Logarithmic plot of the time-activity curve approximates a straight line. From this $T_{\frac{1}{2}}$ values may be calculated. The normal $T_{\frac{1}{2}}$ value from the palpebral aperture is between 2 and 6 min. This indicates that in 2–6 min, one half the activity placed into the palpebral aperture will leave it. (From Hurwitz et al., ref. 3, with permission.)

with insufficient drainage of tears, the etiology is either due to an anatomical problem (and is sorted out by syringing, probing, and DCG) or to a physiologic problem (this can usually be adequately assessed clinically). We perform approximately 20 to 30 lacrimal scans per year. That is, for every lacrimal scan we perform, we perform approximately seven or eight dacryocystograms. The computer quantitative assessment of the images is not routinely performed, but this technique can be useful from a research point of view if one wants to accurately calculate outflow parameters from the palpebral aperture.

In practice, when we use radiologic tests, we use the DCG to give us the maximum anatomical information and the lacrimal scan to give us the maximum physiologic information. It must be emphasized that these tests are *complimentary*, and the lacrimal scan cannot accurately be assessed without some anatomical information, namely, a syringing, and preferably a DCG (9).

The expense is relatively insignificant for these tests. The materials for a DCG are approximately $53 (Canadian), the cost for the staff and equipment is approximately $35, the technical fee is $30, and the professional fee is $11. Therefore, the cost of the DCG is approximately $129. The cost for a CTDCG is approximately $350 (see Chapter 14).

The lacrimal scan materials cost approximately $1.50. The cost for the staff and maintenance and equipment for a lacrimal scan is $28. The technical fee is approximately $100 for a lacrimal scan and the professional fee approximately $50. Therefore, the lacrimal scan cost is approximately $190. Obviously, these expenses vary from province to province and country to country. Nevertheless, these tests are relatively inexpensive and, when one considers the expense of an operation, and if one is able to avoid unnecessary surgery by appropriate testing, there will indeed be a great cost saving to the system (10).

A dacryocystogram can be performed in any hospital

A

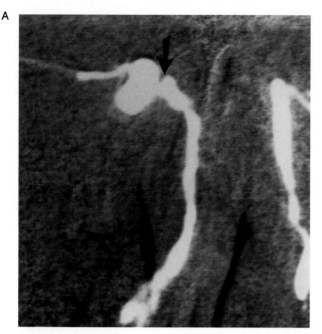

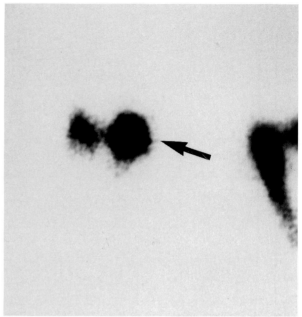

B

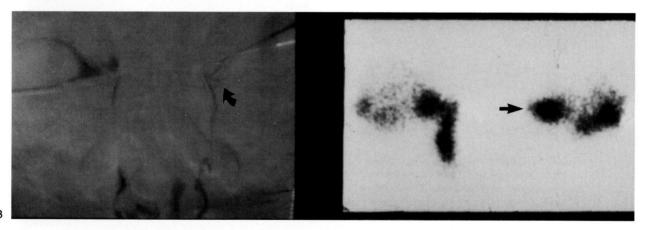

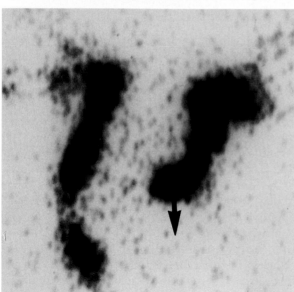

FIG. 7. A(left): Dacryocystogram of a 49-year-old patient referred having had a right dacrocystorhinostomy with tearing and yet a patent system. The dacryocystogram shows a small but patent rhinostomy (*arrow*) and a large, incompletely anastomosed sac. **A(right):** The lacrimal sac on this patient shows that there is no flow past the lacrimal sac (*arrow*). The patient was treated successfully with a repeat DCR. **B(left):** On the *left,* dacryocystogram of a patient with an obstructed left lower canaliculus due to trauma 40 years ago. There is symptomatic epiphora on the left side. The dacryocystogram through the upper canaliculus shows a normal system, although there is no retrograde flow in the lower canaliculus beyond the area of the obstruction, which is 5 mm in from the punctum (*arrow*). **B(right):** The image on the *right* is a nuclear lacrimal scan, which shows that even though the system is patent to syringing and the anatomy is normal except for the obstruction, all the tracer is held up at the inner canthus. **B(bottom):** Following a left dacryocystorhinostomy, flow was increased through the upper canaliculus and the patient was asymptomatic. (From Hurwitz et al., ref. 9, with permission.)

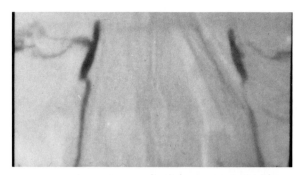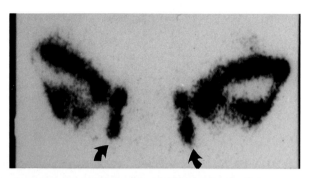

FIG. 8. A dacryocystogram in patient with bilateral tearing appears relatively normal. The nuclear lacrimal scan on the right demonstrates no flow of tracer beyond the sacs for the whole duration of the study, indicating a stenosis between the sacs and the ducts. A bilateral DCR successfully cured the patient's epiphora.

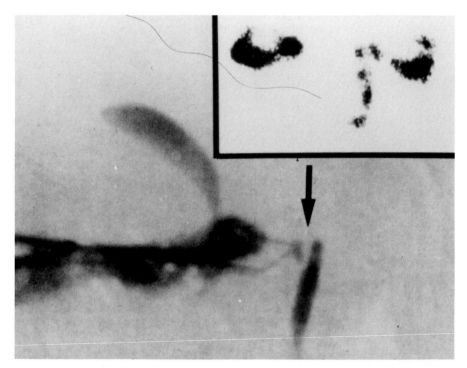

FIG. 9. Patient with right-sided tearing and patency to syringing. The dacryocystogram (*large image*) shows questionable stenosis of the common canaliculus (*arrow*). The nuclear lacrimal scan (*insert*) confirms that there is no flow beyond this questionable area. The patient was treated successfully with a canaliculo-dacryocystorhinostomy operation. (From Hurwitz and Molgat, ref. 10, with permission.)

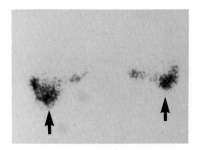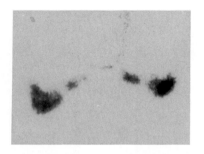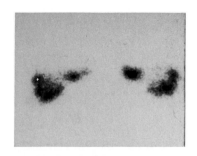

FIG. 10. Patient with bilateral tearing and question of lax lids. The tracer can be seen to pool in the lax lids (*arrow*) and does not flow through the system. The patient was treated successfully with lid-tightening procedures. (From Hurwitz and Molgat, ref. 10, with permission.)

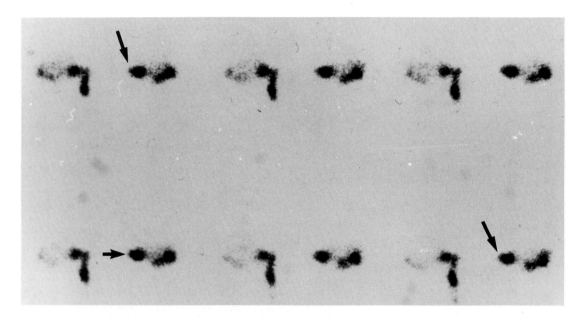

FIG. 11. Patient with left-sided question of punctal stenosis. Even though tracer flows quickly through the right side, it is held up on the left side through the duration of the study at the inner canthus and never gets into the punctum. The patient was treated successfully with a posterior wall punctectomy.

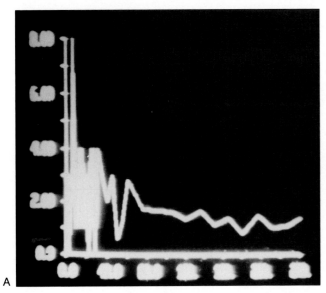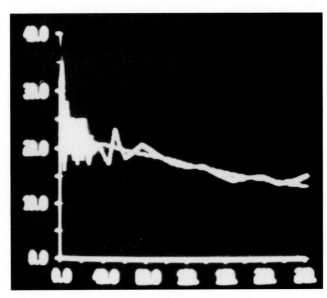

A   B

FIG. 12. Computerized lacrimal scan curves in patient with left-sided facial palsy. **A:** Computer tracing demonstrating fast outflow from palpebral aperture in normal right side. **B:** Computer tracing from side with mild facial palsy shows slower outflow of tracer from the palpebral aperture. (From Rosenstock and Hurwitz, ref. 12, with permission.)

where head and neck imaging is performed. We prefer to use a pediatrics sialography catheter for our DCGs. If a digital subtraction set-up is not available, a conventional DCG can be performed. Similarly, nuclear scanning can be performed in any hospital that has a nuclear medicine department. A standard pinhole collimator can be used. We have used a micropinhole collimator but have not found that it adds much to the physiologic information that one gets from the standard pinhole collimator. We have not found it useful to attempt to visualize the canaliculi with a nuclear scan because even in the best scenario, it is vastly inferior to the visualization of the canaliculi that one gets with a DCG. To do quantitative assessment it is necessary to have a special head holder, which is just the head rest of a standard slit lamp, so that the patient's head can be immobilized during the duration of the test (11).

REFERENCES

1. Hurwitz JJ. Welham RAN. Radiography in functional lacrimal testing. *Br J Ophthalmol* 1975;59:323.
2. Rossomondo RM, Carlton W, Trueblood JH, Thomas RP. A new method of evaluating lacrimal drainage. *Arch Ophthalmol* 1972;88:523.
3. Hurwitz JJ, Maisey MN, Welham RAN. Quantitative lacrimal scintillography. 1. Method and physiological application. *Br J Ophthalmol* 1975;59:308.
4. Von Denffer H, Dressler J, Pabst HW. Lacrimal dacryocyscintigraphy. *Semin Nucl Med* 1984;14:8.
5. Heyman S, Katowitz JA, Smoger B. Dacryoscintigraphy in children. *Ophthal Surg* 1985;16:703.
6. Jacobson ME, Pashby RC, Crawford JS. A new diagnostic method of lacrimal assessment. Poster, American Association of Pediatric Ophthalmology and Strabismus. Phoenix, 1987
7. Doucet TW, Hurwitz JJ, Chin Sang H. Lacrimal scintillography; advances and functional application. *Surv Ophthalmol* 1982;27: 105.
8. Hurwitz JJ, Maisey MN, Welham RAN. Quantitative lacrimal scintillography. 2. Lacrimal pathology. *Br J Ophthalmol* 1975:59: 313.
9. Hurwitz JJ, Welham RAN, Maisey MN. Intubation macrodacryocystography and quantitative scintigraphy: the "complete" lacrimal assessment. *Trans Am Acad Ophthalmol Otolaryngol* 1981;5:75.
10. Hurwitz JJ, Molgat Y. Radiological test of lacrimal drainage. Diagnostic value versus cost effectiveness. In: Miglior M, Van Bijsterveld OP, Spinelli D, eds. *Lacrimal system symposium on the lacrimal system*. Milano: Ghedini Editore; 1993.
11. Chenoweth DR, Hurwitz JJ. A headholder for radionucleotide dacryocystography. *Radiology* 1976;120:730.
12. Rosenstock T, Hurwitz JJ. Functional obstruction of the lacrimal drainage passages. *Canad J Ophthalmol* 1982;17:249.

CHAPTER 14

Computed Tomography and Combined CT-Dacryocystography

Jeffrey Jay Hurwitz, Edward Kassel, and Nasir Jaffer

Dacryocystography (DCG) by itself is limited in its ability to offer information extrinsic to the nasolacrimal drainage system proper. Although displacement of the drainage system may be shown, the exact extent of disease external to the system cannot be directly assessed. High resolution thin section (1.0–2.5 mm slice thickness) computed tomography (CT) imaging in the axial and/or coronal plane may be helpful in assessing those structures intimately associated with the nasolacrimal drainage system, including the lacrimal fossa, adjacent orbit, paranasal sinuses, and nasal cavity. Intravenous enhancement is usually used because CT studies are primarily indicated to assess the presence or extent of inflammatory or neoplastic processes (Figs. 1–3).

The canaliculi are not able to be identified as distinct structures within the medial canthal tissues by intravenous-enhanced CT. The lacrimal sac, however, can be identified as either a tear-filled soft tissue density or air-filled structure normally not exceeding 2 mm in diameter unless distended with air. Enhancement of the venous plexus surrounding the lacrimal sac as well as Horner's muscle help outline the lacrimal sac. The medial orbital septum attaches just posterior to the posterior lacrimal crest. The lacrimal fossa and sac are therefore preseptal

structures. Below the level of the medial palpebral ligament, the lacrimal sac is not enveloped by the orbicularis oculi muscle and therefore is potentially weaker at this site, offering less resistance to intraorbital spread of infection.

The lacrimal sac tapers inferiorly to be continuous with the nasolacrimal duct. The valve-like folds of mucosa separating the lacrimal sac from the nasolacrimal duct are not recognized on CT. The intraosseous component of the duct can be identified as an encircling bony canal inferior to the lacrimal fossa along the medial aspect of the maxilla. The contained membranous duct is usually collapsed and occupies only a small portion of the cross-sectional diameter of the bony canal. The most inferior portion of the nasolacrimal duct, approximately 5 mm in length, is the membranous portion of the canal and may be seen as a slit-like or funnel-shaped foramen beneath the nasal mucosa emptying into the inferior meatus. Coronal CT may better display the longitudinal course of the nasolacrimal duct.

CT may be useful in demonstrating inflammation and dilatation of the lacrimal sac (dacryocystitis) and in differentiating such preseptal pathology from other preseptal inflammatory lesions or from post-septal inflammatory processes such as periorbital abscesses. CT may show inflammatory, neoplastic, or traumatic processes resulting in extrinsic compression or infiltration of the nasolacrimal drainage system resulting in obstruction, enlargement, and dilatation, or compression and infiltration of the lacrimal sac. Lesions arising within the medial canthus, adjacent orbit, paranasal sinuses, or nasal cavity have intimate relationships with the nasolacrimal drainage system and are well visualized on CT.

Primary tumors of the lacrimal sac are rare. Such tumors usually arise from the pseudostratified epithelial lining of the sac and may be missed for months or years.

J. J. Hurwitz: Oculoplastics Program, Mount Sinai Hospital; and Department of Ophthalmology, University of Toronto Faculty of Medicine, Toronto, Ontario M5S 1A8, Canada.

E. Kassel: Neuroradiology Program, Department of Medical Imaging, Mount Sinai Hospital, and Department of Medical Imaging, University of Toronto Faculty of Medicine, Toronto, Ontario M5S 1A8, Canada.

N. Jaffer: Department of Neuroradiology, Mount Sinai Hospital, and Department of Medical Imaging, University of Toronto Faculty of Medicine, Toronto, Ontario M5S 1A8, Canada.

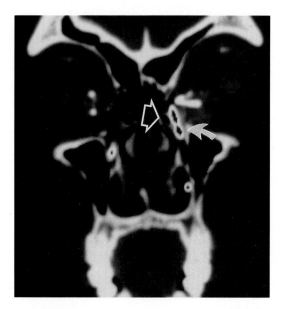

FIG. 1. CT-DCG shows a normal system on the right side and an outlining of a lacrimal stone on the left (*arrow*). (From Hurwitz and Molgat, ref. 3, and Ashenhurst and Hurwitz, ref. 1, with permission.)

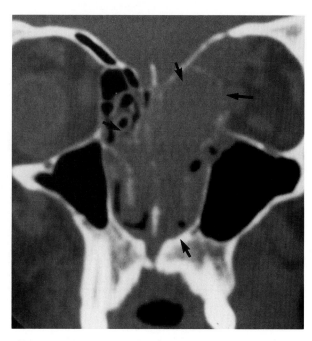

FIG. 2. CT scan showing a large nasal tumor encroaching on the orbit on the left side. Contrast does not pass into the system because of pressure on it by the tumor. (From Hurwitz and Molgat, ref. 3, with permission.)

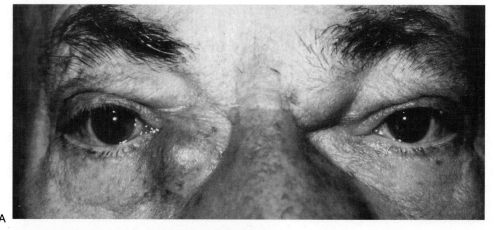

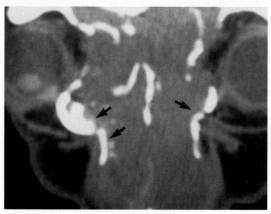

FIG. 3. A: Patient with large lacrimal sac swelling and coexisting tremendous inflammatory process in the nose and lacrimal sinuses. **B:** CT-DCG shows patent systems with a good outlining of the sac and duct on the left side (*1 arrow*) and a significant distortion of the sac laterally on the right (*2 arrows*). (From Hurwitz and Molgat, ref. 3, with permission.)

CT findings of sac enlargement (dacryocystitis) should be distinguished from findings of a solid tumor with possible secondary sac enlargement. CT, in combination with DCG, may help define tumors arising from the lacrimal sac fundus or show the lumen irregularity caused by tumor better than by enhanced CT alone.

COMBINED CT-DACRYOCYSTOGRAPHY (CT-DCG)

By combining CT, with its known capabilities of imaging bone and soft tissue structures of the face and orbit, with DCG, a modality to best show the nasolacrimal drainage system itself, CT-DCG may better demonstrate the relationship between the nasolacrimal drainage system and the surrounding soft tissue or bony structures (1). Such a study may be indicated in the assessment of more complex lacrimal problems such as medial canthal tumors, mid-face trauma, or epiphora following previous sinus or lacrimal surgery. Such combined studies can more confidently show mass lesions to be intrinsic (e.g., dacryolith) or extrinsic to the duct system. Furthermore, the full extent of the extrinsic component of the mass lesion can be more properly defined. Imaging in either the axial or coronal plane may be preferred and frequently are complementary. The location of the osteotomy in patients who have undergone unsuccessful previous dacrocystorhinostomy is extremely helpful and not able to be obtained on DCG alone. CT-DCG may help show the relationship between the bony ostium of the failed DCR and the lacrimal sac filled with radiographic contrast medium. Improper size or location of the osteotomy may be noted or infrequently may show bone regrowth between the lacrimal sac and nasal cavity. CT-DCG studies may also show whether anterior ethmoid air cell resection is required to allow proper mobilization of lacrimal and nasal mucosal flaps and appropriate internal anastomosis and drainage into the nasal cavity. The relationship of surgical clips, sutures, and fixation plates to the lacrimal sac or nasolacrimal duct may also be best noted with CT-DCG. Although CT may be performed following water-soluble contrast medium eye drops placed into the conjunctival cul-de-sac, allowing better patient comfort, tolerance, and ease of procedure, we believe that a more predictable and higher quality of visualization of the contrast medium within the nasolacrimal duct system is attained when contrast medium is injected via cannulation of the appropriate puncta at the commencement of the CT study.

A magnetic resonance (MR) scan may show the lacrimal sac as well, but it does not show the canaliculi and has the same limitations as a standard CT scan in viewing canalicular pathology. Injection of gadolinium may be performed at the same time as doing an MR scan and the canaliculi may be seen (2). Goldberg and his group feel that the test is expensive and they do not recommend it as a routine examination. We have not used MR-DCG, and prefer to use a CT-DCG for the indications outlined above (3).

REFERENCES

1. Ashenhurst ME, Hurwitz JJ. Combined computed tomography and dacryocystography for complex lacrimal obstruction. *Can J Ophthalmol* 1991;26:27.
2. Goldberg RA, Heinz GW, Chiu L. Gadolinium magnetic resonance imaging dacryocystography. *Am J Ophthalmol* 1993;115:738.
3. Hurwitz JJ, Molgat Y. Nasolacrimal drainage system. *Ophthalmol Clin North Am* 1994;7:393.

CHAPTER 15

Ultrasound of the Lacrimal Drainage Pathways

Jeffrey Jay Hurwitz

Ultrasound may be used in two modalities to image the lacrimal drainage pathways: conventional echography and ultrasonic biomicroscopy (see Chapter 16).

CONVENTIONAL OPHTHALMIC ECHOGRAPHY

Standard A scan and B scan ultrasonography allows one to image the enlarged lacrimal sac (1). The advantage of this test is that no intubation of the system is necessary. However, we do not find this to be of great importance because we must still irrigate the lacrimal system to find out if it is obstructed and to localize the obstruction. Potentially, ultrasound may be useful in children if there is a swelling in the medial canthal area to determine whether it is a lacrimal sac mucocele or a tumor (2). This would seem to be a useful indication, but we have not seen a lacrimal sac tumor in a child in whom we would

J. J. Hurwitz: Oculoplastics Program, Mount Sinai Hospital; and Department of Ophthalmology, University of Toronto Faculty of Medicine, Toronto, Ontario M5S 1A8, Canada.

not be able to do an irrigation and, therefore, a subsequent dacryocystogram. Conventional echography does not allow one to determine the site of an obstruction, but one might be able to see a surgically created dacryocysto-rhinostomy (DCR) ostium (3). Practically, we have not been happy with the information obtained with respect to the DCR ostium with ultrasound. If it is imperative to study the bone from a previous DCR, we prefer to use a CT-DCG because this also gives us information as to the integrity of the canalicular passages and accurate visualization of the sac.

Ultrasonography may determine the size of the lacrimal sac in a patient with an obstruction of the common canaliculus. With a dacryocystogram in a patient who has a complete common canaliculus obstruction, one is not able to visualize the sac. Most of the time a medial common canaliculus obstruction is secondary to a primary obstruction at the junction of the sac and the duct. Ultrasonography may be useful in determining the status of the sac that cannot be assessed with DCG in a complete common canaliculus obstruction (4). This last indication is the only time we would use ultrasound in the diagnosis of lacrimal disorders (Figs. 1,2,3).

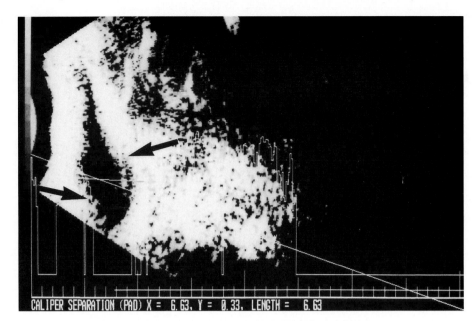

FIG. 1. Ultrasound demonstrating a large tear sac (B scan).

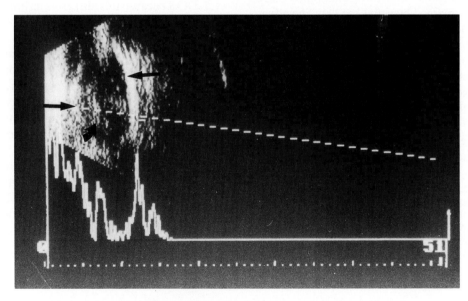

FIG. 2. Ultrasound demonstrating enlarged tear sac in patient with mucocele.

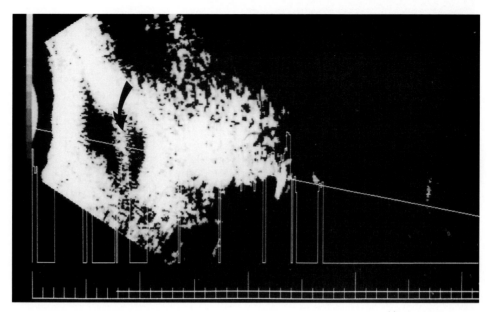

FIG. 3. Patient with obstructed tear sac with filling defects within the sac (*arrow*) indicative of lacrimal stones that were found at surgery.

REFERENCES

1. Vegh M, Nemeth J. Use of ultrasound diagnostics in lacrimal sac diseases. *Int Ophthalmol* 1991;15:397.
2. Vegh M, Nemeth J, Bordas P. Dacryocystography or echography. *Orbit* 1988;7:191.
3. Dutton JJ. Standard echography in the diagnosis of a lacrimal drainage dysfunction. *Arch Ophthalmol* 1989;107:1010.
4. Montanara A, Manino G, Contestabile MT. Macrodacryocystography and echography in diagnosis of the disorders of the lacrimal pathways. *Surv Ophthalmol* 1983;29:33.

CHAPTER 16

Ultrasound Biomicroscopy

Charles J. Pavlin and Jeffrey Jay Hurwitz

Dacryocystography (DCG) is the most useful technique available for imaging the canaliculi, but the best images are obtainable only if there is a complete obstruction. With an incomplete obstruction or a normal canaliculus, the lumen is not distended, and visualization is suboptimal. This is especially a problem in the proximal canaliculus, because the cannula must be inserted at least 4 mm into the canaliculus for the procedure. Conventional ultrasound lacks the resolution to image the canaliculus, but with a new modality of ultrasound, ultrasound biomicroscopy, accurate canalicular visualization becomes a possibility.

Ultrasound biomicroscopy is a new method of examining the eye using high frequency ultrasound (50–100 MHz) (1,2). This method allows subsurface imaging of ocular structures at a resolution approaching 20 m (Fig. 1). The trade-off using ultrasound at these frequencies is limited penetration of approximately 4 to 5 mm depending on the type of tissue being imaged. This method has been helpful in examining various types of pathology of the anterior segment of the eye (3–6) and has also been used to examine ocular adnexal structures (6). Adnexal structures examined include limbal tumors, tumors of the superolateral conjunctival fornix (7), the levator tendon (8), and other lid pathology.

Examination with ultrasound biomicroscopy requires a waterbath technique in which the ultrasound probe is placed directly over the region to be examined (Fig. 2). Examination of lacrimal structures is somewhat limited by difficulty in placing the transducer directly over some regions and limited penetration. The region of the

C. J. Pavlin: Ultrasound Program, Princess Margaret Hospital, Department of Ophthalmology, Toronto Hospital, and Department of Ophthalmology, University of Toronto Faculty of Medicine, Toronto, Ontario, M5S 1A8, Canada.

J. J. Hurwitz: Oculoplastics Program, Mount Sinai Hospital; and Department of Ophthalmology, University of Toronto Faculty of Medicine, Toronto, Ontario M5S 1A8, Canada.

puncta and canaliculi can be imaged by using a waterbath technique and placing the transducer directly over these structures. Usually the conventional eye cup used for ocular examination can be used by applying it with light pressure to the region. A viscous fluid such as 2% methylcellulose should be used as a couplant to minimize fluid loss from the irregular surface. A full waterbath using an operative drape may be helpful in some circumstances. It may be necessary to move the desired structures into the field of view using a cotton swab.

The canaliculi are normally in a collapsed state if internal fluid expansion is not present. This limits the ability to image canalicular channels. The presence of any fluid in the system provides a separation of the walls by a more weakly reflective medium. This allows visualization of the punctal orifice and internal canaliculus and canalicular diameter can be measured. Fluid can be present secondary to pathologic processes or can be introduced to provide contrast. A viscous substance such as methylcellulose or sodium hyaluronate can be used in the latter mode.

Lacrimal ultrasound biomicroscopy had been used initially in patients with suspected or proven canaliculitis. Canaliculitis is a condition in which the canaliculus becomes obstructed, dilated, and filled with material including mucus, debris, and concretions. The punctum may not always be seen to be pouting on clinical examination, and discharge is not always present (Fig. 3). The dilation of the canaliculus with internal debris in this condition allows imaging of the punctum (Fig. 4) and internal canaliculus (Fig. 5) by ultrasound biomicroscopy. The internal material in Fig. 5 has a medium reflectivity consistent with mucus. The posterior wall of the canaliculus is not imaged because of sound attenuation. The canaliculus in the example shown in Fig. 5 is dilated to a diameter of approximately 3 mm. The punctal orifice may be seen to have discharge exuding from the internal canalicular orifice, as illustrated in Fig. 6. Occasionally small regions of higher reflectivity with

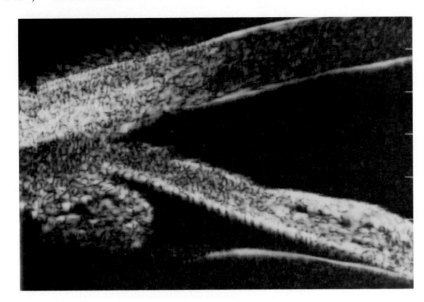

FIG. 1. A typical anterior segment examination in a normal eye shows the resolution that can be obtained with ultrasound biomicroscopy.

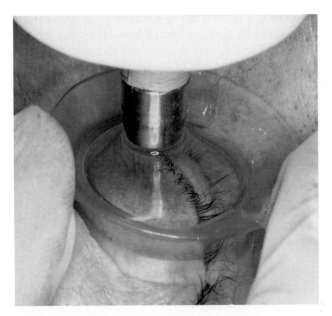

FIG. 2. Ultrasound biomicroscopy is performed in an eye cup filled with methylcellulose placed above the region to be examined.

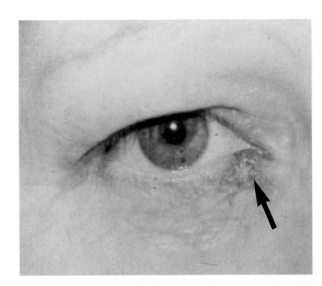

FIG. 3. Clinical photograph of the canaliculus in a patient with localized swelling in the canalicular region.

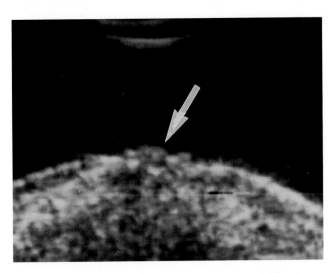

FIG. 4. The punctum is imaged by ultrasound biomicroscopy. The orifice is closed (*arrow*).

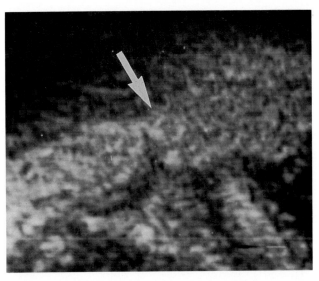

FIG. 6. Ultrasound biomicroscopic image of the canalicular orifice in a patient with discharge from the punctum. The discharge can be seen exuding from the dilated inner canaliculus (*arrow*).

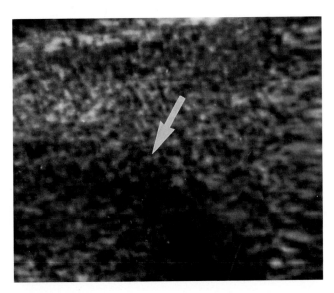

FIG. 5. Ultrasound biomicroscopy shows a dilated canaliculus with medium reflective internal material (*arrow*).

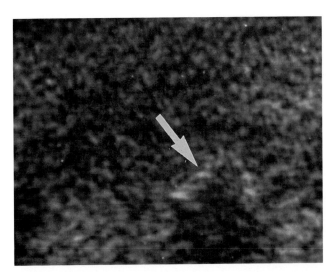

FIG. 7. Ultrasound biomicroscopic cross-section of the canaliculus shows a small concretion in the medium reflective material. The concretion (*arrow*) has a higher reflectivity with shadowing behind it.

shadowing behind them can be imaged (Fig. 7). These likely represent concretions.

Ultrasound biomicroscopy is capable of providing information on the internal state of the proximal canaliculus. Currently, research is being undertaken to determine the value of this technique in differential diagnosis of canalicular lesions and in the localization of canalicular obstructions.

REFERENCES

1. Pavlin CJ, Sherar MD, Foster FS. Subsurface ultrasound microscopic imaging of the intact eye. *Ophthalmology* 1990;97:244–250.

2. Pavlin CJ, Sherar MD, Harasiewicz K, Foster FS. Clinical use of ultrasound biomicroscopy. *Ophthalmology* 1991;98:287–295.

3. Pavlin CJ, Harasiewicz K, Foster FS. Ultrasound biomicroscopy of anterior segment structures in normal and glaucomatous eyes. *Am J Ophthalmol* 1992;113(4):381–389.

4. Pavlin CJ, McWhae J, McGowan H, Foster FS. Ultrasound biomicroscopy of anterior segment ocular tumors. *Ophthalmology* 1992:99(8):1220–1228.

5. Pavlin CJ, Foster FS. High-frequency ultrasound biomicroscopy: imaging the eye at microscopic resolution. *Ophthalmol Clin North Am* 1994;7:509–522.

6. Pavlin CJ, Foster FS. *Ultrasound biomicroscopy of the eye.* New York: Springer-Verlag; 1994.

7. Molgat YM, Pavlin CJ, Hurwitz JJ. Ultrasound biomicroscopy as a diagnostic tool in space-occupying lesions of the supero-temporal conjunctival fornix. *Orbit* 1993;12:121–126.

8. Hosal BM, Pavlin CJ, Hurwitz JJ. Clinical use of ultrasound biomicroscopy in involutional blepharoptosis. *Orbit* 1994;13:167–171.

CHAPTER 17

Endoscopy

Nasal and Sinus

Ian J. Witterick, Michael Hawke, and Jeffrey Jay Hurwitz

The nasal endoscope is a useful diagnostic tool for the lacrimal surgeon. Because of the popularity of endoscopic sinus surgery, and its potential involvement of lacrimal structures, the lacrimal surgeon should fully understand this procedure.

HISTORY AND PHILOSOPHY

Conventional "radical" sinus surgery for chronic inflammatory disease targets the mucosa of the affected sinus(es) because it is believed the mucosa is irreversibly damaged. Most of these operations involve removal of the sinus mucosa in the hope that healthy mucosa will regenerate. In addition, an opening is made from the sinus into the nose to promote drainage and allow ventilation of the sinus. In some cases, this surgically created opening is at a different location than the natural sinus ostium, which may not allow drainage even though the opening is patent. This was eloquently demonstrated by Hilding in animal experiments in which surgically created inferior meatal antrostomies were circumvented by mucus as the mucus was preferentially transported to the natural ostium by the cilia (1). In humans, middle meatal antrostomy (fenestration) has also been found to be superior to inferior meatal antrostomy but has not been

I. J. Witterick: Department of Otolaryngology, Mount Sinai Hospital, and Department of Ophthalmology, University of Toronto Faculty of Medicine, Toronto, Ontario M5S 1A8, Canada.

M. Hawke: Department of Otolaryngology, St. Joseph's Hospital, Mount Sinai Hospital, Toronto, Ontario M5S 1A8, Canada.

J. J. Hurwitz: Oculoplastics Program, Mount Sinai Hospital; and Department of Ophthalmology, University of Toronto Faculty of Medicine, Toronto, Ontario M5S 1A8, Canada.

popularized until recently because of the difficulty in visualizing the middle meatus and the close proximity (and potential for injuring) the orbit. The alternative approach with some conventional sinus operations is to remove the mucosa and "obliterate" the sinus cavity with various substances such as adipose tissue in an attempt to prevent the mucosa from regenerating.

Intranasal surgery to facilitate the drainage of purulent secretions was initially reported in the late 19th century. The development of the endoscope came from the desire and necessity to visualize the crucial structures. In 1909, Hirschman made the first attempts at nasal and sinus endoscopy using a modified cystoscope (2) but Messerklinger is credited with being the first to develop and establish a systematic endoscopic diagnostic approach to the lateral wall of the nose. His work began in Austria in the 1950s but was not published in the English literature until 1978 (3); his revolutionary concepts and techniques were not introduced to North America until 1985 (2,4). Messerklinger demonstrated the critical areas of frontal and maxillary sinus drainage in the narrow spaces of the lateral nasal wall in the anterior ethmoid sinus. This important area has been termed the "ostiomeatal complex" (OMC). Primary disease in the OMC can indirectly involve the larger frontal and maxillary sinuses by blocking their drainage and ventilation (Fig. 1).

Messerklinger focused on changes in the lateral wall of the nose with the use of rigid nasal endoscopes and tomography of the sinuses. He observed that the eradication of primary anterior ethmoidal disease resulted in healing of the larger paranasal sinuses and this led to the development of endoscopic surgical procedures directed at the OMC to establish drainage and ventilation of the larger sinuses through their natural ostia. Even limited removal of disease in the OMC was noted to reverse mas-

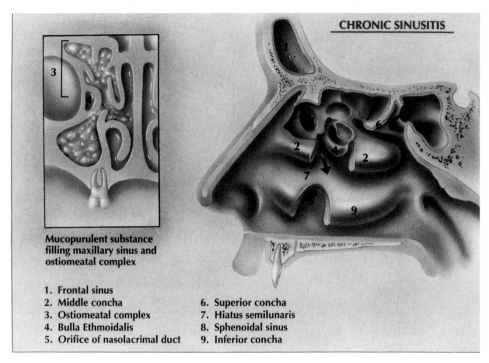

FIG. 1. Inflammatory disease in the ostiomeatal complex leads to chronic sinusitis involving the anterior ethmoid, maxillary, and frontal sinuses. (Courtesy of Dr. Michael Hawke, Toronto.)

sive mucosal pathology in the adjacent sinuses. Messer-klinger's concepts have improved and revolutionized the techniques used for the diagnosis and treatment of chronic inflammatory sinus disease. This "functional endoscopic sinus surgery" (FESS), as termed by Kennedy (2,4), removes disease from anterior to posterior in the

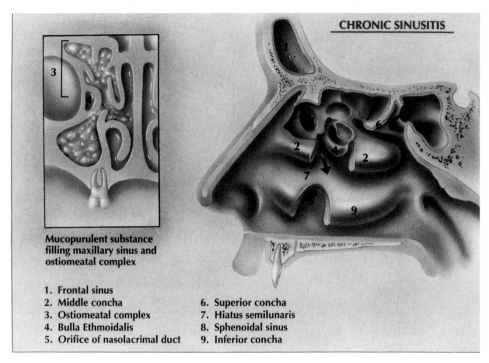

FIG. 2. Viral rhinitis from the "common cold" leads to mucosal edema and obstruction of the ostiomeatal complex with secondary sinusitis. (Courtesy of Dr. Michael Hawke, Toronto.)

OMC and limits the operation only to those areas involved. The technique was popularized in Europe by Stammberger (5) and in North America by Kennedy, Stammberger, and others (6). Endoscopic sinus surgery was originally developed for the treatment of recurrent acute sinusitis and chronic sinusitis. The concepts and techniques have been applied to other nasal/sinus problems including the biopsy or surgical removal of some benign neoplasms, drainage of abscesses, repair of cerebrospinal fluid leaks, and control of epistaxis (Fig. 2).

DIAGNOSTIC NASAL ENDOSCOPY

Diagnostic nasal endoscopic examination is a routine component of the clinical evaluation of patients with a history suggestive of chronic, recurrent sinusitis. Traditional anterior rhinoscopy with a nasal speculum and headlight is of limited value because of the restricted view of the anterior nose and the difficulty in visualizing the middle meatus well. Fiberoptic telescopes (rigid or flexible) inserted transnasally greatly enhance the evaluation of the nose and in particular the middle meatus and lateral nasal wall (Fig. 3). The rigid nasal telescope gives a wider field of view and comes in a variety of diameters (e.g., 2.7 and 4 mm) and angles of view (e.g., 0°, 30°, 70°, 120°). The most useful rigid scopes for endoscopic diagnosis are the 4-mm 0° and 30° telescopes, but when the nasal passages are narrow, the 2.7-mm telescopes may be required (Fig. 4). The examination is greatly enhanced if the nasal mucosa is topically decongested and anaesthetized. A single drug (e.g., 4% or 5%

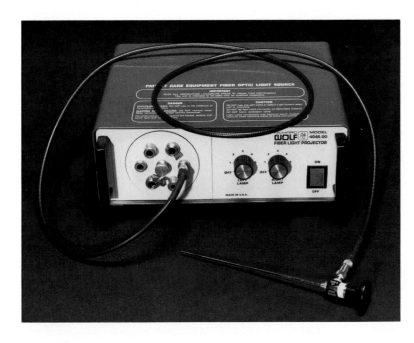

FIG. 3. Halogen light source with 0° 4-mm rigid nasal telescope.

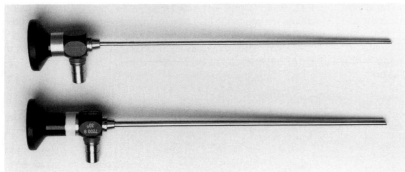

FIG. 4. Comparison of the 30° 2.7-mm (*top*) and 4-mm (*bottom*) diameter rigid nasal telescopes.

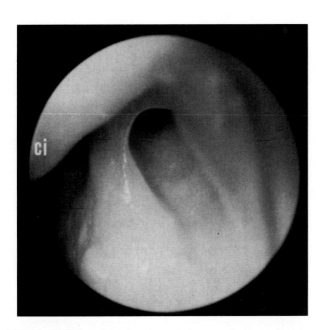

FIG. 5. Well-developed ostium of the nasolacrimal duct in a left inferior meatus (*ci,* inferior turbinate). (From Stammberger and Hawke, ref. 9, with permission.)

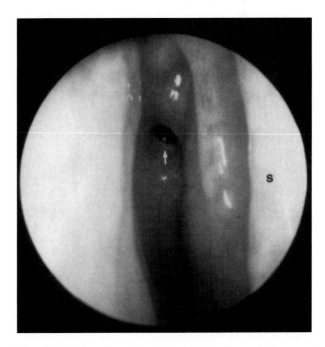

FIG. 6. Right sphenoid sinus ostium (*arrow*) (*s,* nasal septum). (From Stammberger and Hawke, ref. 9, with permission.)

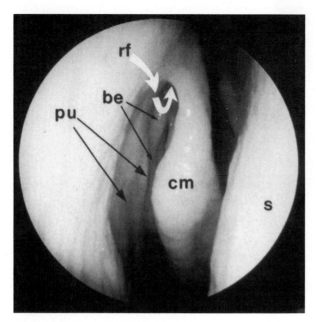

FIG. 7. View into a normal right middle meatus. The *white arrows* indicate the path into the frontal recess behind the insertion of the middle turbinate. *rf*, frontal recess; *be*, ethmoidal bulla; *pu*, uncinate process; *cm*, middle turbinate; *s*, nasal septum. (See also Colorplate 4 following page 142.) (From Stammberger and Hawke, ref. 9, with permission.)

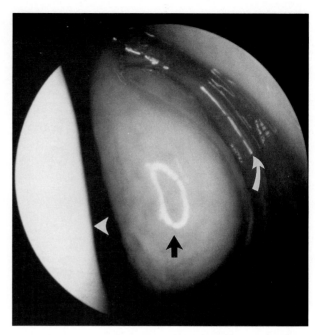

FIG. 9. Enlarged left middle turbinate (*black arrow*) closing off the middle meatus. Thick mucus can be seen in the middle meatus (*curved white arrow*; nasal septum = *white arrowhead*). The corresponding coronal CT scan is shown in Fig. 12. (Courtesy of Dr. Michael Hawke, Toronto.)

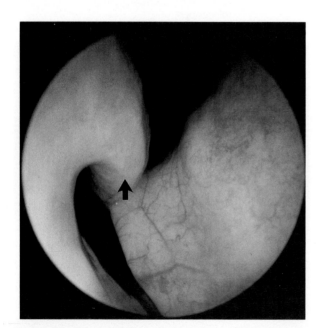

FIG. 8. Deviated nasal septum to right impinging on right inferior turbinate (*black arrow*). (Courtesy of Dr. Michael Hawke, Toronto.)

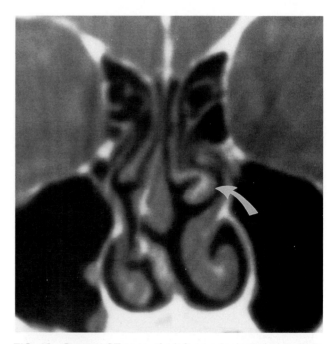

FIG. 10. Coronal CT scan of a left paradoxically bent middle turbinate (*curved white arrow*). The middle turbinates should normally be scrolled toward the lateral nasal wall but in this case they are scrolled toward the nasal septum. Paradoxically bent middle turbinates narrow the ostiomeatal complex and can lead to recurrent or chronic sinusitis.

cocaine) or drug combination (e.g., phenylephrine and xylocaine) can be used. Patients may be examined supine or sitting as long as their head is supported to prevent movement.

The endoscopic examination of the nasal cavity and lateral nasal wall is performed in a systematic fashion and usually involves three steps or "passes" with the telescope. The first pass provides a general survey and orientation and visually inspects the nasal vestibule, nasopharynx, inferior turbinate, and inferior meatus. The opening of the nasolacrimal duct can sometimes be observed near the highest point of the roof of the inferior meatus (Fig. 5). In the second pass, the telescope is directed medial to the posterior end of the middle turbinate to evaluate the sphenoethmoidal recess and superior nasal meatus (Fig. 6). The third pass evaluates the middle meatus and lateral nasal wall (Fig. 7 and see Colorplate 4 following page 142). It is easier to enter the middle meatus by rolling the scope under the posterior end of the middle turbinate than try to enter the middle meatus anteriorly. The bulla ethmoidalis and uncinate process can usually be seen in the healthy nose but rarely can the maxillary sinus ostium be seen. In approximately 25% of patients, accessory ostia can be seen leading into the maxillary sinus.

Common endoscopic abnormalities that are readily identified include nasal septal deviations (Fig. 8) and abnormalities of the middle turbinate and uncinate process. Anatomic variations of the middle turbinate predis-

posing to OMC obstruction include pneumatization of the middle turbinate (concha bullosa), enlarged (Fig. 9) and anterior extending middle turbinate, and a paradoxically bent middle turbinate (Fig. 10). Common abnormalities of the uncinate process include a medial (Fig. 11) or lateral bend and enlargement or elongation.

DIAGNOSTIC IMAGING

Diagnostic endoscopy and computed tomography (CT) of the lateral nasal wall and sinuses precisely localize underlying anatomical and inflammatory abnormalities responsible for recurrent or chronic sinus disease and thus aid the clinician in planning appropriate therapy. It is important to identify radiologically abnormalities that may result in surgical morbidity if not recognized before the procedure.

Plain sinus x-rays show the maxillary and frontal sinuses well but poorly visualize abnormalities in the OMC and lateral nasal wall. Conventional tomograms give more information but this technique has been largely replaced by CT scans. CT scans of the sinuses are an essential component of the diagnostic investigation in identifying anatomic variations or discrete areas of diseased mucosa compromising ventilation of the sinuses responsible for recurrent or chronic sinusitis. Many of these abnormalities will not be evident or only suspected following careful diagnostic endoscopy. In addition, CT scans provide valuable information about the presence of potential hazards during endoscopic sinus operations. These include dehiscence of the lamina papyracea, a low-lying ethmoid roof and cribriform plate, adhesions of the uncinate process to the medial orbital wall, proximity of the orbit to areas of disease, and location of the internal carotid artery and optic nerve. In addition, the CT scan provides information about abnormal size and shape of the sinuses, septations within the sinuses, and whether the sinus is formed at all.

Thin slices in the coronal plane are taken through the major area of interest, the OMC. Coronal images are more helpful to the surgeon because they show the anatomical detail of the OMC better than axial scans and show the anatomy as the surgeon would see it during endoscopic sinus operations. Axial images can also provide important information, particularly the relationship of the posterior ethmoid sinuses to the optic nerve and the lateral wall of the sphenoid sinus to the internal carotid artery and optic nerve. Many centers use a screening CT protocol leading to more extensive CT investigation if abnormalities are detected or need to be clarified from the screening CT.

Important anatomical variations of the OMC that should be looked for on the coronal CT images include an enlarged ethmoid bulla, abnormalities of the middle turbinate and uncinate process (hypertrophy, pneumatization, paradoxically bent), Haller's cells (air cells along inferomedial orbital floor that can block the natural os-

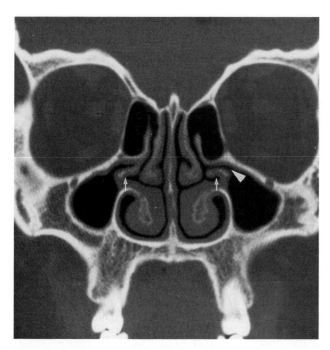

FIG. 11. Coronal CT scan of bilateral medially bent uncinate processes (*straight white arrows*) that may lead to obstruction of the ostiomeatal complex. The entrance to the left infundibulum is shown by the *white arrowhead*. The right medially bent uncinate process has caused some slight narrowing (opacification) in the right infundibulum.

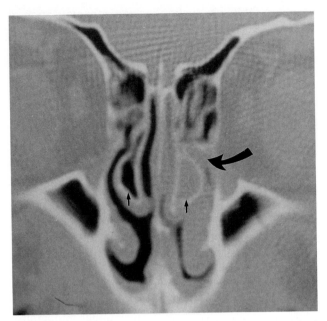

FIG. 12. Coronal CT scan of bilateral concha bullosa (*black arrows*) with opacification of the left ostiomeatal complex (*curved black arrow*) from persistent inflammation leading to chronic left-sided maxillary and ethmoid sinusitis. (Courtesy of Dr. Michael Hawke, Toronto.)

tium of the maxillary sinus), septal deviations, and agger nasi cells (when present and enlarged, can obstruct the frontal recess). Inflammatory changes are characterized by thickened mucoperiostium and opacification of the OMC (Fig. 12). Areas of increased attenuation in a diseased sinus are suggestive of fungal infection. Magnetic resonance imaging (MRI) can be diagnostic of fungal infection demonstrating decreased signal intensity on T1- and T2-weighted sequences.

TECHNIQUE, RESULTS, AND COMPLICATIONS OF FUNCTIONAL ENDOSCOPIC SINUS SURGERY

The procedure is performed under local or general anaesthesia. Apart from the increased cardiorespiratory risks of general anesthesia, local anesthesia has the advantages of excellent hemostasis, earlier recovery, and the fact that intraoperative pain can be an early warning of impending injury to the roof of the ethmoid sinus, orbit, or optic nerve. The nose is decongested (e.g., topical 1:1,000 epinephrine on cotton pledgets) and the lateral nasal wall is infiltrated with a local anesthetic/adrenalin mixture (e.g., 1% xylocaine with 1:100,000 epinephrine). The surgeon performs the procedure looking through the rigid nasal telescope or alternatively projects the images on to a television screen with a small camera attached to the telescope. The preferred endoscope for surgical procedures is the 0° (straightforward viewing). The 30° and

70° telescopes are used in special situations such as viewing the frontal recess or maxillary ostium. Specifically designed instruments in a variety of shapes and angles to access the narrow area of the OMC have been developed and continue to be refined.

Most procedures proceed from an anterior to posterior direction in the OMC and target only those areas that have been identified as diseased either clinically or radiologically. Critical landmarks such as the insertion of the middle turbinate and maxillary ostium are constantly checked to avoid getting lost with the potential for catastrophic injury to the orbit and skull base. There is no "standard" or "routine" endoscopic sinus procedure but, in general, the uncinate process is resected to gain access to the infundibulum and ethmoidal bulla. This is followed by removal of the anterior ethmoidal air cells (including the ethmoidal bulla) and the area of the frontal recess is opened. The natural maxillary ostium is identified and, if narrowed, the natural ostium is widened. If there is disease in the posterior ethmoids or sphenoid sinuses, these areas are opened and the diseased mucosa removed. Care is required to avoid injuring the optic nerve and carotid artery. If an abnormality of the middle turbinate is present such as a concha bullosa, then a portion or all the middle turbinate can be resected. Mucoceles in the ethmoid, frontal, and maxillary sinuses can be treated effectively by establishing drainage by endoscopic sinus surgery techniques.

A variety of lasers (e.g., carbon dioxide, potassium titanyl phosphate) have been used to assist in the endoscopic dissection (5,6). Complications including postoperative bleeding, creation of synechiae, and thermal injury to nasal skin have been seen (7). Laser-assisted endoscopic sinus surgery has not gained wide acceptance because it offers few advantages over conventional techniques and has the potential for thermal or direct laser injury to adjacent structures (e.g., medial rectus muscle, optic nerve) (6).

Packing is usually not required at the conclusion of the case. Temporary stents (e.g., Silastic) are sometimes placed in the middle meatus to stabilize a weakened middle turbinate or prevent adhesions between opposing areas of denuded mucosa. Systemic antibiotics are commonly given for 1 to 2 weeks postoperatively to prevent infection of the open mucosal surfaces. Several endoscopic cleanings of clots, secretions, and crusts are performed as an outpatient in the first few weeks postoperatively. There is generally little pain after surgery, but reactive swelling of the nasal mucous membranes may cause some temporary nasal obstruction. The goal of endoscopic sinus surgery is not to create a large smooth cavity connecting all the sinuses but to remove obstructing mucosal or structural variations in key locations. Normal mucosa is preserved as much as possible. In experienced hands, this technique will cure or dramatically improve patients with recurrent or chronic sinusitis 80% to 85% of the time (8,9). The best results are obtained in patients with anatomical variations that can be corrected. Less satisfactory results are obtained in patients with diffuse polyposis and nonallergic rhinitis with eosinophilia syndrome (NARES) because of the sometimes quick regrowth of polypoid mucosa despite adequate surgery and postoperative topical nasal steroid medication.

Endoscopic sinus surgery carries the potential for major complications because of the close proximity of important structures. Potential major complications include intraorbital bleeding, injury to the orbit contents or optic nerve (potential for diplopia and blindness), penetration of the skull base with resultant cerebrospinal fluid leak (potential for meningitis, brain abscess, pneumocephalus, and death) and carotid artery injury (potential for severe neurologic impairment and death). With care and proper training, these complications are extremely unlikely.

The nasolacrimal system may be damaged by intranasal procedures that involve manipulations in either the inferior or middle meatus. Maxillary inferior meatal antrostomy (nasoantral window) is a procedure that can be performed by itself or as part of the Caldwell-Luc procedure to provide ventilation and possibly drainage to the maxillary sinus. The inferior meatal antrostomy is placed at least 1 cm posterior to the anterior end of the inferior turbinate and preferably mid-way along the length of the inferior turbinate. If it is placed too anteriorly, it may directly damage the nasolacrimal duct as it exits in the inferior meatus (10). During endoscopic sinus operations, the natural maxillary ostium in the middle meatus is often enlarged. If the enlargement is too aggressive anteriorly, nasolacrimal injury may result (11). The duct lies approximately 9 mm (range 0.5–18 mm; standard deviation ±3 mm) from the natural ostium of the maxillary sinus (12). The protective bony covering over the nasolacrimal duct can be thin and offers little protection from surgical injury. It is important to avoid this complication by not enlarging the natural ostium anteriorly beyond the uncinate process or attachment of the middle turbinate. The incidence of unrecognized lacrimal system injury following endoscopic surgery is not known, but preliminary investigations suggest it is not uncommon and minor injuries invariably heal without complication (13). Postoperative epiphora requiring some form of intervention develops in approximately 0.3% to 1.7% of patients (14,15).

NASAL ENDOSCOPY AND THE LACRIMAL SYSTEM

The nasal endoscope may have a role in the assessment and treatment of lacrimal patients.

Pre-Operative Nasal Examination

1. Further assessment of the nose in the lacrimal patients if pathology is found in the nose on anterior rhinoscopy, which may be the cause of the tearing.
2. Further assessment of the nose, if on anterior rhinoscopy structural or anatomical abnormalities are found which may affect proposed lacrimal surgery.
3. More sophisticated interpretation of Jones' fluorescein dye test.

Endonasal Laser DCR (see Chapter 39)

The endoscope allows for viewing the light pipe within the lacrimal sac, and aids in placement of the laser intranasally.

Following Lacrimal Surgery (see Chapters 36 and 39)

1. To view the size and location of the DCR opening.
2. To view the nasal position of a Jones' tube.
3. Failed lacrimal surgery.
   To determine any compromise of the opening.
   To diagnose any lesion obstructing the opening such as granulomas, fibrous tissue, polyps, synechiae, etc.

Revision Lacrimal Surgery (see Chapter 39)

1. Endoscopic visualization greatly facilitates endoscopic revision of a DCR. Fibrous and granulomatous tissue may be visualized and excised to reopen the anastamosis.
2. Endoscopic visualization allows the surgeon to view the nasal end of a Jones' tube in a reinsertion, and to remove any potentially obstructing tissue (fibrous, granulomatous, middle turbinate, ethmoids, etc.).

REFERENCES

1. Hilding AC. Experimental sinus surgery: effects of operative windows on normal sinuses. *Ann Otol* 1941:50;379–392.
2. Kennedy DW, Zinreich SJ, Rosenbaum A, Johns ME. Functional endoscopic sinus surgery. Theory and diagnostic evaluation. *Arch Otolaryngol* 1985:111;576–582.
3. Messerklinger W. *Endoscopy of the nose.* Baltimore: Urban and Schwarzenberg; 1978.
4. Kennedy DW. Functional endoscopic sinus surgery. Technique. *Arch Otolaryngol* 1985:111;643–649.
5. Levine HL. Endoscopy and the KTP/532 laser for nasal sinus disease. *Ann Otol Rhinol Laryngol* 1989:98;46–51
6. Ossoff RH, Coleman JA, Courney MS, et al. Clinical applications of lasers in otolaryngology-head and neck surgery. *Lasers Surg Med* 1994:15;217–248.
7. Papel IR, Scott JC, Fairbanks DNF. Complications of nasal surgery and epistaxis management. In: Eisele DW, ed. *Complications in head and neck surgery.* St. Louis: CV Mosby: 1993:447–457.

8. Stammberger H. Endoscopic endonasal surgery: concepts in treatment of recurring rhinosinusitis. Part I and Part II. Anatomic pathophysiologic considerations and surgical technique. *Otolaryngol Head Neck Surg* 1986:94;143–156.

9. Stammberger H, Hawke M. *Essentials of functional endoscopic sinus surgery.* St. Louis: CV Mosby; 1993:193–198.

10. Meyers AD, Hawes MJ. Nasolacrimal obstruction after inferior meatus nasal antrostomy. *Arch Otolaryngol* 1991:117;208–211.

11. Serdahl CL, Berris CE, Chloe RA. Nasolacrimal duct obstruction after endoscopic sinus surgery. *Arch Ophthalmol* 1990:108;391–392.

12. Calhoun K, Waggenspack GA, Simpson CB, et al. CT evaluation of paranasal sinuses in symptomatic and asymptomatic populations. *Otolaryngol Head Neck Surg* 1991:104;480–483.

13. Bolger WE, Parsons DS, Mair EA, Kuhn FA. Lacrimal drainage system injury in functional endoscopic sinus surgery: incidence, analysis and prevention. *Arch Otolaryngol Head Neck Surg* 1992:118:1179–1184.

14. Kennedy DW, Zinreich SJ, Kuhn FA, et al. Endoscopic middle meatal antrostomy: theory, technique and patency. *Laryngoscope* 1987:97;1–9.

15. Davis WE, Templer JW, Lamear WR, et al. Middle meatus antrostomy: patency rates and risk factors. *Otolaryngol Head Neck Surg* 1991:104;467–472.

CHAPTER 18

Endoscopy

Canaliculus

Jeffrey Jay Hurwitz

J. J. Hurwitz: Oculoplastics Program, Mount Sinai Hospital; and Department of Ophthalmology, University of Toronto Faculty of Medicine, Toronto, Ontario M5S 1A8, Canada.

Whereas nasal endoscopy has been adapted for use in patients with tearing, lacrimal imaging can be performed through the punctum and canaliculus. Ashenhurst, Hurwitz, and Katz presented the prototype of a lacrimal canaliculoscope at the European Society of Ophthalmic Plastic and Reconstructive Surgery in May 1990 (1). The endoscope is similar in rigidity and size to a Crawford probing set (No. 28-0185, Jed Med, Clearwater, Florida) (Fig. 1). The external diameter of the device is less than 1 mm and is equivalent to #0 lacrimal probe. This passes nicely through the canalicular system (2).

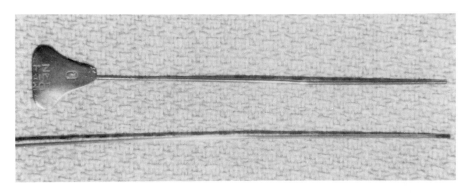

FIG. 1. Photograph of a canaliculoscope. The canaliculoscope (*lower image*) is less than 1 mm in diameter and is equivalent to the #0 lacrimal probe (*upper image*). (From Ashenhurst and Hurwitz, ref. 2, with permission.)

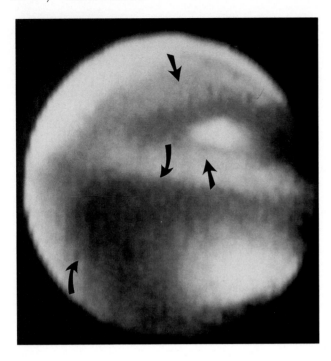

FIG. 2. The image through a canaliculoscope demonstrates the junction of the upper and lower canaliculus as one approaches the common canaliculus. *Arrows* represent canalicular walls. (From Ashenhurst and Hurwitz, ref. 2, with permission.)

Thus far we perform canaliculoscopy out of interest and in a research capacity, and it is not a routine part of our investigation protocol. However, with further developments and refinements, it may prove to be an important adjunct in lacrimal diagnosis (Fig. 2 and see Colorplate 5 following page 142).

REFERENCES

1. Ashenhurst ME, Hurwitz JJ, Katz A. Proceedings of the European Society of Ophthalmic Plastic and Reconstructive Surgery. Vienna, 1990.
2. Ashenhurst ME, Hurwitz JJ. Lacrimal canaliculoscopy: development of the instrument. *Can J Ophthalmol.* 1991;26:306.

CHAPTER 19

Imaging

Other Techniques

Jeffrey Jay Hurwitz

THERMOGRAPHY

The measurement of temperature at the external surface of the tear sac and in the area around the tear sac may be done by thermography (1) or by inserting a thermocouple through the canaliculus into the lacrimal sac (2). The thermographic equipment that has been used is that employed in breast evaluation. However, nowadays the thermographic machine is not used in mammography and the equipment has become obsolete. For this reason, thermography is no longer used in our investigation protocol. Thermography was useful because it could indicate the temperature in the area around the tear sac and would give evidence as to whether a subacute or chronic dacryocystitis was present. One would theoretically, like any infection or inflammation within the tear sac eradicated before a definitive drainage procedure would be performed. Thermography was able to give this information (Figs. 1 and 2 and see Colorplate 6 following page 142). Thermography was able to determine the efficacy of antibiotic treatment for a dacryocystitis. In our investigation protocol, with the thermography machinery being obsolete, we do not perform this assessment.

J. J. Hurwitz: Oculoplastics Program, Mount Sinai Hospital; and Department of Ophthalmology, University of Toronto Faculty of Medicine, Toronto, Ontario M5S 1A8, Canada.

CHEMILUMINESCENT EVALUATION OF THE LACRIMAL SYSTEM

The use of a chemiluminescent material Cyalume (American Cyanamid) has been used experimentally in human cadavers (3). On injection into the lacrimal system the Cyalume can be seen when the lights are turned out because it illuminates through the skin. A delineation of the pathways as is seen in dacryocystography is obtained (Fig. 3). The material itself does not seem to be toxic in rabbits experimentally if it stays within the drainage pathways (4). Unfortunately, the material has not been used in humans in the clinical setting because no approval has been yet obtained for human usage.

PRESSURE ASSESSMENT WITHIN THE LACRIMAL SYSTEM

The insertion of pressure transducers into the nasolacrimal system may demonstrate a change in pressure within the canaliculi and sac if the system was open or totally or partially blocked (5). As well, mini-pressure transducers inserted into the system would show pressure changes as the patient blinked, in patients who had normal and abnormal lids (6,7). These techniques are extremely interesting from a physiologic point of view and demonstrate the validity of the lacrimal pump theory. However, we have not used these techniques in practice, and they are not part of our treatment protocol. We have

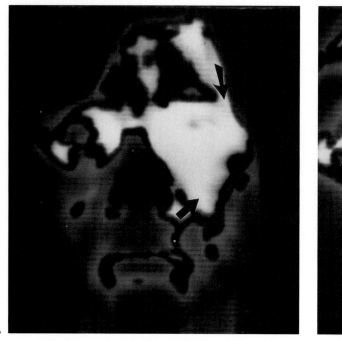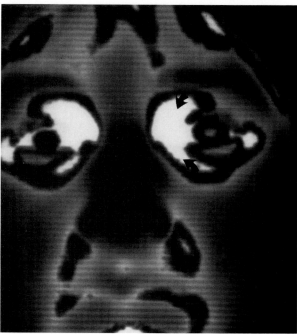

A B

FIG. 1. A: Thermogram of patient with left-sided dacryocystitis outlining area of increased heat. The right side is normal. **B:** The patient has been treated with penicillin. Clinically the infection is gone and the thermographic patterns are symmetrical. (From Rosenstock et al., ref. 8, with permission.)

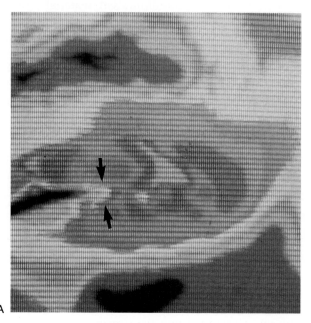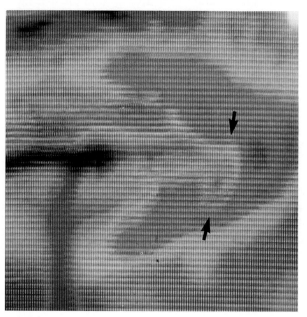

A B

FIG. 2. A: Thermogram of normal patient before cold water is injected into the lacrimal sac (*arrows*). **B:** Thermogram demonstrating that when cold water is injected the cold radiation from within the sac may be seen to increase (*arrows*). (From Rosenstock et al., ref. 8, with permission.)

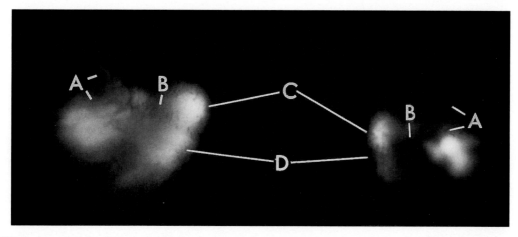

FIG. 3. Image of Cyalume in the lacrimal system when injected into a cadaver. *A,* palpebral aperture, *B,* canaliculi, *C,* lacrimal sac, and *D,* nasolacrimal duct. (From Raflo and Hurwitz, ref. 3, with permission.)

not felt that it was necessary to use a determination of intrasac or intracanalicular pressure readings to help us determine what the treatment should be in any specific patient with a watery eye.

REFERENCES

1. Raflo GT, Chart P, Hurwitz JJ. Thermographic evaluation of the human lacrimal drainage system. *Ophthal Surg* 1982;13:119.
2. Billington B, Hurwitz JJ, Galbraith D, Gentles W. A mini-probe for the assessment of lacrimal sac temperatures. *Ophthal Surg* 1984;15:680.
3. Raflo GT, Hurwitz JJ. Assessment of the efficacy of chemilumines-cent evaluation of the human lacrimal drainage system. *Ophthal Surg* 1982;13:36.
4. Vettese T, Hurwitz JJ. Toxicity of the chemilumescent material Cyalume in anatomic assessment of the nasolacrimal system. *Can J Ophthalmol* 1983;18:131.
5. Callahan WP, Forbath PG, Besser WDS. A method of determining the patency of the nasolacrimal apparatus. *Am J Ophthalmol* 1965;60:476.
6. Hill JC, Bethell W, Smirmaul HJ. Lacrimal drainage—a dynamic evaluation. Part 1 Mechanics of tear transport. *Can J Ophthalmol* 1974;9:411.
7. Hill JJ, Apt R, Smirmaul HJ. Lacrimal pump pressure patterns. *Can J Ophthlmol* 1975;10:25.
8. Rosenstock T, Hurwitz JJ, Chart P. Inflammation of the lacrimal drainage system— assessment by thermography. *Ophthal Surg* 1982;13:119.

CHAPTER 20

"Functional Obstruction" of the Lacrimal Drainage Passages

Jeffrey Jay Hurwitz

The term "functional obstruction" of the lacrimal drainage passages has been used by a number of authors to refer to a situation in which the lacrimal system is patent to syringing in a patient complaining of tearing (1). From the previous chapters on lacrimal investigation, it is obvious that if a system is patent to syringing, it certainly does not mean that it is normal. All that one can say from syringing is that if the system is not blocked it is open, but not necessary open in a normal manner. If a system is patent to syringing, one must determine whether indeed the system is normal or whether it is stenotic. This is absolutely mandatory if the ophthalmologist is to determine if the patient has a problem with tear flow and what, if any, surgery would be appropriate in this specific patient. To determine whether the anatomy is indeed normal, that is to say, if lacrimal drainage surgery would be the treatment indicated, one must perform an anatomical test. That anatomical test is the dacryocystogram. The dacryocystogram in many older patients and in the majority of younger patients who have tearing with patency of the duct will be shown on dacrocystography (DCG) to have an incomplete obstruction. This incomplete obstruction often will be significant enough that a lacrimal drainage operation can and should be planned, if the patient wishes to try to be relieved of the symptoms of epiphora. Even if the system is 100% patent to syringing, there may still be an incomplete obstruc-

TABLE 1. *Protocol for the work-up of the tearing patient*

History: lacrimal, ophthalmic, periocular, general, medical
Physical examination
Adnexa
    Face, eyelids, medial canthus, conjunctiva, globe
Clinical tests
    Tests of secretion
        Fluorescein tear film test
        Corneal fluorscein test
        Punctal fluorescein test
        Schirmer's test
    Tests of lacrimal excretion: anatomical
        Syringing
        Probing to hard stop or soft stop
        Probing to measure canalicular obstruction
    Tests of lacrimal excretion: physiologic (functional)
        Fluorescein dye disappearance
        Fluorescein and nose blowing
        Fluorescein and inspection of nose for appearance of fluorescein
Radiologic tests
    Dacryocystography:
        Obstructed to syringing
        Patency to syringing: if anatomical stenosis is suspected
        Trauma
        Suspected tumor or stone
        Failed DCR
    CTDCG:
        If nasal sinus or periocular trauma and/or tumors suspected
    Nuclear lacrimal scanning
        To quantitate suspected stenosis on syringing and/or DCG
        To document tear flow abnormality if anatomy totally normal
Nasal examination (endoscopy)

J. J. Hurwitz: Oculoplastics Program, Mount Sinai Hospital; and Department of Ophthalmology, University of Toronto Faculty of Medicine, Toronto, Ontario M5S 1A8, Canada.

tion, significant enough so as to warrant lacrimal surgery. We have found this especially to be true in younger patients, in whom the tear film and lids are usually normal. In older patients in whom the tear film and lids may be abnormal, if the system is indeed 100% patent to syringing, it is less likely that a stenosis within the drainage pathways will be found on DCG, but it certainly is possible that there might be some anatomical abnormalities.

A physiologic test is in our opinion not of any value unless it is confirmed that the anatomy of the system is indeed normal. The only situation in which the Jones dye test would provide additional information in a normal-looking DCG, and that a DCR *might* be indicated, would be a negative primary dye test and a positive secondary dye test. This would suggest that an "atonic sac" exists whereby the sac is normal anatomically but functionally does not drain. This situation in our experience is very rare. If indeed an atonic sac does exist, we have usually found an abnormality on the DCG, whereby there is a distended but patent sac and, therefore, we would do a DCR. We do not feel that, on the basis of a negative primary dye test and a negative secondary dye test (in which all the dye is held up in the palpebral aperture), one can plan a treatment protocol because there may be a problem with the lid, punctum, canaliculi, or even the sac (stones, tumor). We feel that it is imperative that if more physiologic information is required, a dacrocystogram and/or sophisticated lacrimal scan gives more information and helps the surgeon decide whether and what kind of surgery is indicated (2).

Therefore, when we consider the term "functional obstruction," we would suggest that if the term "obstruction" is used, it should imply an anatomical blockage within the lacrimal drainage pathways. If the term "functional" is being used, it should apply to a situation in which the anatomy is completely normal and there is a physiologic dysfunction (i.e., there is a problem with the position of the punctum, and/or the pumping of tears through the system via the orbicularis action in the eyelids and/or the lacrimal sac diaphragm). The term itself is misleading and we propose that, in these situations with epiphora and patency to syringing, the term "functional obstruction" be dropped from our terminology.

In a recent survey, a question was asked as to how one

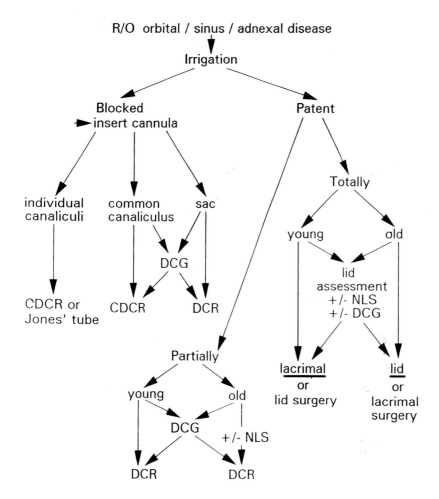

FIG. 1. Evaluation of epiphora.

would treat a "functional obstruction." The example given was a 60-year-old patient who presented with chronic epiphora for 6 months in whom the external examination was normal (3). What was obvious from this survey were a number of items. Analysis of answers suggested:

1. the work-up of the tearing patient was not standardized
2. there was no prevailing consensus as to what adjunctive tests to order and when to order them
3. certain procedures were being performed to see "what would happen," and then if the procedure did not work another type of procedure would be attempted
4. a particular type of procedure would not necessarily be performed in correlation with the supposed pathology determined on the investigation.

Wobig states in his editorial comment following the survey that the survey "points out a number of inconsistencies in the work-up for lacrimal excretory system problems" (4). Wobig also states "this paper is excellent in revealing the poor quality of work-up in evaluating the lacrimal excretory obstructions, especially the functional block." We would therefore like to propose a protocol for the work-up of the patient with tearing (Table 1). In this fashion a rational plan for investigating patients with tearing can be undertaken. This will suggest the nature of treatment to be instituted, and if surgery is planned, the approach can be appropriately determined (Fig. 1).

REFERENCES

1. Silver B. Ophthalmic plastic surgery. *American Academy of Ophthalmology manual*, 3rd ed; 1977.
2. Rosenstock T, Hurwitz JJ. Functional obstruction of lacrimal drainage passages. *Can J Ophthalmol* 1982;17:249.
3. Conway ST. Evaluation and management of "functional" nasolacrimal blockage: results of a survey of the American Society of Ophthalmic and Reconstructive Surgery. *Ophthal Plast Reconstruct Surg* 1994;10:185.
4. Wobig J. Editorial comment. *Ophthal Plast Reconstruct Surg* 1994;10:188.

CHAPTER 21

Dry Eye

Raymond Stein and Jeffrey Jay Hurwitz

In the management of dry eye patients, it is important to identify which component of the precorneal tear film is disturbed and to what severity. A careful history and diagnosis is required to determine the underlying causes before initiating therapy. The therapy and the dosage involved must be related to a specific condition.

DRUGS

Systemic medications may result in a diminished tear film and dry eye symptoms. Beta-blocking agents used in the treatment of hypertension can result in a significant decrease in the tear film. In addition, the benzodiazepines, antidepressants, and neuroleptics can produce a dry eye.

A reduction in tear film stability as measured by the break-up time has been shown to be decreased in cigar smokers compared to nonsmokers. It is therefore apparent that cigarette smoking may influence the tear film negatively.

ENVIRONMENTAL DISTURBANCES

Before initiating therapy with topical medication, it is important to rule out possible environmental disturbances. Both dust and smoke may cause aggravating symptoms. If the air humidity declines, as is frequently experienced in overheated rooms during the winter months, then irritative symptoms can develop. A heating system using a fan blower as frequently seen in motor vehicles can cause an increase in drying of the eyes if the air is directed at the face. It is important to know the

R. Stein: Cornea and External Disease Program, Mount Sinai Hospital, Toronto, Ontario M5G 1X5, Canada.

J. J. Hurwitz: Oculoplastics Program, Mount Sinai Hospital; and Department of Ophthalmology, University of Toronto Faculty of Medicine, Toronto, Ontario M5S 1A8, Canada.

patient's occupation and whether the patient is exposed to chemical irritants or toxic substances.

PHARMACEUTICAL TREATMENT

If the clinician is not successful in identifying a cause or underlying irritative factors of dry eye, a medication should be initiated to improve the subjective and objective symptoms.

The objective is to normalize the tear film over the corneal surface. The ideal artificial tear should be well tolerated, without toxicity, have a long retention period, not interfere with vision, and not inhibit tear secretion or mucous production.

ARTIFICIAL TEAR PREPARATIONS

The mainstay of therapy for dry eyes is replacement tears. A wide variety of artificial tear preparations exist today. In general, patients are able to tolerate nonviscous products better. A newer type of artificial tear preparation (Bion Tear) employs a unique electrolyte-based formulation that has shown to be beneficial to the ocular surface. Another new product, Aqua-Site, employs a viscous drop that is reported to act as a reservoir replenishing the tear film for a sustained period.

The development of nonpreserved artificial tears over the past few years has been a significant advance in the treatment of dry eyes. Long-term use of artificial tears with preservatives may lead to sensitivity to these chemicals. Preservatives may result in toxic or allergic symptoms that may be noted only after significant epithelial changes have occurred. Bromhexine hydrochloride is a mucolytic agent based on an herbal plant that has shown promise in Europe as a tear stimulant. The drug is felt to increase tear production by working on the central nervous system at the level of the brain stem. Clinical trials in the United States are currently taking place.

METHYLCELLULOSE

Cellulose derivatives are water-soluble polymers that are available in commercial eyedrops as a 0.5% to 1% solution. The synthetic polymer has a stable pH value, is chemically inert and nontoxic, and the refractive index is similar to that of the natural tear film. This type of substitute has a short retention period and disintegrates after less than 20 minutes. Therefore, patients using this form of eyedrop will require frequent application.

HYDROXYPROPYL METHYLCELLULOSE

Hydroxypropyl methylcellulose is a cellulose derivative that is more viscous and considered superior to other methylcellulose preparations. Unfortunately, this viscous drop does not enhance tear film stability.

These viscous substances tend to slow the elimination of tear fluid as a consequence of their high molecular structure. Treatment results have been somewhat disappointing as the surface tension is relatively high, which limits surface activity of the substance (1). The tear film retention time of preparations containing methylcellulose is longer than that based on polyvinyl alcohol. Methylcellulose drops are generally best suited for moderate to severe cases of dry eyes (2).

POLYVINYL ALCOHOL

Polyvinyl alcohol is a hydrophilic polymer with only moderate viscosity but good lubricating function. This agent has been shown to be of value in the treatment of keratitis sicca. The properties of polyvinyl alcohol solutions reduce surface tension without compromising visual acuity.

TEAR GELS

To improve the retention period of artificial tear agents, gel-type substances have been developed. Gel-based tear substitutes are particularly suitable for the long-term treatment of medium to advanced forms of keratitis sicca. These agents have positive influence on the tear film break-up time for up to 60 minutes. In severe cases of dry eyes, four applications per 24-hour period is usually sufficient to produce significant therapeutic effectiveness.

HYALURONIC ACID

Hyaluronic acid is a viscoelastic that can bind water and has significant adhesion to cell surfaces. It is obtained from the comb structures of roosters. Its high price has restricted the use of hyaluronic acid solutions in the management of dry eye patients.

CHONDROITIN SULFATE

Chondroitin sulfate is another viscoelastic substance that has been used in the treatment of dry eyes.

These solutions have an excellent affinity to the corneal surface and prevent tear film break-up. Preliminary studies with this type of solution appear promising (3).

INSERTS

Inserts were developed to improve the retention time for tear substitutes and to decrease the frequency of drop applications. The inserts are soft polymers that are inserted into the cul-de-sac and take several hours to dissolve. The inserts tend to be preferred by patients with advanced keratitis sicca, with mild to moderate dry eye patients preferring frequent use of eyedrops. The inserts may result in a foreign body sensation and commonly are lost.

MUCOLYTIC AGENTS

Mucolytic agents are restricted to cases of keratitis sicca in which an excessive accumulation of mucus occurs in the precorneal tear film.

Acetylcysteine has been shown to be of value in breaking down or dissolving mucus. It is usually used in the form of 10% eyedrops. Acetylcysteine used three or four times a day is effective in dissolving excess mucin in the tear film and improving corneal wetting.

EYE OINTMENTS

In cases of keratitis sicca where there is corneal involvement, ointments may have a significant value. Ointments, however, may damage the precorneal tear film and reduce the break-up time. If ointment is used during the day, a considerable reduction in vision can occur. Ointments are generally used overnight to improve lubrication of the anterior surface of the eye.

GOGGLES

A pair of tightly fitted protective goggles can protect against the loss of humidity from the tear film. When properly fitted, these goggles can approximate a moist chamber. The goggles provide a relatively damp chamber and improve the level of comfort for the dry eye patient.

INFUSION PUMPS

In advanced cases of dry eyes, spectacles can be constructed with an infusion pump. A continuous flow of fluid is ensured by a pump operated by a motor installed on the side arm. The tears are passed via a plastic tube into the lower conjunctival fornix. At a flow rate of 1 to 3 mm over a 12-hour day, patients can note significant relief when other therapeutic measures have been unsuccessful (4).

SURGICAL TREATMENT OF THE DRY EYE

Closure of a portion or the entire upper and lower eyelids by a tarsorrhaphy may improve comfort but is generally cosmetically unacceptable. This is generally undertaken only with a nonhealing epithelial defect or a melt secondary to exposure. A small lateral tarsorrhaphy can reduce the amount of surface exposure by more than 50% without significantly affecting the vision.

TEMPORARY OCCLUSION OF THE PUNCTA

Temporary occlusion of the lacrimal puncta can be performed using a variety of commercially available silicone plugs (Fig. 1). These are generally simple to insert in the office under topical anesthesia. The early plugs were designed from gelatin, which would temporarily block

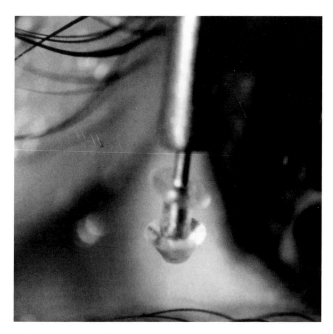

FIG. 1. Punctal plug being inserted into lower canaliculus. The plug is held on the end of an inserter and placed within the dilated punctum. It has a flange on the end which holds it onto the punctum without the need for a suture.

tear flow along the punctum, and then later dissolve. The improvement of the symptoms, with the plugs in place, would give the clinician the information to determine whether permanent occlusion might be beneficial. However, absorption of the gelatin is variable, and studies using lacrimal scanning suggest that tracer can flow along the canaliculi, past the plugs, as if they were not even there (5).

Silicone plugs, later developed, did a better job in temporarily obstructing the punctum while in place, and our studies have shown that plugs in the upper and lower puncta can be effective in blocking tear flow. If symptoms improve with the plugs in place, it might be surmised that permanent occlusion of the puncta might be useful. There is little chance that permanent occlusion would help if the plugs did not.

The plugs are meant to be temporary, but some patients are so happy with the improvement in symptoms that they wish the plugs to be left in place long term. However, the plugs may migrate down the canaliculi, and necessitating another operation for their removal (6,7). If plugs are to be left in for a longer period of time, the patients should be followed closely.

If one is to insert a plug, should it be in the upper punctum, the lower punctum, or both? Certainly it would seem prudent to determine whether the lacrimal system is patent before inserting a plug. Obviously, with a blocked system, a plug could not be expected to do much good. It is known that both the upper and the lower canaliculi have a role in tear flow (8). Blocking one punctum would therefore decrease the total flow into the sac, with only one punctum functional rather than two. However, it has been shown that one punctum alone is probably sufficient to carry the tears to the lacrimal sac (9). There is even the possibility that flow is augmented through the one remaining punctum.

We suggest permanent occlusion of one punctum at a time. Perhaps one punctum can be occluded, symptoms assessed, and if still symptomatic, a plug could temporarily be placed in the other punctum. If the plug helps, sealing the second punctum could be considered.

In some patients, repeated wiping of the eye causes the lid to be lax. Lid laxity may help symptoms by decreasing flow through the puncta (lacrimal pump dysfunction), but may increase symptoms by increasing the height of the palpebral aperture and cause more thinning of the tear film. Therefore, it is unpredictable whether tightening a loose lid will help symptoms of dry eye.

PERMANENT OCCLUSION OF THE PUNCTA

If there is a long-term history of severe dry eyes with the Schirmer's test of less than 5 mm, then consideration could be given to permanent occlusion of the lacrimal puncta and canaliculi. A handheld cautery can be used to perform this procedure. It is not uncommon for spontaneous opening to occur after heat cautery of the punctum. Therefore, we prefer to insert the needle tip of a Hyfrecator or Ellman Radiosurgical Surgitron™ into the canaliculi, but not as far as the common canaliculus. When the current is turned on, the needle can be withdrawn in a circling motion, removing a scroll of canaliculus mucosa. The surface of the punctum can then be cauterized. This seems to decrease the chance of the punctum reopening.

If permanent obstruction has been performed and the patient still has symptoms, one must determine whether the system has partially reopened. The punctum may be somewhat assessed on slit lamp examination regarding patency, but the canaliculus can be best assessed by lacrimal scintillography.

More permanent occlusion occurs from sealing the canaliculus as well as the punctum. For this reason we prefer needle cautery obliteration within the canaliculus, rather than surface occlusion with cautery or laser (10). We advise injecting local anesthetic around the canaliculus so that the procedure can be done with minimal discomfort.

SALIVARY TRANSPLANTATION

Transplantation of the parotid duct into the conjunctival fornix may increase secretions but the ptyalin in the gland may be irritating to the eye. Sublingual gland tissue transplanted into the conjunctival cul-de-sac (11) will grow with time and increase secretory function. Further studies will determine the role of this exciting new development in patients with dry eye syndrome (11).

REFERENCES

1. Lemp MA, Holly FJ. Ophthalmic polymers as ocular wetting agents. *Ann Ophthalmol* 1972;4:15–20.
2. Krishna N, Mitshell B. Polyvinyl alcohol as an ophthalmic vehicle. *Am J Ophthalmol* 1965;59:840–864.
3. Limberg MB. Topic application of hyaluronic acid and chondroitin sulfate in the treatment of dry eye. *Am J Ophthalmol* 1987;103:104–107.
4. Dohlmann CH. Mobile infusion pumps for continuous delivery of fluid and therapeutic agents to the eye. *Ann Ophthalmol* 1971;3:126–128.
5. Hurwitz JJ, Maisey MN, Welham RAN. Quantitative lacrimal scintillography. *Br J Ophthalmol* 1975;59:308–313.
6. Levinson JE, Hofbaver J. Problems with punctal plugs. *Arch Ophthalmol* 1989;107:493–495.
7. McGuire H, Bartley GB. Complications associated with a new smaller size Freeman punctal plug. *Arch Ophthalmol* 1989;107:960–965.
8. Rabinovitch J, Hurwitz JJ, Chin-Sang H. Canalicular flow patterns. *Orbit* 1985;3:263–266.
9. Linberg JV, Moore CA. Symptoms of canalicular obstruction. *Ophthalmology* 1988;95:1077–1079.
10. Rashid R. Modification of the Rashid argon dye canalicular occlusion procedure. In: Miglior M, Van Bijsterveld OP, Spinelli D, eds. *The lacrimal system.* Milan: Kugler and Ghedini; 1990:73–78.
11. Murube-del-Castillo J, Murube-Jiminez I. Transplantation of sublingual salivary gland to the lacrimal basin in patients with dry eye. Histological postoperative study. In: Miglior M, Van Bijsterveld OP, Spinelli D, eds. *The lacrimal system.* Milan: Kugler and Ghedini; 1990:63–72.

CHAPTER 22

Diseases of the Sac and Duct

Jeffrey Jay Hurwitz

OBSTRUCTION OF THE NASOLACRIMAL SAC AND DUCT

It is convenient to consider obstructions of the nasolacrimal sac and duct separately from obstructions of the punctum and canaliculi. The mucosal lining of the punctum and canaliculi is nonkeratinizing stratified squamous epithelium, and that of the sac and duct is stratified columnar epithelium. The stratified columnar epithelium of the sac, as it descends into the membranous nasolacrimal duct, tends to become ciliated and has some of the characteristics of nasal mucosa and respiratory epithelium close to the inferior turbinate and the lining of the nose.

Obstructions of the nasolacrimal sac and duct may be divided into congenital and acquired obstructions. In the adults, untreated congenital obstructions may persist and cause tearing into adulthood. The acquired obstructions may be divided into those that are nonspecific and those that are specific. The nonspecific obstructions are related to pathologic changes involving the epithelium, vascular plexus, and adnexal structures surrounding the nasolacrimal duct. The specific causes of obstructions may be related to infections, specific inflammations, trauma, tumors, and those related to surgery. Dacryolithiasis and dacryocystitis are commonly occurring sequelae of nasolacrimal sac and duct obstructions.

Congenital Obstruction into Adulthood

The etiology of congenital obstruction of the nasolacrimal system is felt by most people to be due to an imperforate valve of Hasner within the inferior meatus (1).

J. J. Hurwitz: Oculoplastics Program, Mount Sinai; and Department of Ophthalmology, University of Toronto Faculty of Medicine, Toronto, Ontario M5S 1A8, Canada.

As well, there are some abnormalities in the nose on a congenital basis that may contribute to obstructions; namely, septal deviation (2), congenital malformations with flattening of the inferior turbinate against the lateral wall of the nose, and other congenital facial and maxillary bone maldevelopments (3).

Patients may, for one reason or another, not be treated in the early childhood years and reach adulthood having had tearing all their lives. These patients may be treated by probing of the nasolacrimal system as one would do in a child. However, the older the patient gets, the less the chance that a probing will work (4). Past the age of 5 or 6 years, the success of probing (even with tubes) decreases so much that we prefer to treat the obstruction with a dacrocystorhinostomy (DCR).

Acquired Obstruction

Nonspecific Obstruction of the Nasolacrimal Sac and Duct

Pathologic studies of the nasolacrimal sac and duct in cadavers (5) and during the time of DCR in which a lacrimal duct biopsy is performed (6) have shown that there are changes that are invariably seen in the "normal" and "abnormal" states. The mucosa of the nasolacrimal duct is a stratified columnar epithelium that, in the upper end of the duct, has a loose connective tissue structure around the mucosa. Within this structure is a rich vascular network, mainly venous, some collections of lymphocytes, and loose fibrous tissue (6). The attachment of the mucosal lining of the duct at its upper end is much looser than its lower end as it approaches the valve of Hasner. As well, in the lower end there are some goblet cells and also some cilia, and indeed the mucosal lining of the lower end resembles the inferior turbinate mucosa and the respiratory epithelium lining the nose. Because of this, it might be postulated that some of the nonspecific inflammatory, edematous, allergic, and atrophic conditions that afflict the nasal mucosa may also afflict the mucosa of the lower end of the nasolacrimal duct. We know that the valve of Hasner becomes patent during the first year of life in at least 90% of patients (1), and the level of patency will vary from patient to patient. We know that the valve of Hasner must be flaccid in many patients because it is not uncommon for certain patients to be able to blow air from the nose through into the palpebral aperture. In these patients, the valve of Hasner (and also the valve of Rosenmuller) must not be functioning to their normal capacities. It might be supposed that with a patulous valve of Hasner some of the diseases of the nose may affect the diseases of the lower end of the nasolacrimal duct and thereby cause an obstruction.

Many of these biopsy specimens show inflammation with vascular congestion, lymphocytic infiltration, and edema. Many of the specimens show some fibrosis developing, and it would be assumed that the fibrosis is the consequence of inflammatory edema. It could be postulated that the inflammatory reaction and congestion in the thick venous network around the mucosa might cause some extrinsic pressure on the membranous lining and incite either a partial or a complete obstruction. Certainly the stagnation could lead to tears pooling in the site, with the possibility of secondary bacterial contamination. We confirmed the findings of Linberg that it is uncommon to find organisms in the biopsies of the lacrimal sacs and nasolacrimal ducts. This is probably because at the time of lacrimal surgery, the infection has usually subsided and one is left just with fibrosis and an obstruction. Certainly, it has been our plan to avoid performing a lacrimal drainage operation in the face of

acute infection. With chronic inflammation, there is change in the epithelium of the duct and squamous metaplasia may ensue. Occasionally one finds oncocytic change of the epithelium (7).

Linberg has correlated the intervals between the onset of symptoms and the biopsies, and has described three stages: early (active) inflammatory phase, intermediate phase, and later (fibrotic) phase (8). During the early active inflammatory phase, there is often not a complete obstruction but just a lot of edema of the mucosa and of the tissues around the mucosa. There is not a significant amount of active inflammation. Presumably, these findings, in the face of incomplete obstruction, may be reversible. In the intermediate phase, there is proliferation of periductal connective tissue with a move toward fibrosis and low grade chronic inflammation around the venous plexus. The late fibrotic phase shows scar tissue and granulation tissue developing, and one must assume that in this phase the process is irreversible. The pathogenesis of nonspecific acquired nasolacrimal sac and duct obstruction is crucial to the understanding of this condition and the formulation of a plan for investigation and treatment of these patients (Figs. 1–3). Presumably, steroid treatment in these early stages *might* reverse the process. This postulate requires a long-term study.

Predisposition to Nonspecific Acquired Nasolacrimal Sac and Duct Obstruction

The pathophysiologic changes described in nonspecific acquired nasolacrimal sac and duct obstruction are observed once the obstructing process begins, but are

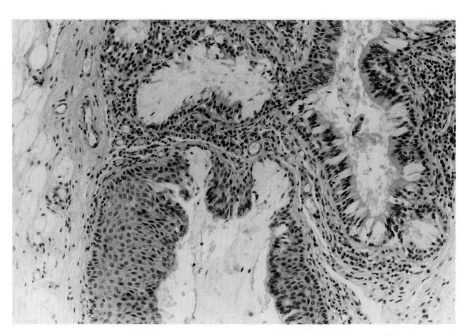

FIG. 1. Photomicrograph demonstrating inflammatory edema, chronic cellular infiltration, and mucosal changes of the lacrimal sac taken during DCR surgery.

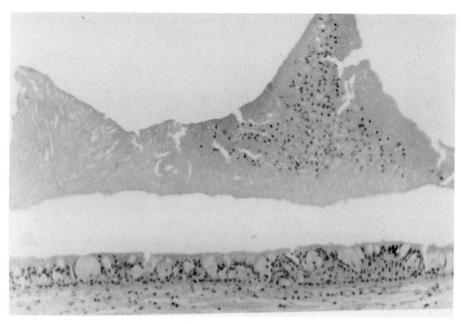

FIG. 2. Photomicrograph of a stone taken at DCR surgery with nasolacrimal obstruction secondary to previous sinus surgery. Inflammation in sac mucosa is evident.

there predisposing factors that may lead a patient to the development of this condition?

Age of the Patient

It would seem that the older a patient gets the more the chance of developing this condition (9). It must be remembered that since tear secretion decreases with age,

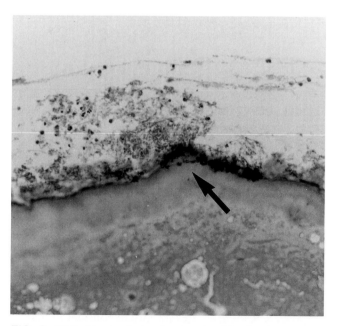

FIG. 3. High power photomicrograph of lacrimal sac, mucosa, and submucosal tissues. Particles are seen that have a high concentration of titanium on the microspectral analysis suggestive of make-up fragments (*arrow*).

many older people will have nasolacrimal sac and duct obstruction with no symptoms. Dalgleish (10), in a series in which he syringed a large series of asymptomatic patients, found that approximately 9% of males and 10% of females over the age of 40 years had nasolacrimal sac and duct obstructions. The site of the obstruction was usually at the junction of the nasolacrimal sac and the nasolacrimal duct. At age 90 years approximately 35% to 40% of all the patients had obstructions.

Racial Incidence

This condition occurs much more commonly in Whites than Blacks, and occurs more commonly in Asian patients than black patients (11). It has also been suggested that the disease is more common in Whites of Mediterranean origin than Whites of more northern climates (9).

Sex Incidence

Most authors have suggested that obstruction is more common in females than males (12,13). The shape and the length of the bony nasolacrimal canal is different in men than in women: women have a more oval opening of the superior aspect of the canal than do men. Also, the canal in women is more angulated and smaller. As well, the bones of women are often smaller and the lacrimal bones and maxillae may be somewhat underdeveloped. It has also been suggested that women may have on the average flatter noses than men and may be predisposed to more nasolacrimal obstructions. Even though a hereditary and familial tendency has been described in the past (14), it is probably due to hereditary structural configuration of the face.

Social Conditions

Many authors have noted the fact the people from lower socioeconomic levels and people whose cleanliness is a problem are more predisposed to have nasolacrimal duct obstructions. This may be because more bacteria and debris may get into the nasolacrimal canal, and if there is some partial compromise, these people may be more at risk for developing complete obstructions (11).

Nasal Conditions

It has been suggested that turbinate swelling due to a form of rhinitis may cause obstruction (15). Patients often mention that they develop nasolacrimal symptoms when they have upper respiratory tract infections with colds, stuffy noses, and sinus infections. Perhaps the inflammation in the nose secondarily causes obstruction of the valve of Hasner and/or extrinsic compression on the lower aspect of the nasolacrimal duct (16). The question of sinusitis causing nasolacrimal obstruction is a difficult one. The lacrimal bone is as thin as tissue paper and often becomes absorbed with age. Immediately adjacent to the lacrimal bone is the anterior ethmoidal air cell complex, and the absorbtion of the bone would put the ethmoidal cells in direct proximity to the nasolacrimal sac. It has not been our experience that treating a *sinus* infection (even a subclinical one) has any effect on the symptoms of tearing or the nasolacrimal obstruction, but if there is a *nasal* problem, treating this may help symptoms of tearing.

Certainly patients who have allergic conditions with inflammation of the nasal mucosa may indeed develop some extrinsic compression of the nasolacrimal duct. However, it has been our experience that more often these patients have symptoms of itchiness of the eyes as well as those symptoms of tearing. This would lead one to believe that there is an oversecretion of tears rather than an incomplete removal of tears. This is usually substantiated by the fact that these patients have a nasolacrimal system that is completely patent to syringing.

Lacrimation

There is a theory that increased secretion of tears leads to stagnation of tears in the sac, which may become secondarily infected and lead to obstruction (11). Even though this may be possible, it is probably unlikely because it is so rare to culture or find organisms within the mucosa.

Specific Acquired Nasolacrimal Sac and Duct Obstruction

Sarcoidosis

Sarcoidosis (17) may involve the nasal passages and the nasal bone. The swelling over the bridge of the nose has a characteristic appearance that is suggestive of sarcoidosis. The inflammatory response may involve the inferior aspect of the nasolacrimal duct and ultimately cause a secondary obstruction of the duct. These patients are often treated with steroids. They also are somewhat immunocompromised. For this reason, secondary infection and dacryocystitis is not unusual. These patients may be treated once the infection subsides, with a standard DCR. The success rate of the surgery is high, but it is probably a good idea to keep these patients on systemic antibiotics as well as systemic steroids (often they have previously been on these medications) during the postoperative period. If the patients are not on steroids, we do not generally place the patients on steroids unless there has been a tremendous amount of bogginess and inflammation of the mucosa. Even though certain authors have implicated sarcoidosis as a cause for failure of a DCR (17), we have not experienced this problem. We routinely biopsy the sac and nasal mucosa of suspected sarcoid patients and if we find that there is granuloma formation, we follow the patient closely and put them on steroids much more liberally than if the biopsies are negative.

Inflammation in the tear sac may also be related to other inflammatory conditions such as Crohn's disease, and although one may try systemic steroids, a therapeutic DCR is recommended (18).

Wegener's Granulomatosis

It is well known that people with Wegener's granulomatosis, those with the full blown syndrome of renal, pulmonary, and sinus involvement, as well as those with only orbital involvement, may get secondary obstruction of the nasolacrimal canal. Because of the immunocompromised state, in that these patients are often on steroids and/or immunosuppressive agents, secondary dacryocystitis is frequent. These patients may be treated with a DCR once the infection subsides. However, one must be careful because wound healing may be a problem. The development of a fistula between the nose and the skin has been described by Jordan et al. (19). We have also seen this complication as well as wound necrosis, which Jordan and his co-workers also described. At the time of DCR there are two important considerations:

1. making sure that the wound is tightly closed with a series of long-lasting sutures in the subcutaneous layer, and perhaps silk sutures in the skin, which will

cause an intensified inflammatory reaction and possibly help wound healing

2. using systemic corticosteroids and perhaps an intensified immunosuppressive regime during the immediate postoperative period.

Even though a dacryocystectomy has been reported as a form of treatment in these patients (20), we prefer to perform a DCR for a few reasons: (a) we feel that it is impossible to remove all the infected material with a dacryocystectomy, and these patients may develop tearing and/or infection later on, and (b) the complications of wound breakdown and fistula formation still exist with a dacryocystectomy.

Infections

Many organisms have been incriminated in the development of dacryocystitis in a patient who has a pre-existing nasolacrimal duct obstruction. It would seem that the nasolacrimal obstruction predates the secondary infection and dacryocystitis in most situations. The exception to this rule would be infections that may be systemic or those that are primarily located in the nose and perhaps the sinuses. We have found the common commensal organisms in the sac to be *Staphylococcus, Pneumococcus,* and rarely *Actinomyces.* We feel that the most common organism causing dacryocystitis is *Staphylococcus,* and secondly *Streptococcus.* This would be in keeping with the work of Coden et al. (21). In fact, these organisms are so frequently the cause of dacryocystitis that we routinely treat these patients with Cloxicillin, and most of the patients will have a resolution of the infective process (22). However, other organisms such as *Pseudomonas, Haemophilus influenzae,* and *Proteus vulgaris* are common gram-negative organisms that may be present. Coden et al. (21) found *Pseudomonas* to be present in 8.7% of their patients, *H. influenza* in 5.8% of their patients, and *P. vulgaris* in 4.1% of their patients. Of interest is that Coden et al. also found anaerobic organisms such as *Propionibacterium acnes* present in 4.7% of their patients. They found fungus organisms present in only 1.2%, and these were identified as *Candida albicans.* It has been our experience and also the experience of Bartley (23) that fungal infections due to *Actinomyces* are not that uncommon. Classically, these organisms are present in canaliculitis, but we and Bartley have found these to be present in patients with nasolacrimal duct obstructions. In one study in which we performed biopsies in a large series of patients undergoing DCRs, the sacs in a surprisingly large number of these patients, especially those with dacryolithiasis, also harbored *Actinomyces* organisms (24). Other organisms such as *Mycobacterium fortuitum* have been described in this condition (25). Another organism causing more

trouble is *Eikenella corrodens,* which has been recently described by Duahs et al. (26).

Viruses may also cause secondary dacryocystitis. In fact, the Epstein-Barr virus of infectious mononucleosis has been described (27). The human papilloma virus has been described in epithelial tumors of the lacrimal sac and it is of interest to know whether this virus may lie dormant in the sac and not cause any trouble, or may cause infection and/or a tumor (28). Parasitic infections due to ascaris in the lacrimal system have also been reported (29).

Systemic infections such as trachoma, leprosy, tuberculosis, and rhinosporidiosis that occur in the nasal-sinus region have also been implicated in causing secondary obstruction of the nasolacrimal system in conjunction with dacryocystitis.

Foreign Bodies

Foreign bodies may be present in the nose and gain entrance through the valve of Hasner to the nasolacrimal canal and cause an obstruction. An eyelash has been described as the cause of a stone that secondarily caused an obstruction (30). Other foreign bodies such as casts of topical epinephrine may lodge in the nasolacrimal duct and cause obstruction (31).

Trauma

Trauma in the region of the maxillary sinus because of its close proximity to the nasolacrimal duct may cause obstruction. This may be due to a direct tear to the nasolacrimal duct by the bone surrounding the membraneous passage or to indirect trauma with secondary edema, congestion, inflammation, and closure of the system. Nasoethmoidal fractures, especially those with telecanthus, are most likely to produce nasolacrimal duct obstruction (32). Iatrogenic trauma may be caused by rhinoplasty (33) following orbital decompression for Graves' disease (34), and also following endoscopic sinus surgery (35).

Other causes of iatrogenic trauma producing nasolacrimal dysfunction may be due to punctal occlusion causing acute dacryocystitis (36), a granuloma following insertion of a plomb into the system (37), or after a standard silicone intubation for a congenital nasolacrimal duct obstruction (38).

Neoplasms

Neoplasms involving the nasolacrimal sac and duct may be primary (arising from the tissues from the sac and duct) or secondary (invading the sac and duct from outside). The most common primary neoplasm is a papilloma, with others being squamous cell carcinomas, hemangiopericytomas, fibrous histiocytomas, oncocytic adenocarcinomas, and melanomas. Those that may invade from outside are specifically maxillary and ethmoidal sinus tumors, basal cell carcinomas, and midline granulomas. We have had some patients with neurofibromatosis who have had secondary obstructions from lesions in the face compressing the ducts. As well, lymphomas may start in the exterior of the sac or the duct and grow in through the mucosa. Of note is the fact that dacryocystitis may sometimes be related to a primarily existing tumor of the lacrimal sac such as a malignant lymphoma (39).

DACRYOCYSTITIS

Acute Dacryocystitis

For dacryocystitis to develop there must be some impedance to the flow of tears through the nasolacrimal sac and duct, such as a stenosis, stone, infection with edema, or foreign body. There exists within the mucosa of the lacrimal sac secretory granules with mucinous and serous glands (Fig. 4). These are found in pathologic specimens to be in varying degrees from individual to individual (40). It may be presumed that in certain individuals microbial contamination of the sac may cause an irritation to these glands that may hypersecrete and cause a build-up of fluid and, possibly, if infected, pus within the system. As the sac expands, it can expand laterally quite easily, but it cannot distend well superiorly or medially. The superior extension of the sac expansion is limited to a certain extent by the anterior limb of the medial canthal tendon. However, one certainly can see swelling above the medial canthal tendon in a patient with dacryocystitis. The sac is limited in its medial expansion by the bone of the lacrimal fossa. However, the lacrimal bone itself, which may undergo absorption in older pa-

tients, may undergo pressure erosion because of some expansion medially of the sac. However, the sac has no restriction in expanding inferolaterally, and this is usually what occurs in a patient with acute dacryocystitis and swelling. There may be some compression because of the fine nerve endings around the sac causing a tremendous amount of pain. As well, there may be some expansion into the area of the inferior oblique muscle that indeed may cause some pain on movement of the eye. We have had patients with kidney stones and also dacryocystitis, and these patients informed us that the dacryocystitis is as equally painful as the renal colic. We have performed studies in which the temperature of the sac is measured and, when external thermography is used (41) or when a miniprobe has been placed into the lacrimal sac to measure the temperature (42), it has found that in dacryocystitis, the temperature within the lacrimal sac increases dramatically. In fact, with thermographic assessment it can be shown that the temperature increase will spread all the way to the back of the head and the ear. This is certainly consistent with our experience that patients complain of dacryocystitis pain going around the side of the head and sometimes down to the teeth because of intraorbital nerve involvement, but also back to the ear. This indeed is the "syndrome of acute dacryocystitis."

Classification

The classification of the three clinical syndromes of dacryocystitis will help one develop a management plan.

Dacryocystitis Localized to the Sac (Fig. 5)

A palpable painful mass is present in the lacrimal sac fossa. There will be a swelling that is usually nonreducible. The obstruction is due to an obstruction at the junc-

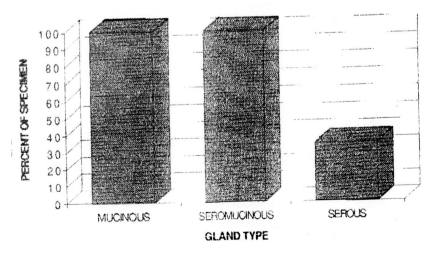

FIG. 4. Gland types in lacrimal sacs specimens. It may be seen that most cadaver specimens, when the lacrimal sacs were assessed, had mucinous and seromucinous glands present. About half the specimen had serous glands present. (From Cowen et al., ref. 7, with permission.)

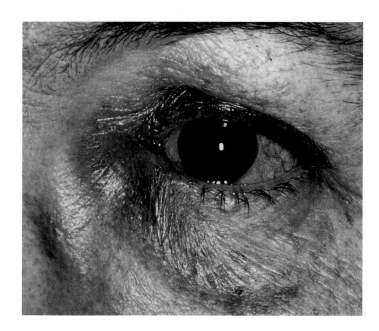

FIG. 5. Dacryocystitis localized to the sac. (From Hurwitz and Rodgers, ref. 22, with permission.)

tion of the lacrimal sac and duct. The patient may have had a period of time in which there was a history of pressure over the sac, of expressing fluid through the puncta into the palpebral aperture, or of expressing fluid down the nasolacrimal duct into the nose. However, when the dacryocystitis develops, the lateral expansion of the sac tends to kink the common canaliculus so the common canaliculus becomes S-shaped instead of straight (see Chapter 12, Fig. 4). This prevents the reducibility of the sac and allows for build-up and stagnation of material within the sac. The chronic state presumably predisposes to infection due to extrinsic organisms, or more likely due to replication of the pre-existing organisms in the normal flora of the sac that then become pathogenic. These patients usually have had such severe pain that they have not slept and indeed look quite sick. There may be a history of a pre-existing upper respiratory tract infection as well as repeated attacks of dacryocystitis. There is no question that some of these patients may have resolution of the attack, disappearance of the epiphora, and may never have another attack again. Our experience has been that about 40% of patients with one attack of dacryocystitis will not have another attack. However, of this 40%, half these patients will have an ongoing nasolacrimal duct obstruction and will eventually come to lacrimal surgery. Of the other 60%, recurring dacryocystitis attacks are common unless the patients are so dismayed after the first attack that lacrimal surgery is requested.

Dacryocystitis with Pericystitis (Fig. 6)

The lacrimal sac mucosa is surrounded by a thin fascial layer laterally that is an expansion of the orbital septum posteriorly and a reflection of the periorbita. This is separate from the lacrimal sac mucosa with a small pocket between the two layers. With increasing infection and edema of the sac, bacterial contamination may secondarily occur in this space between the sac mucosa and the surrounding tissues. This leads to a pericystitis and causes quite a degree of redness and congestion in the area of the nasolacrimal sac, and into the eyelids. In the immunocompromised patient there may be rapid deterioration in the condition once this occurs.

Dacryocystitis with Orbital Cellulitis

Following the pericystitis, there may be percolation of the inoculum anteriorly through the tissues, as there is

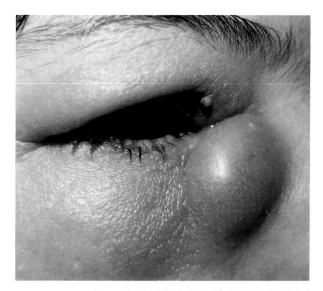

FIG. 6. Dacryocystitis with pericystitis. The infection has broken through the lacrimal sac and lies in the surrounding tissues.

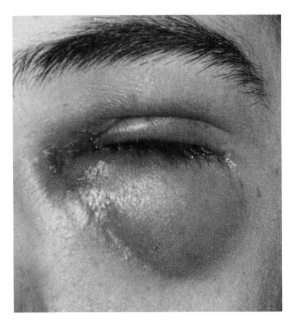

FIG. 7. Patient with dacryocystitis and anterior orbital cellulitis. There is spread of the infection anterior to the orbital septum around the eyelids. The ocular function itself is normal. (From Hurwitz and Rodgers, ref. 22, with permission.)

ity disturbance but may develop signs of optic neuropathy with color vision defect, field defect, and visual loss with a relative afferent pupillary defect (Fig. 8). The motility may be grossly restricted and there may be increased resistance to retropulsion of the globe, indicating increased orbital pressure. This constitutes a dire medical emergency. One must always keep in mind the possibility of an orbital abscess (Figs. 9 and 10), and indeed this is where dacryocystitis may become a life-threatening condition (43). There have been few reports in the literature regarding this, but another alarming report was published by Alan et al. (44) describing orbital cellulitis secondary to dacryocystitis following a four-lid blepharoplasty. Certainly in the preantibiotic area, acute dacryocystitis complicated with posterior orbital cellulitis and/or orbital abscess could lead to optic atrophy, blindness, cavernous sinus thrombosis, meningitis, and death.

Chronic Dacryocystitis

Chronic dacryocystitis may be the end stage of an acute (or subacute) dacryocystitis, but more often it presents as a low grade smoldering, almost subclinical, infection secondary to a nasolacrimal duct obstruction. These patients may present with a red eye with constant watering, tearing, and matting of the eyelashes. There may be a swelling in the lacrimal sac fossa, and if there is one it is usually reducible so that pressure on the swelling will cause discharge to come into the palpebral aperture, or to be decompressed through the nasolacrimal duct into the nose. The organisms involved in a chronic dacryocystitis are usually those that are commensal organisms within the duct such as *Staphylococcus* and *Streptococcus*. The chronic low grade infection within the sac may cause an enlarging mucocele (Fig. 11) to develop because of irritation presumably of the glandular structures within the sac that increase their secretion into the sac and cause the enlarging mucocele. It is if and when the common canaliculus becomes kinked than an "acute dacryocystic retention syndrome" might secondarily develop.

not much of a plane to prevent spreading anterior to the orbital septum along the eyelid tissues (Fig. 7). The edema of the eyelids may induce a ptosis and produce chemosis as well. With anterior orbital cellulitis (infection anterior to the septum), the orbit is still not yet involved.

With posterior orbital cellulitis (infection posterior to the orbital septum), the orbit may become involved (43). It is unusual for the sac that lies separate from the orbit itself to be the culprit in the evolution of orbital cellulitis. However, there may be a posterior perforation of the membrane that attaches to the posterior lacrimal crest. This membrane is comprised of the orbital septum and slips from the periorbita that run to the posterior lacrimal crest posteriorly. If this occurs, the infection from the sac and the pericystic area have direct access to the orbit at large. These patients initially may develop motil-

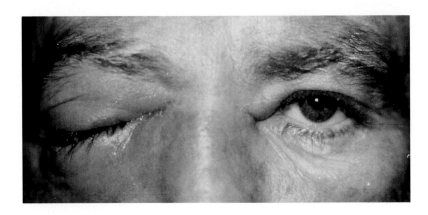

FIG. 8. Patient with dacryocystitis and posterior orbital cellulitis. There is proptosis and motility restriction, and the vision has decreased to counting fingers vision. (From Molgat and Hurwitz, ref. 43, with permission.)

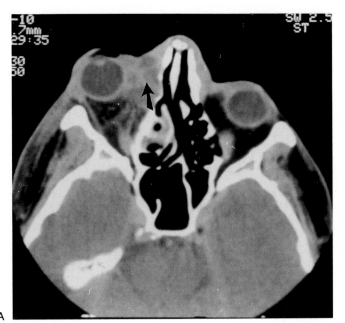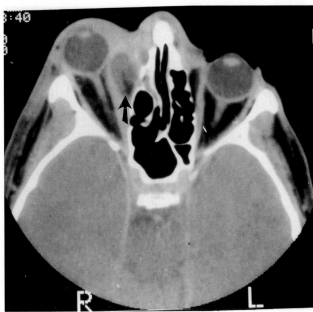

A   B

FIG. 9. **A:** CT scan of patient in Fig. 8. A diffuse orbital infiltration is present. **B:** CT scan of patient in Fig. 8. An orbital abscess lateral to the lacrimal sac has developed. (From Molgat and Hurwitz, ref. 43, with permission.)

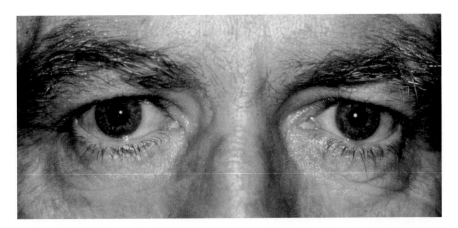

FIG. 10. Three months following DCR and orbital abscess drainage. Vision and motility have returned to normal. There is no epiphora. (From Molgat and Hurwitz, ref. 43, with permission.)

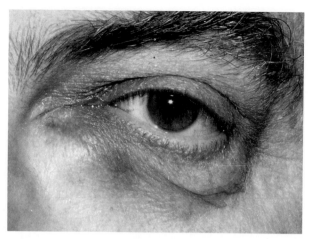

FIG. 11. Patient with chronic dacryocystitis and mucocele of the tear sac. (From Hurwitz and Rodgers, ref. 22, with permission.)

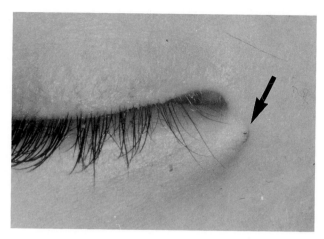

FIG. 13. Congenital lacrimal sac fistula. Notice dimple around the fistula.

Fistula

The result of an increase in swelling within the sac, usually in the acute dacryocystitis condition, may cause the sac to perforate through the skin, and there will be discharge of the pus and debris, and often blood, through the skin (Fig. 12). This usually results in an immediate relief of pain and partial resolution of the condition. The fistula may be left alone, and indeed when a DCR is performed, the fistula usually closes and does not need to be ligated. It is our feeling that when a large DCR opening is performed, there is no flow through the fistula, as all the flow goes through the DCR into the nose and the fistula ultimately closes. We have only had one situation in which we operated on the fistula at the time of a DCR, and that was to close the skin that had been widely macerated, to try to improve the ultimate cosmetic appear-

ance. In no other situation were there any cosmetic sequelae of the fistula having not been addressed at the time of DCR surgery.

Congenital fistulae have a small dimple in the skin with a raised mound around it (Fig. 13). These may be cauterized or ligated. If there is an obstruction at the valve of Hasner, a probing often is therapeutic. A fistula due to trauma will be usually located in the center of a scar (Fig. 14). A fistula due to an ethmoidal mucocele has constant drainage through the skin, regardless of whether or not one presses on the sac (Figs. 15 and 16).

Granuloma (Pyogenic)

Occasionally when the sac perforates into the subcutaneous tissues, there will be a build-up of debris and a

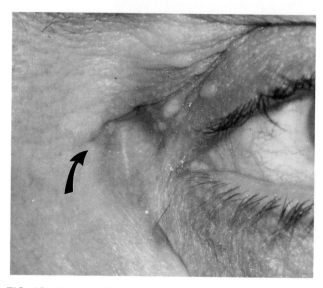

FIG. 12. Acquired fistula following acute dacryocystitis and rupture through the skin.

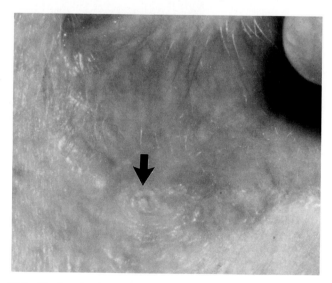

FIG. 14. Lacrimal sac fistula due to trauma. The full thickness scar goes from the skin down to the lacrimal sac. The fistula is present in the scar.

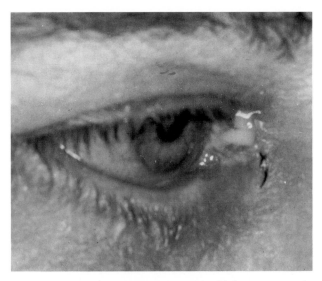

FIG. 15. Patient with fistula from ethmoidal sac mucocele. There is a constant drainage of mucus through the skin at the medial canthus. There are no symptoms of tearing.

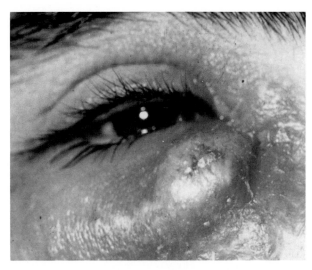

FIG. 17. Patient with dacryocystitis and secondary granuloma formation beside the sac. The granuloma spontaneously subsided within 6 weeks following a DCR.

granuloma or multiple granulomas will develop (Fig. 17). We specifically have not removed these at the time of DCR surgery because we find that usually if the DCR is open and there is no longer any epiphora, the granulomas will resolve on their own. There certainly is a temptation to remove the granulomas and one would think it would probably be a worthwhile endeavor, but we feel that unless the patient requests it, we tell the patient that the granulomas will eventually resolve and we rarely operate on them.

Differential Diagnosis of Dacryocystitis

Patients with abscesses in their skin or immediately under their skin (boils, furuncles) may present with acute swellings in the medial canthal region (Fig. 18). However, these patients have no history of tearing and are patent to syringing. It must be remembered that older patients may, in fact, even with a blocked tear duct and dacryocystitis, have no symptoms of tearing. Therefore, the test that definitively determines whether dacryocystitis is present or not is syringing of the lacrimal passages. Acute ethmoiditis may also mimic a dacryocystitis. In

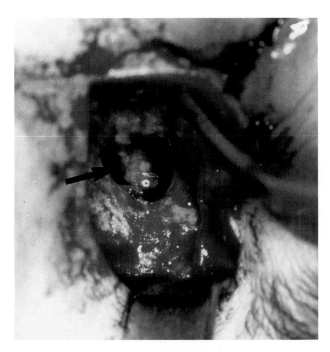

FIG. 16. Surgery of the patient in Fig. 15 reveals an ethmoidal sac mucocele. The fistulous tract was excised.

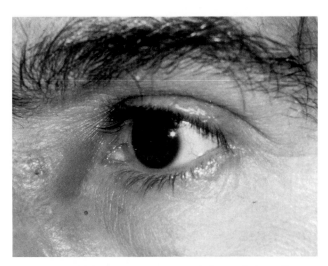

FIG. 18. Patient with swelling at left medial canthus— "pseudodacryocystitis." The patient has an infected subepithelial inclusion cyst. There is nothing wrong with the lacrimal system.

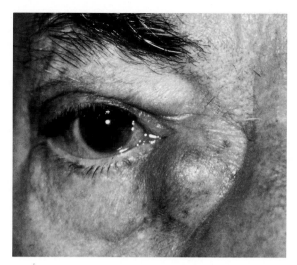

FIG. 19. Patient with swelling at medial canthus due to ethmoidal mucocele.

ethmoiditis there may be a fistula that discharges into the lacrimal area. However, this fistula may be seen to expel fluid on a constant basis without pressure over the lacrimal sac, and this drainage may even be seen to be contingent on the patient breathing in and out through the nose. A swelling above the medial canthal tendon suggests an ethmoidal mucocele, but this may also present below the tendon (Fig. 19).

Other nonlacrimal lesions of the sac such as dermoids (45), cavernous hemangioma (46), and fibromas may mimic mucoceles of the lacrimal sac (Fig. 20). These will be nonreducible lesions on palpation. The ducts may also be blocked to syringing. Dacryocystography can be useful in making the differentiation between a lacrimal sac swelling and a space-occupying lesion of the lacrimal fossa. As mentioned, tumors of the lacrimal sac must also be considered in the differentiatial diagnosis.

Osteomyelitis

There always is the question as to whether osteomyelitis in the area may be a consequence of acute dacryocystitis. Certainly for any surgeon doing reconstruction in the mid-face it would be important to know whether an osteomyelitis would be possible secondary to a nasolacrimal duct obstruction. Studies examining the bones of patients undergoing DCR showed conclusively that there was no element of osteomyelitis even when the DCR procedures had been done in sacs that had not been completely free of clinical infection. This would suggest that osteomyelitis must indeed be very rare as a consequence of a dacryocystitis, and that the bone would not otherwise be infected (47). We have seen situations in which infected implants in the mid-face and orbital floor have caused compression of the nasolacrimal system and obstruction, but we do not feel that it was osteomyelitis that had caused the secondary obstruction. Other bony conditions such as Paget's disease and osteopetrosis (48) (Fig. 21) can also cause bony lesions in the area of the sac with nasolacrimal obstruction. Usually the bony impingement is lower down in the nasolacrimal duct. causing a lacrimal obstruction without a secondary swelling in the lacrimal sac, unless secondarily a lacrimal sac mucocele develops.

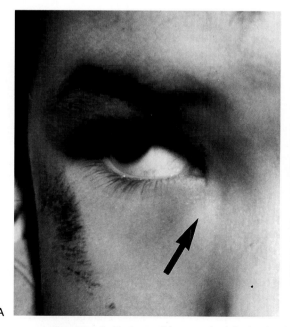

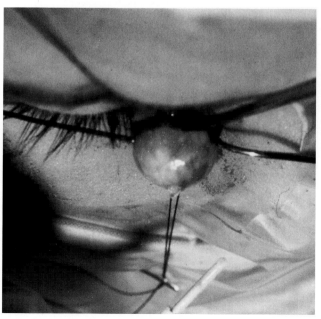

A   B

FIG. 20. A: Patient with mass in right lacrimal sac fossa. There is no tearing. **B:** Mass at surgery is a dermoid. (From Hurwitz et al., ref. 45, with permission.)

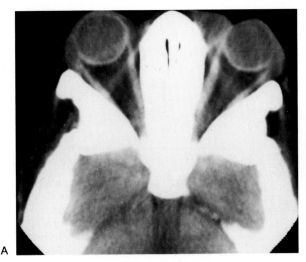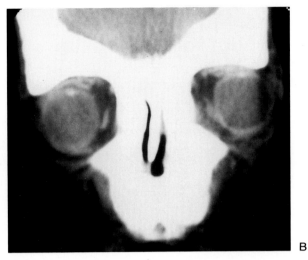

FIG. 21. A: Patient with osteopetrosis. Axial CT scan shows tremendous obliteration of the ethmoids and medial orbits. **B:** Coronal CT scan of patient with osteopetrosis. The DCR was extremely difficult. (From Hurwitz, ref. 88, with permission.)

Swelling of the Sac due to Air (Pneumatocele) (49)

Swelling of the sac is caused by air getting into the nasolacrimal duct and sac after a bout of coughing or sneezing. Usually there is a wide nasolacrimal ostium without a Hasner valve. This may also be seen after sneezing or blowing the nose following a DCR, where the valve of Rosenmuller is intact. Pressure over the sac may cause a squeaking noise. We have not intervened on any patient with this condition.

Dacryolithiasis

Stones found within the lacrimal sac on DCR have been reported in varying series to occur in 5% to 20% of patients (50). Veirs described two types of dacryoliths: those that contain amino acids and that were hydrophobic such as cystine, lysine, histidine, glutamic acid, lysine etc., and those that did not contain any amino acid (51). The stones are variable in consistency, from being mush to amorphous to hard stones. Typically, patients who present with stones are younger females having a history of intermittent tearing, intermittent swelling of the lacrimal sac, and intermittent dacryocystitis. Typically these patients may be patent to syringing on one day and completely obstructed on another. The dacryocystitis with these patients is a noninfectious dacryocystitis and is due to the build-up of pressure within the sac when there is edema of the common canaliculus and/or distention of the sac so that the common canaliculus becomes kinked. This condition has been termed the "acute dacryocystic retention syndrome" (52). It is our feeling, however, that this syndrome is usually characteristic of dacryolithiasis in the noninfectious state. The pathogenesis is probably

stagnation secondary to a partial or a complete (but usually partial) nasolacrimal stenosis. There is a build-up of calcium salts within the amorphous material (50). In fact, most of the stones in the study of Herzig and Hurwitz were found to be calcium and phosphate stones, with some urea stones. The stones sometimes form around foreign bodies within the lacrimal passages such as eyelashes, but may occur de novo. The question of a hypersecretion of calcium within the tears was looked into by Herzig and Hurwitz, and it was found that in no case of patients with stones was there a hypersecretion of calcium into the tears, nor was there any patient with a hypercalcemic state. None of these patients had histories of renal stones or gall stones, although renal stones are more closely related to lacrimal calculi than are gall stones. Although stones associated with actinomycosis are common in the canaliculus (53), there have been few reports of fungus in the lacrimal sac stones. *C. albicans* and Pityrosporum species (54) have been reported in lacrimal sac stones. Heathcote et al. (55) have done an extensive analysis of stones and lacrimal sac mucosa in patients who have stones. They felt that the fundamental step in the formation of a dacryolith is squamous metaplasia of the sac epithelium as a result of chronic (even if subclinical) dacryocystitis. Continued desquamation of the altered epithelium associated with sloughing of nonmetaplastic epithelium from inflamed mucosa results in growth of the stone. Fungi and bacteria may accentuate the process, perhaps by forming a nucleus for growth, as may irritation by chemical agents such as foreign bodies. As well, Cowen et al. (7) have shown that in a high percentage of cadavers, stones were found within the mucosa of the sac itself, within the lumen, and within the serous and mucus gland of the lacrimal sac mucosa (Fig. 22). Perhaps these stones may ultimately develop clinical

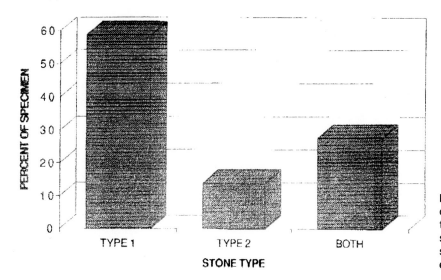

FIG. 22. Stones found within specimens of cadaver lacrimal sacs. Type 1 stones are those present in the sac lumen and Type 2 stones are those present in serous glandular structures within the sac wall. (From Cowen et al., ref. 7, with permission.)

dacryoliths. Heathcote et al. also found that within the lacrimal sac of any of the female patients, when the stones were assessed with x-ray microanalysis, there was a high percentage of patients who had titanium and iron present, elements that are normally not present in the lacrimal sac (Fig. 23). It is reasonable to expect that there had been some exposure of these patients to these elements. It is well known that titanium dioxide is a white powder that is commonly found in cosmetics. It is usually inert and has a long retention time within the body ($T_{\frac{1}{2}}$ is greater than 320 days). Studies were performed on various sorts of cosmetics and found the concentration

of titanium to be the highest of all the elements. The patients with high titanium in their lacrimal sac biopsies were questioned about their make-up histories and there was a high correlation between the titanium and the fact that these biopsies were from women who used a lot of cosmetics. The women who did not use any cosmetics had a high correlation of having little if any titanium in their lacrimal sac biopsies. Those patients who had the high iron content within their biopsies, by and large, were from the male population. It is known that iron is also an element in make-up, but only one of the men questioned used a lot of facial creams around his eyes

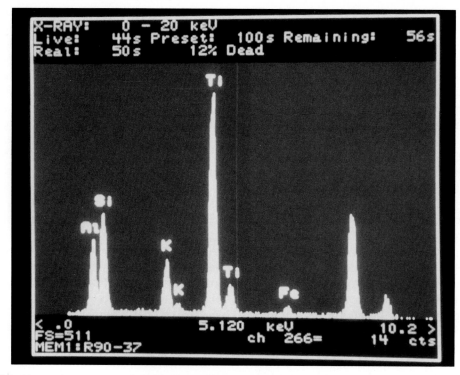

FIG. 23. X-ray microanalysis of fragments within sac biopsies in patients at the time of DCR surgery. A high concentration of titanium (T_1) suggests the presence of make-up.

and this man indeed had a large iron concentration. All the other men with high iron concentrations were factory workers, specifically in iron and steel factories or in shops, and, therefore, this could explain the high iron concentration. It is therefore questioned whether indeed make-up may play a role as a foreign body lodging in the nasolacrimal sac and/or duct mucosa and just as an eyelash may be the nidus of a stone as may a foreign body, the titanium may be involved in the development of a stone.

The diagnosis of dacryolithiasis can be made from history of intermittency of symptoms, signs, and patency, or obstruction, to syringing. The definitive diagnosis can be made with dacryocystography, which will show in a patent system a deflection of the contrast material around a space-occupying lesion within the sac and duct (Fig. 24). Other causes of stones may be due to foreign material such as topical adrenaline applied in glaucoma where a black dacryolith can be found within the system. Another potential nidus for the development of a stone is a lacrimal sac diverticulum. It is well known that lacrimal sac diverticula may develop within the sac or within the duct alone. It might be postulated that there may be chronic stagnation of fluids and possibly debris within the lacrimal sac diverticulum that may predispose to stones (56). Dacryoliths are more common in women than in men. This may be due to the anatomical predisposition for women to develop nasolacrimal obstruction because of the shape of the bony nasolacrimal system. It also may be because women wear make-up more than men and may have more titanium in their nasolacrimal sacs. It may also be due to hormonal influences. We have looked for estrogen receptors, as others have done, but our results have been inconclusive. As well, Werb (57)

has described epiphora due to nasolacrimal obstruction in women who take oral contraceptives, whereby the obstruction and the epiphora resolved after cessation of the hormones.

We have been impressed how often women will come in having had an acute attack of "acute dacryocystitic retention" that has been spontaneously relieved, and they bring in a stone that they have blown out of the nose through the nasolacrimal system. Even when the stones have been sitting around for a number of days, we have still been able to culture actinomyces within the stones. This had led us to postulate whether patients can be temporarily (if not permanently) relieved of their symptoms by having them expel their stones through the duct and out the nose.

Orbital Cyst of Lacrimal Derivation

Diverticulae of the sac or duct may become "pinched off" from the septum and undergo cystic degeneration (58). The size of the cyst will not change with pressure over the lacrimal sac. The sac is lined with lacrimal sac epithelium (Figs. 25 and 26). Treatment consists of excision of the cyst. If there is communication with the lacrimal sac, so that the sac wall must be opened, a DCR is, in our opinion, indicated. If not, a DCR is not necessary.

MANAGEMENT OF NASOLACRIMAL SAC AND DUCT OBSTRUCTION IN THE ADULT

Management of Acquired Dacryocystitis

Acute Dacryocystitis Localized to Sac

These patients are treated with systemic Cloxicillin, which will presumably combat a penicillin-resistant staphylococcus. We give 500 mg immediately and then 250 mg every six hours for 1 week. We do not use hot compresses if the dacryocystitis is localized to the sac because we do not want to cause a fistulization through the skin, which so often occurs in a star-shaped pattern from hot compresses. If the swelling increases we prefer to do a dacryocystotomy and produce a surgical linear scar.

Dacryocystotomy

A dacryocystotomy is a stab incision through the skin into the lacrimal sac. This procedure is done in the office. For anesthesia 5% xylocaine gel is rubbed on the skin of the inflamed sac and the patient is left for approximately 20 to 30 minutes. This allows adequate penetration of the xylocaine subcutaneously. It is difficult to inject the area with xylocaine, and indeed it is extremely painful. In fact, the pain of opening up the sac with a knife is

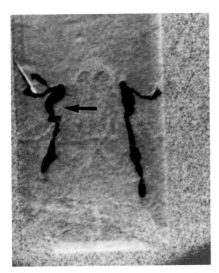

FIG. 24. Dacryocystogram of patient with a stone showing deflection of ribbon of contrast material within the sac due to the stone.

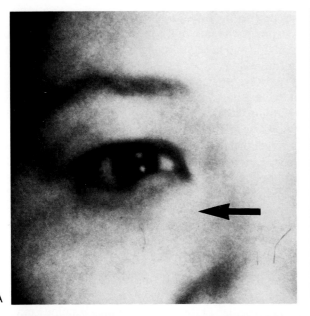

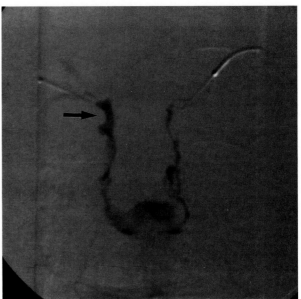

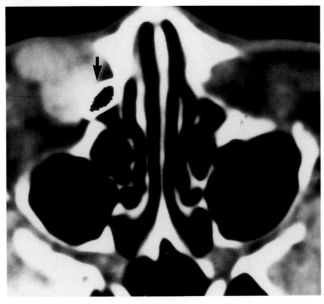

FIG. 25. A: Patient with right medial canthal lesion. (Courtesy of Drs. B. Hosal, J.J. Hurwitz, and D. Howarth.) **B:** Dacryocystogram shows slightly enlarged sac with filling defect within the sac (*arrow*) and medial displacement of the contrast. **C:** Axial CT-DCG demonstrates a lobulated soft tissue mass lateral to the nasolacrimal sac (*arrow*). The lesion at surgery proved to be a lacrimal sac cyst.

usually less painful than injecting xylocaine under the skin. A #11 blade with a sharp point is used to go through the skin and into the sac in one stab and the stab is enlarged as the blade is withdrawn. Cotton-tipped applicators can be used to squeeze out some of the debris and the area can be curetted with a chalazion curette. The wound is left open to drain. This usually leads to resolution of the rapid resolution of the infection (Fig. 27).

Most of the time it is not necessary to do a dacryocystotomy, and the infection will resolve on the medication. We also use decongestant nasal spray on the pretext that there is some swelling of the valve of Hasner. We use Naphazoline spray 0.1%, two puffs directed toward the inferior meatus three times a day for 5 days. If the patient has any allergic history at all, we suggest that the patient take some Chlortripolon Maleate, 2 mg three times a

day. We tell these patients not to drive because they will be drowsy when they are on this medication, but if they do have a lot of pain this medication will also help them to sleep. If these patients do not get better and we need a culture, we do a percutaneous stab through the skin with a #22 needle and aspirate. We do not believe in inserting a cannula through the punctum into the sac because, as mentioned, the compressed common canaliculus may be S-shaped and we worry about perforating the common canaliculus. It is much easier to go through the skin to get a sac culture and, if one wants, one can actually inject some antibiotic into the sac itself (59), although this is usually not necessary. We do not irrigate the system until 3 to 4 weeks after the resolution of a dacryocystitis and then we determine whether the system is patent or not. If the system is patent we do not do anything

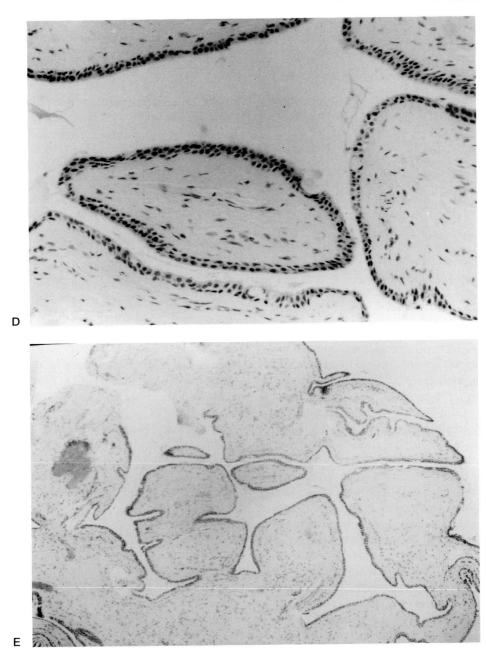

FIG. 25. (*Continued*) **D:** Histologic section showing the cystic structure lined by pseudostratified columnar and cuboidal epithelium with interspersed goblet cells. **E:** Histologic section showing broad-based papilla protruding into the lumen of the cyst.

with the patient because the epiphora might resolve. If the system is obstructed, we wait for at least 2 to 3 months to see if the dacryocystitis recurs, or if the patient is troubled enough with the epiphora to request a dacryocystorhinostomy.

Dacryocystitis with Pericystitis

We treat these patients the same as we would a patient with dacryocystitis localized to the sac except that we use hot compresses to localize the infection to the sac. Once

the pericystitis resolves and the dacryocystitis is localized to the sac, we stop the hot compresses. These patients are treated as outpatients but are followed closely for the potential development of orbital cellulitis. Once they localize to the sac they are treated the same as the patients with dacryocystitis localized to the sac.

Dacryocystitis with Orbital Cellulitis

Dacryocystitis with *anterior* orbital cellulitis (anterior to the orbital septum) is treated the same as a dacryocys-

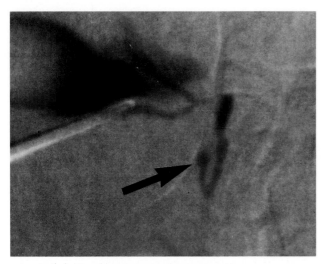

FIG. 26. Dacryocystogram with a diverticulum. It is from these diverticuli that a cyst may develop.

titis with pericystitis. Hot compresses are used until the obstruction localizes within the sac, and then the hot compresses are stopped. If a *posterior* orbital cellulitis develops (especially in an immunocompromised patient) the patient must be admitted, and we feel that a CT scan must be performed because there may be an orbital abscess. These patients are often very sick, losing vision, and may develop an impending cavernous sinus thrombosis. The CT scan must be obtained as an emergency. The patient must be treated on maximum intravenous antibiotic therapy. We prefer to use Cefuroxime sodium 750 mg every 8 hours, and Vancomycin hydrochloride 500 mg every 6 hours. A CT scan must be performed urgently and surgery undertaken. A modified Lynch approach is used to gain access to the ethmoids whereby a partial ethmoidectomy may be performed as necessary. It may be postulated that the infection has entered the orbit and the lacrimal sac through the ethmoids, but we usually find the ethmoids to be quite clear and the lacrimal sac to be the culprit. The lacrimal sac can be easily identified, a DCR performed, and the orbital abscess (which is subperiosteal) identified and evacuated. The patient must be maintained on high dose intravenous antibiotics.

As with all patients with dacryocystitis, there is significant pain and we prefer to use acetaminophen with codeine and not acetylsalicylic acid (ASA). ASA is contraindicated if surgery is to be undertaken within 2 weeks of presentation because of its tendency to increase bleeding at the time of surgery.

Management of Chronic Dacryocystitis

Although historically dacryocystitis has been treated by probing and dilatation, we prefer to employ a DCR to open and drain the sac into the nose. This has an extremely high success rate (12). With chronic dacryocystitis, the membrane that closes off the nasolacrimal duct and the sac-duct junction may also envelop the inner walls of the lacrimal sac. If the lateral wall of the lacrimal sac becomes fibrotic, it may close off the common internal punctum and there may be a secondary common canaliculus obstruction. This medial end of common canaliculus obstruction is usually secondary to a primary obstruction of the sac-duct junction. Besides a DCR, these patients also need a common internal punctoplasty whereby the membrane is excised and the system is temporarily intubated (6–12 weeks) (60).

Management of Dacryolithiasis

When we suspect dacryolithiasis, we treat the patient with Naphazoline nasal spray 0.1%, two puffs three times, and ask the patient to spray with the tip in the external nares directed backward toward the inferior lobe of the ear. This will allow the spray to get into the inferior aspect of the nasolacrimal duct at the valve of Hasner. We then have the patient blow the nose hard and inspect the tissue for any stones. Often the patient will expel a stone onto the tissue through the decongested valve of Hasner. We have found this to be something that we can do nonsurgically for this condition. We have also done experimental work to dissolve stones with biochemical materials that have been used on renal stones,

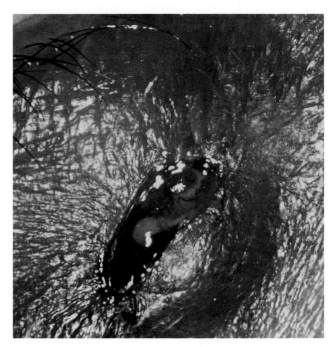

FIG. 27. Patient with dacryocystitis after dacryocystotomy and drainage of mucopus through the skin. (From Hurwitz and Rodgers, ref. 22, with permission.)

such as renacidin (61). We have done this experimentally in rabbits but found the biochemicals to be too toxic and, therefore, we would not advocate this in humans. One may try forced syringing and probing to wash out the dacryoliths (62). We have also tried forced irrigation of the duct as a diagnostic (therapeutic) endeavor, but have followed this with decongesting the nasal mucosa with Naphazoline as well. Dilation of the system with a balloon catheter has also been attempted (63).

Those measures may occasionally help but the condition, without definitive treatment, often recurs. However, we ultimately treat dacryolithiasis and the "acute dacryocystic syndrome" in the same way as we do with chronic dacryocystitis and chronic nasolacrimal duct obstruction, that is, with a DCR. At the time of the DCR, when there is a clinical and radiologic suspicion of stones, it is important to remove some of the bone from the roof of the nasolacrimal bony canal to gain access to the membranous canal. The reason for this is that stones often lodge within the superior aspect of the canal and one must remove the stones not only to relieve the epiphora, but to eliminate the intermittent dacryocystitis. There also may be folds within the distended sac and common canaliculus where stones may lodge. These must be looked for and the stones removed. A wide DCR must be performed. It is unusual for these patients to return later with epiphora and/or symptoms of dacryocystitis.

Management of Acquired Lacrimal Sac and Duct Obstruction

Although nonsurgical methods and techniques may be used in the management of acquired nasolacrimal sac and duct obstructions in the adult, usually surgery is the treatment of choice.

Observation

In patients who have had symptoms for only a short period of time (less than a month), one could argue to wait and see whether the obstruction resolves on its own. We have occasionally found this to happen, but we use the initial visit to explain to the patient the operation of a DCR, so that if the symptoms do not go away, the patient will be well informed and return with confidence for a DCR procedure.

Medications

As mentioned in the section under "dacryocystitis," if the symptoms have been present for less than a month or two, we might try some nasal decongestants such as Naphazoline spray. However, we do not use spray for more than 5 days at a time for fear of developing an atrophic rhinitis. The Naphazoline (which may also be used topically) is used to shrink the swollen mucosa of the system, which may be contributing to the obstruction.

Decreasing Lacrimal Secretion

Drugs

It is well known that certain drugs may affect the lacrimal glands by decreasing lacrimal secretion. Certainly drugs that block the parasympathetic pathways to lacrimal secretion may have an effect on decreasing tear secretion, but these drugs are not used clinically because of other ocular side effects. Antihistamines (both systemic and topical) have been known to decrease lacrimal secretion. However, keratinized epithelium of the cornea and conjunctiva and chronic vascular changes may preclude the prolonged use of topical antihistamines. Systemic antihistamines also produce drowsiness, etc. Our use of botulinum toxin for chronic blepharospasm has produced decreased tear secretion in some of our patients. However, we have not felt that it would be worthwhile to employ botulinum toxin in the long term with repeated injections to treat epiphora, when other modalities are more definitive.

Palpebral Lobectomy

Attempts to decrease lacrimal secretion in patients with epiphora have been attempted through the years. Removal of the accessory lacrimal glands was suggested by Wheeler in 1915 (64). Because of the fear of producing a dry eye, Jameson in 1937 described cutting the lacrimal gland ductules (65). The procedure has been resurrected by Taira and Smith (66). In this procedure under local anesthesia the superotemporal conjunctiva and lacrimal gland (palpebral lobe) just above the superior tarsus is clamped and excised. We have seen four patients with persisting epiphora who have had this operation, and in all cases we were able to identify that there was indeed a site of lacrimal obstruction and we were able to cure these patients with appropriate lacrimal surgery. We have used this procedure in two patients whom we felt had true hypersecretion (no cause for epiphora), but tearing persisted. It is our feeling that there are few indications for this surgery.

SURGICAL TREATMENT OF SAC-DUCT OBSTRUCTIONS

DCR

The classic operation that provides the highest success rate is Toti's operation (67), which describes the exteriorizing of the lacrimal sac into the nose. Many modifications of this operation have been performed over the years, but the DCR provides a success in well over 90% of cases (12). Modifications of the procedure have allowed the DCR to be performed under local anesthesia (68) as well as in the outpatient setting (69).

Alternatives to DCR in the Treatment of Acquired Sac-Duct Obstructions

Dacryocystectomy

Dacrocystectomy, removal of the lacrimal sac, has been around for centuries. Whereas removal of the lacrimal sac does have a role in the management of lacrimal sac tumors (70), nowadays there are few indications for the removal of the lacrimal sac if a tumor is not present. Presumably in an elderly patient with dacryocystitis, negligible symptoms of tearing, and potentially with a tear film deficiency, a dacryocystectomy could be performed. However, it is often difficult (if not impossible) to remove all the infected tissues so that dacryocystitis will not later recur. By removing a sac full of infected pus and debris, the reflex arc back to the secretors of the lacrimal gland via the trigeminal nerve may be relieved of irritants that cause oversecretion of the tears. It has been said that in 50% of dacryocystectomies the tear secretion will decrease (71). By removing the toxins that potentially stimulate tearing, symptoms of epiphora may be lessened. However, we feel that a DCR provides a better chance of a complete and long-lasting cure of epiphora. Whereas the symptoms of tearing are usually not predominant in the face of a rampant dacryocystitis, when the dacryocystitis may be improved by removal of the sac, persistent symptoms of tearing may become more obvious to the patient and become problematic, necessitating further reconstructive surgery. Also, because it is often impossible to remove all the epithelial lacrimal sac tissue, the sac may regenerate and another episode of dacryocystitis may recur in a lacrimal sac that had supposedly been removed (72). A dacryocystectomy may also be attempted in patients who have disease in which one would want to avoid opening into the nose, such as Wegener's granulomatosis (73). However, we have found that with certain modifications of the DCR procedure in patients with Wegener's granulomatosis, we usually attempt a curative DCR.

Dacryocystoductorhinostomy

Procedures whereby the lacrimal sac may be opened and a tube placed from the sac into the nose (inferior meatus) may be attempted as well when one does not want to open into the middle meatus (74). Others have attempted to put in an artificial device that sits as a funnel at the inner canthus much like a Jones' bypass tube (75), to drain into the sac and then down through the nasolacrimal duct without an opening into the nose (76). However, we feel that this procedure necessitates an artificial device, the same magnitude of surgery as a DCR, and certainly one would not anticipate that the long-term success rate would be better than that of a DCR in the treatment of a sac obstruction.

Probing and Syringing

Probing may open up an intracanalicular membrane and may be tried before formal surgery. We limit this to the patient with canalicular (not sac) obstruction. We are also worried that probings may turn incomplete obstructions into complete obstructions. Syringing with antibiotics seems to be useful if canaliculitis (not dacryocystitis) is present.

Silicone Intubation

The passing of bicanalicular tubes through the lacrimal system with a loop at the inner canthus and the two free ends tied to each other within the nose has been used over the years to avoid a DCR procedure. These tubes may be passed from the punctum down into the nose (77). One may also attempt to pass these tubes from the nose toward the punctum (78). The concept of passing tubes through the pathology underlying a primary nasolacrimal sac and duct does not alleviate or circumvent the underlying process. As well, it is important that before one can be sure that a "success" is achieved, a long follow-up period must be observed (79). Again for this reason, we prefer in the most cases to perform a DCR in an acquired sac-duct obstruction rather than intubation.

Balloon Dilatation of the Sac and Duct

More recently, attempts have been made by ophthalmologists and by radiologists to dilate the nasolacrimal system using a balloon catheter (80). However, their success rates were low and the authors state "the high failure and recurrence rates in a study are not encouraging." Further attempts at the balloon dilatation in conjunction with stents in the system did yield higher success rates (81). However, the success rates reported by these authors were not in the "acceptable" success rates from the DCR procedure, and presumably their increased success rate using the balloon catheter in their second study as opposed to their first study was because they did use stents in the system. This would lead to suggest that balloon dilatation of the duct, which indeed is encased in a rigid bony system, especially without the use of stents, could not be expected to yield acceptable success rates.

Endonasal Surgery

Performing a procedure to open the sac into the nose via an intranasal approach has been around longer than the standard DCR approach. However, with the advent of the nasal endoscope, the procedure has been resurrected (82). The advantage of this procedure is that it can be done without an external scar in the skin. However, our experience thus far has suggested that we cannot be as sure of providing an opening of the lacrimal sac into the nose that would stay patent long term, as we are with a standard external DCR. In fact, if the scar is perceived as being a big problem, the DCR procedure may be performed through a smaller incision (83), and certainly the use of traction sutures during the DCR procedure will give adequate access without compromising the size of the opening. Thus far we have limited the use of endonasal surgery to those patients presenting with previously unsuccessful nasolacrimal surgery where the pathology lies within the wall of the nose.

Endonasal Laser DCR

The use of the laser to make an opening into the nose rather than bone punches that one uses the endonasal approach had a surge of enthusiasm in the early 1990s (84). However, it would seem that it would be difficult to perform a laser opening into the sac if there were large ethmoidal air cells and/or previous trauma with impaction of bone. It has always been our philosophy to preserve the nasal mucosa and lacrimal sac mucosa and treat them as atraumatically as possible. This obviously would not be the case if one burned a hole from the nose through the bone and into the sac. It would seem that even some of the surgeons who performed the laser surgery early on in its inception do not have the same enthusiasm for this procedure at this time (85). Perhaps with future refinements the morbidity will decrease and the success rates increase.

Transcanalicular Thermal Recanalization

Attempts to destroy membranes by passing a thermal instrument along the canaliculus have been attempted (86,87). It is yet to be determined whether the transcanalicular laser approach has anything to add over the endonasal laser approach. It is our feeling that with assistance of a canaliculoscope, this procedure might be useful in treating canalicular membranes.

REFERENCES

1. Kushner BJ. Congenital nasolacrimal system obstruction. *Arch Ophthalmol* 1982;100:597.

2. Garfin SW. Etiology of dacryocystitis and epiphora. *Arch Ophthalmol* 1942;27:167–188.

3. Avasth IP, Misra RM, Sood AK. Clinical and anatomical considerations of dacryocystitis. *Int Surg* 1971;55:200–203.

4. Hurwitz JJ, Welham R. The role of dacryocystography in the management of congenital nasolacrimal duct obstruction. *Can J Ophthalmol* 1975;10:346–349.

5. Walker D, Heathcote G, Hurwitz JJ. The pathology of lacrimal obstruction. *Proceedings of University of Toronto, Ophthalmology Research Day*; 1987.

6. Linberg JV, McCormick SA. Primary acquired nasolacrimal duct obstruction: a clinical pathological report and biopsy technique. *Ophthalmology* 1986;93:1055.

7. Cowen D, Nianiaris N, Howarth D, Hurwitz JJ. *Lacrimal stone histopathology and lacrimal stone formation—new insights: symposium of the European Society of Dacriology.* Milan: Ghedini; 1995 (in press).

8. McCormick SA, Linberg JV. Pathology of nasolacrimal duct obstruction. In: Linberg JV, ed. *Lacrimal surgery.* New York: Churchill Livingstone; 1988.

9. Duke-Elder S. The ocular adnexa. In: Henry Kimpton, ed. *System of ophthalmology*, vol. XIII, part II, 1974;700.

10. Dalgleish R. Idiopathic acquired lacrimal drainage obstruction. *Br J Ophthalmol* 1967;51:463.

11. Santos Fernandez J. De la disposition anatomica del canal naso en el negro, que explicasumenor predisposicion a las afeccicions de las dias lagrimales. *Arch Oftal Hisp-Am* 1903;3:193.

12. Hurwitz JJ, Rutherford S. Computerized survey of lacrimal surgery patients. *Ophthalmology* 1986;83:14.

13. Meller J. Disease of the lacrimal apparatus. *Trans Ophthal Soc UK* 1929;49:233.

14. McKenzie J. *A practical treatise on the disease of the eye*, 3rd ed. Duke Elderis: London, 1840;700.

15. Saundermann R. Beitraj Zur Pathologie Und Therapie Den Dakryocystitis Phlegmonosa. *Kline Monapsbl Augenheilk* 1923;70:692.

16. Veirs ER. Lacrimal disorders. St Louis: CV Mosby; 1976.

17. Weingarten R, Goodman EF. Late failure of a dacryocystorhinostomy from sarcoidosis. *Ophthal Surg* 1981;12:343.

18. Mauriello JA, Mostafavi R. Bilateral nasolacrimal obstruction associated with Crohn's disease successfully treated with dacryocystorhinostomy. *Ophthal Plast Reconstruct Surg* 1994;10:261.

19. Jordan DR, Miller D, Anderson RL. Wound necrosis following dacryocystorhinostomy in patients with Wegener's granulomatosis. *Ophthal Surg* 1987;18:800.

20. Holds JB, Anderson RL, Wolin MJ. Dacryocystectomy for the treatment of dacryocystitis patients with Wegener's granulomatosis. *Ophthal Surg* 1989;20:443.

21. Coden DJ, Hornblass A, Haas BD. Clinical bacteriology of dacryocystitis in adults. *Ophthal Plast Reconstruct Surg* 1993;9:125.

22. Hurwitz JJ, Rodgers KJA. Management of acquired dacryocystitis. *Can J Ophthalmol* 1983;18:213.

23. Bartley GB. Acquired lacrimal drainage obstruction: an etiologic classification system, case report, and a review of the literature. Part 1. *Ophthal Plast Reconstruct Surg* 1992;8:237.

24. Walker D, Hurwitz JJ, Heathcote G. The pathology of lacrimal sac obstruction. Abstract section *Can J Ophthalmol* 1989;24.

25. Artenstein AW, Eiseman AS, Campbell GC. Chronic dacryocystitis caused by *Mycobacterium fortuitum*. *Ophthalmology* 1993;100:666.

26. Duahs J, Paterson A, Smith FW, Scott GB, Forrester HV. Dacryocystitis caused by *Eikenella corrodens*. *Am J Ophthalmol* 1988;106:238.

27. Steel RJ, Meyer DR. Nasolacrimal duct obstruction and acute dacryocystitis associated with infectious mononucleosis (Epstein Barr virus). *Am J Ophthalmol* 1993;115:265.

28. Madreperla FA, Green WR, Daniel R, Shaw KV. Human papilloma virus in primary epithelial tumours of the lacrimal sac. *Ophthalmology* 1993;100:569.

29. Kaplan CS, Freedman L, Elsdon-Dewr. A worm in the eye: a familiar parasite in an unusual situation. *South Afr Med J* 1956;37:91.

30. Baratz K, Bartley J, Campbell R, Garrity J. An eyelash nidus for dacryoliths of the lacrimal excretory and secretory systems. *Amer J Ophthalmol* 1991;11:624.

31. Spaeth GL. Nasolacrimal duct obstruction caused by topical epinepherine. *Arch Ophthalmol* 1967;77:355.
32. Nik NA, Hurwitz JJ, Gruss JS. Management of lacrimal injury after naso-orbito-ethmoid fracture. *Adv Ophthal Plast Reconstruct Surg* 1984;3:307.
33. Flanagan JC. Epiphora following rhinoplasty. *Ann Ophthalmol* 1978;2:1239.
34. Colvard DM, Waller RR, Neault RW, Desanto LW. Nasolacrimal duct obstruction following transantral-ethmoidal orbital decompression. *Ophthal Surg* 1979;10:25.
35. Serdahl Cl, Berris CE, Choele RA. Nasolacrimal duct obstruction after endoscopic sinus surgery. *Arch Ophthalmol* 1990;108:391.
36. Glatt H. Acute dacryocystitis after punctal occlusion for keratoconjunctivitis. *Am J Ophthalmol* 1991;111:769.
37. Vaughan-Schmidt W. Lipogranuloma after treatment of the nasolacrimal duct. *Folia Ophthalmol* 1988;13:279.
38. Hawes MJ, Dortzbach RK, Segrest DR. Lacrimal canalicular trauma. In: Dortzbach RK ed. *Ophthalmic plastic surgery—prevention and management of complications.* New York: Raven Press; 1994:233.
39. Karesh JW, Perman KI, Rodrigues MM. Lymphoma of the lacrimal sac. *Ophthalmology* 1993;100:669.
40. Nianiaris N, Cowen DE, Howarth D, Hurwitz JJ. *Lacrimal sac histopathology and lacrimal sac stones formation: New insights. In Proceedings of Ophthalmology Research Day,* University of Toronto; 1993.
41. Raflo GT, Hurwitz JJ, Chart P. Thermographic assessment of the human lacrimal drainage system. *Ophthal Surg* 1982;13:119.
42. Billington B, Hurwitz JJ, Galbraith D, Gentles W. A mini-probe for assessment of lacrimal sac temperatures. *Ophthal Surg* 1984;15:680.
43. Molgat Y, Hurwitz JJ. Orbital abscess due to acute dacryocystitis. *Can J Ophthalmol* 1993;28:181.
44. Alan MV, Cullen KL, Grimson BS. Orbital cellulitis secondary to dacryocystitis following blepharoplasties. *Ann Ophthalmol* 1985;17:498.
45. Hurwitz JJ, Rodgers KJA, Doucet TW. Dermoid tumours involving the lacrimal drainage pathway. *Ophthal Surg* 1982;3:377.
46. Ferry A, Kaltreider SA. Cavernous hemangioma of the lacrimal sac. *Am J Ophthalmol* 1990;110:316.
47. Hinton P, Hurwitz JJ, Cruickshanks B. Nasolacrimal bone changes and diseases of the lacrimal drainage system. *Ophthal Surg* 1984;15:516.
48. Silvia D, Patrinely JR. Dacryocytorhinostomy and osteopetrosis. *Ophthal Surg* 1991;22:396.
49. Rochels R, Bleier R, Nover A. Compressive pneumatocele of the lacrimal sac. *Klin Mbl Augenagilk* 1989;195:174.
50. Herzig S, Hurwitz JJ. Lacrimal sac calculi. *Can J Ophthalmol* 1979;14:17.
51. Viers ER. *Lacrimal disorders.* St. Louis: CV Mosby; 1976.
52. Gonnering RS, Bosniak SL. Recognition and management of acute non-infectious dacryocystic retention. *Ophthal Plast Reconstruct Surg* 1989;5:27.
53. Fine M, Raring WS. Mycotic obstruction of the nasolacrimal duct (*Candida albicans*). *Arch Ophthalmol* 1947;38:39.
54. Wolter JR. Pityrosprum species associated with dacryoliths in obstructive dacryocystitis. *Am J Ophthalmol* 1977;84:806.
55. Heathcote G, Veloudias A, Holmyard DP, Hurwitz JJ. The pathogenesis of dacryolithiasis. *Ophthalmology* (accepted for publication).
56. Bullock JD, Goldberg SH. Lacrimal sac diverticuli. *Arch Ophthalmol* 1989;107:756.
57. Werb A. Unusual causes of epiphora. *Br J Ophthalmol* 1971;55:559.
58. Hornblass A, Gross ND. Lacrimal sac cyst. *Ophthalmology* 1987;94:706.
59. Carreras Y, Matas M, Garcia MM. Our experience with conservative therapy of chronic dacryocystitis employing Penicillin lavage of the lacrimal sac. *Rev Esp Otoneuro Ofial* 1966;25:93.
60. Doucet TW, Hurwitz JJ. Canaliculodacryocystorhinostomy in the treatment of canalicular obstruction. *Arch Ophthalmol* 1982;100:306.
61. Jacobs SC, Gittes RF. Dissolutions of residual renal calculi with Hemiacidrin. *J Urol* 1976;115:532.
62. Smith B, Tenzel RR, Buffam SV, Boynton JR. Acute dacryocystic retention. *Arch Ophthalmol* 1976;94:1903.
63. Becker BB, Berry FD. Balloon catheter dilatation in lacrimal surgery. *Ophthal Surg* 1989;20:1930.
64. Wheeler JM. Removal of the lacrimal sac and accessory lacrimal gland. *Int J Surg* 1915;28:106.
65. Jameson PC. Subconjunctival section of the ductules of the lacrimal gland as a cure for epiphora. *Arch Ophthalmol* 1937;17:207.
66. Taira C, Smith B. Palpebral adenectomy. *Am J Ophthalmol* 1973;75:461.
67. Toti A. Dacriocystorhinostomia. *Mag Ophthalmol* 1910;23.
68. Kratky V, Hurwitz JJ, Anathanarayan C, Avram DR. Dacryocystorhinostomy in elderly patients: regional anesthesia without Cocaine. *Can J Ophthalmol* 1994;29:13.
69. Dresner SC, Klussman KG, Meyer DR, Linberg JV. Outpatient dacryocystorhinostomy. *Ophthal Surg* 1991;22:222.
70. Hornblass A, Jakaobiec FA, Bosniak S, Flanagan JC. The diagnosis and management of epithelial tumours of the lacrimal sac. *Ophthalmology* 1980;87:476.
71. Mosher HP. The combined intranasal and external operation on the lacrimal sac. *Ann Otorhinol Laryngol* 1923;32:8.
72. Rizk SNM, Dark AJ. Regeneration of the lacrimal sac *Trans Ophthal Soc UK* 1967;87:695.
73. Hardwig TW, Bartley GB, Garrity JA. Surgical management of nasolacrimal duct obstructions in patient with Wegener's granulomatosis. *Ophthalmology* 1991;99:133.
74. Actis G, Bellan B, Kuba I, Malinverni W. Dacryocystoductorhinostomy. *Orbit* 1985;4:65.
75. Jones LT. Conjunctivodacryocystorhinostomy. *Am J Ophthalmol* 1965;59:773.
76. Reinecke RD, Carroll JM. Silicone lacrimal tube implantation. *Trans Am Acad Ophthalmol Otolaryngol* 1969;73:85.
77. Psilas K, Eftaxias V, Kaseanioudakis J, Kalogeropoulos C. Silicone intubation as an alternative to dacryocystorhinostomy for nasolacrimal drainage obstruction in adults. *Eur J Ophthalmol* 1993;3:71.
78. Steinkogler FJ, Huber E, Kuchar A, Karnel F. Retrograde dilatation of the post saccal lacrimal stenosis. *Ann Otol Rhinol Laryngol* 1994;103:110.
79. Jones LT, Wobig JL. The lacrimal dilemma. In: Jones LT, Wong JL, eds. *Surgery of the eyelids and lacrimal system.* Birmingham, AL: Aesculapius Co., 1976.
80. Song HY, Ahn HS, Park CK, Koon SH, Kim CS, Chou KC. Complete obstruction of the nasolacrimal system. Part I treatment with balloon dilatation. *Radiology* 1993;186:367.
81. Song HY, Jin Yh, Kim JH, Sung KB, Han YM, Cho NC. Nasolacrimal duct obstruction treated nonsurgically with use of plastic stents. *Radiology* 1994;195:35.
82. Rich DA. Endoscopic intranasal dacryocystorhinostomy results in four patients. *Arch Otolaryngol Head Neck Surg* 1990;116:1061.
83. Dortzbach R, Woog JJ. Small incision techniques in ophthalmic plastic surgery. *Ophthal Surg* 1990;21:615.
84. Massaro BM, Gonnering RS, Harris GJ. Endonasal laser dacryocystorhinostomy. A new approach to nasolacrimal duct obstruction. *Arch Ophthalmol* 1990;108:1172.
85. Gonnering RS. Dacryocystorhinostomy and conjunctival dacryocystorhinostomy. In: Dortzbach RK, ed. *Ophthalmic Plastic Surgery Prevention and Management of Complications.* New York: Raven Press; 1994.
86. Silkiss RZ. Nd:Yag nasolacrimal duct recanalization. *Ophthal Surg* 1993;24:772.
87. Silkiss RZ, Axelrod RN, Iwach AG, Vassiliadis A, Hennings DR. Transcanalicular Nd:Yag dacryocystorhinostomy. *Ophthal Surg* 1992;23:351.
88. Hurwitz JJ. Dacriocystoplasty. In: Ghedini, ed. *The lacrimal system 1994.* 1995;in press.

CHAPTER 23

Canalicular Diseases

Jeffrey Jay Hurwitz

The punctum and canaliculus must be treated as separate structures. Certainly some diseases involve both the punctum and the canaliculus, but many involve either one or the other. The common canaliculus may be discussed in conjunction with the afflictions of the canaliculi.

It is convenient to divide canalicular obstructions into those that are nonsuppurative and those that are suppurative.

NONSUPPURATIVE CANALICULAR OBSTRUCTIONS

Nonsuppurative canalicular obstructions may occur from diseases that cause inflammation of the lining of the canaliculi (intracanalicular obstruction) or from conditions that cause scarring of the outer walls of the canaliculi, with secondary extrinsic compression and obstruction (pericanalicular obstruction). This consideration is important when one attempts to formulate a treatment plan. Certainly, one could anticipate that if an intubation is performed of the canaliculi in an *intracanalicular* obstruction, where the epithelium is not damaged, the success rate might be acceptable. As well, intubation might help in a situation in which a *temporary pericanalicular* process is going on (such as radiation), and that if the tubes are removed once the process has resolved, a patent system might be anticipated. However, it is more difficult to understand why a progressive *permanent pericanalicular* etiology for obstruction should be helped with silicone intubation.

J. J. Hurwitz: Oculoplastics Program, Mount Sinai Hospital; and Department of Ophthalmology, University of Toronto Faculty of Medicine, Toronto, Ontario M5S 1A8, Canada.

ETIOLOGY OF NONSUPPURATIVE CANALICULAR OBSTRUCTION

Trachoma

In populations where trachoma is endemic, canalicular stenosis and subsequent epiphora is common (1). This is characterized by a pericanalicular swelling that has been said to be present in 37% of patients with trachoma. Secondary dilations of the canaliculus might occur, leading to secondary bacterial infections. The punctum often becomes stenotic and treatment might be undertaken by opening up the canaliculus with a snip and injecting antibiotics as determined on culture. However, most of the patients we see with trachoma are chronic and burnt out, and there is no active infection. The epiphora due to canalicular obstruction has to be treated by more formal canalicular surgery.

Viral Infections

Herpes simplex has been implicated in obstruction of the punctum and the proximal canaliculus (2). However, patients who have been treated with antivirals such as idoxuridine for herpes simplex have also been found to have canalicular stenosis; it has been felt that the stenosis is on the basis of the antiviral treatment (3). However, canalicular obstruction may certainly occur in herpes simplex where patients have not been treated with antivirals. Herpes zoster may also cause canalicular obstruction (4), as may vaccinia (5).

Chicken pox and small pox have been implicated as etiologic factors in canalicular obstructions. We have seen a number of cases of chicken pox obstructions and the treatment usually necessitates lacrimal bypass surgery (6), rather than simple methods (7).

Cicatrizing Diseases

Ocular pemphigoid and Stevens-Johnson syndrome cause subepithelial fibrosis of the conjunctiva with subsequent symblepharon formation and may cause obstruction of the canaliculus and/or punctum (Fig. 1). Some of these patients, because of scarring of the ductules of the lacrimal glands, will not have symptoms of epiphora because of decreased tear secretion even though the canaliculi are obstructed. Obviously these patients do not need any treatment of the canalicular obstructions. One may attempt to probe the obstructions and insert indwelling stent tubes, but there is a tendency for fibrous tissue formation around any artificial device that may lead to further problems on removal of the tubes, and subsequent closure. With proximal canalicular obstruction, one may try to cut down on the canaliculus to determine whether there is some more distal patent part of the canaliculus. One may then try to probe retrogradely through the canaliculus and put in some sort of a stent (8). We have tried this but have not had good results in obtaining long-lasting patency. We have also tried to do this and marsupialize the medial end into the lacrimal lake. However, we have not been happy with this treatment either. More formal canaliculodacryocystorhinostomy surgery may be attempted if the obstructions are located in a more distal location within the canalicular system (9). However, if the obstructions are more proximal, a bypass procedure such as with a Jones tube (6) is the only hope of relieving the epiphora. However, one must also be aware of the fact that there may be excess fibrous tissue formation around even a Jones tube (10), which may lead to further problems.

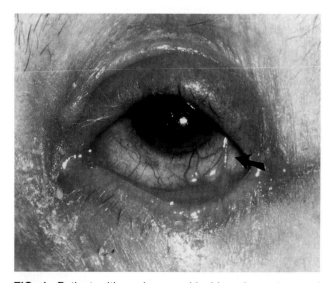

FIG. 1. Patient with ocular pemphigoid, and punctum and canalicular obstruction. Symblepharon formation is present (*arrow*).

Canalicular Stenosis Due to Drugs

Many glaucoma drugs such as phospholine iodide (11), epinephrine (12), and less rarely other antiglaucoma medications can cause canalicular stenosis. Idoxuridine and other antivirals have been implicated as well.

Certain drugs such as penicillin may cause canalicular obstruction by initially causing a Stevens-Johnson syndrome (13). Chemotherapeutic agents such as fluorouracil are known to cause fibrosis of the punctum and the canaliculus (14).

Burns (Radiation, Thermal)

Radiation effects may produce stenosis of the canaliculi and indeed the whole nasolacrimal system (15). Patients with tumors in the area of the inner canthus when radiation has been used may develop canalicular obstruction. This may be seen following radiation for basal cell carcinomas (16). Radiation to the sinus and periorbital region related to maxillary and ethmoidal tumors may cause obstruction of the canaliculus following radiation, but indeed may occur when radical surgery has been performed without radiation (17). Radiation usually causes a pericanalicular obstruction, and we have found that the only treatment that works is excising the stenotic canaliculus and reconstructing the ends (9), or bypassing the whole system with an artificial bypass tube (6). One may try to prophylactically prevent stenosis by inserting tubes into the system before the radiotherapy and leaving them for a period of time afterward (3–6 months). We have done this in a few patients with variable results. Desmet et al. (18) have had some success in preventing permanent radiation-induced obstruction when medial canthal tumors were to be treated with radiotherapy.

Tumors of the Canaliculus

Neoplasms rarely arise from the canaliculus. Papilloma formation may occur in the nasolacrimal system (19) (Fig. 2). Even less rarely, basal cell carcinomas may arise from the lacrimal canaliculus (20).

Common Canalicular Obstruction

Common canalicular obstruction may be divided into two groups:

1. medial end of common canalicular obstruction (at junction with nasolacrimal sac)
2. lateral common canalicular obstruction (at the junction of the upper and lower canaliculus).

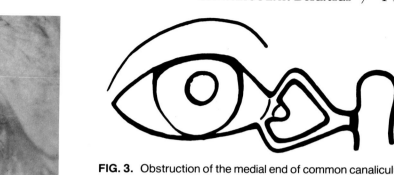

FIG. 2. Patient with papilloma of the canaliculus projecting from the punctum.

FIG. 3. Obstruction of the medial end of common canaliculus with its junction with the lacrimal sac. (From Hurwitz, ref. 43, with permission.)

When common canalicular obstruction occurs at the junction of nasolacrimal sac it is almost always secondary to an obstructing membrane secondary to a primary nasolacrimal sac-duct obstruction. The fibrotic membrane that closes off the junction of the sac and the duct pathologically will also scar off the opening at the common internal punctum level. At surgery one finds a membrane overlying the common internal punctum that is found once the sac is open at the time of dacryocystorhinostomy (DCR) surgery. It is necessary to perform, in conjunction with the DCR, a common internal punctoplasty whereby the membrane is excised (21). When this common internal punctoplasty has been performed, it is necessary to intubate the system temporarily with a Silastic tube to prevent closure of the common internal punctum (9).

Lateral common canalicular obstructions generally have the same etiology as individual canalicular obstructions. One must search for an etiology and treat the patient appropriately.

Iatrogenic

Certainly the canaliculus can be transected at the time of excising a basal cell carcinoma at the medial canthus (22). Fortunately, many of these older patients have decreased tear secretion because of their age, or because they have had previous radiotherapy, and tearing is absent, even though the punctum and canaliculus have been excised. Certainly if the lid reconstruction is satisfactory, the remaining canaliculus in most patients will carry enough of the tears to keep the patients symptom free.

A snip procedure or an iatrogenic slit canaliculus from a Silastic tube have been implicated in causing canalicular obstruction and secondary epiphora. However, we have found that this etiology is indeed very rare, and that

even if patients do have a slit or snipped lower punctum and canaliculus, if the rest of the system is normal the patients usually do not have epiphora (23).

Postmenopausal Women

It has been suggested that there is a form of idiopathic canaliculus stenosis that develops most frequently in postmenopausal women (24). We have looked for estrogen receptors but have not been able to come to any conclusions. Certainly it is possible that the common canaliculus becomes more stenotic with age as one might demonstrate when dacryocystography is performed.

Idiopathic

There is indeed a canalicular obstruction that may be idiopathic. Perhaps the patient had a pre-existing congenital punctal stenosis or canalicular stenosis that has, with chronic wiping and chronic tearing, led to a permanent obstruction. However, there are some patients with

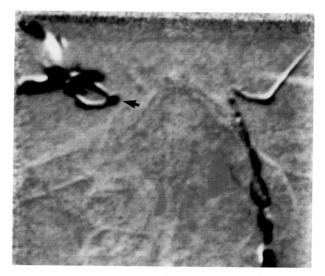

FIG. 4. DCG of right medial common canalicular obstruction. (*arrow*).

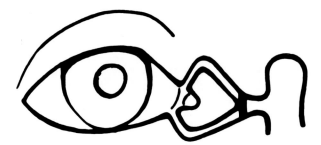

FIG. 5. Obstructed common canaliculus at its lateral end where it meets the upper and lower canaliculi. (From Hurwitz, ref. 43, with permission.)

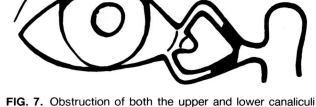

FIG. 7. Obstruction of both the upper and lower canaliculi with more than 8 mm of each remaining. (From Hurwitz, ref. 43, with permission.)

normal puncta and lids and no other causes of a definitive etiology of canalicular obstruction, who definitely present with a blocked canaliculus.

There is often a history of a subacute or acute episode of conjunctivitis or discharge preceding the evolution of a canalicular obstruction. After the red eye and discharge disappears, the patient may be left with the watery eye. The infection may presumably be an adenovirus or some other supposedly innocuous virus. On careful questioning of the patient with a so-called idiopathic canalicular obstruction, one is often able to get this sort of a history.

TREATMENT OF NONSUPPURATIVE CANALICULAR OBSTRUCTION

1. Common canalicular obstruction at the medial end (Figs. 3 and 4): the obstructing membrane is within the sac overlying the common internal punctum and secondary to a primary sac-duct obstruction. The treatment consists of a DCR, removal of the membrane, and temporary silicone intubation for approximately 8 weeks (9).

2. Common canalicular obstruction at the lateral end (Fig. 5): this usually requires a canaliculodacryocystorhinostomy (9).

3. Obstruction of an individual canaliculus (Fig. 6): the treatment of this condition, if the other punctum,

canaliculus, and rest of the system is normal, and the lid is in good apposition, can be treated merely by performing a straightforward DCR (silicone intubation optional). It has been shown that a straightforward DCR will decrease the resistance at the lower end of the system to allow tears to flow through to the nose through the one remaining canaliculus (9). Also with the sac being opened up into the nose, the effect of respiration will probably have more of a role of draining the tears from the common internal punctum directly into the nose (25).

4. Medial obstruction of the canaliculi (more than 8 mm remaining) (Fig. 7): the scar tissue between the upper and lower canaliculus and the common canaliculus may be excised and a canaliculodacryocystorhinostomy performed (9).

5. Less than 8 mm of obstruction (distal obstruction) (Figs. 8–10).

A canaliculodacryocystorhinostomy is extremely difficult to perform and the success rate decreases the more lateral the obstruction is in the system (26) (Fig. 8). To relieve the epiphora, it is usually necessary to bypass the lacrimal system totally and drain the tears directly from the palpebral aperture into the nose. The standard treatment is a conjunctivodacryocystorhinostomy with the placement of a Lester Jones' glass bypass tube (6), and

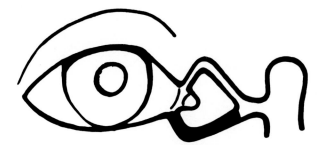

FIG. 6. Obstructed lower canaliculus where the rest of the system is normal. If the lids are normal, this patient can be cured with a standard dacryocystorhinostomy. (From Hurwitz, ref. 43, with permission.)

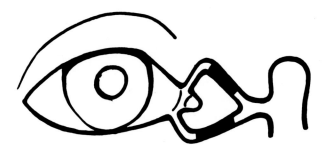

FIG. 8. Lateral canalicular obstruction in the upper and lower canaliculi. There are less than 8 mm left and a Jones' tube procedure is recommended. (From Hurwitz, ref. 43, with permission.)

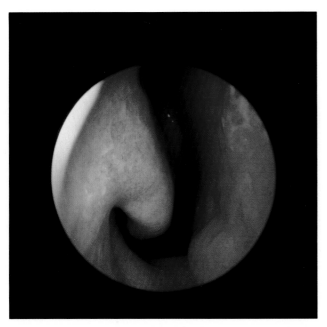

FIG. 1. Endoscopic visualization of normal nasal structures. (Courtesy of Dr. Michael Hawke, Toronto.)

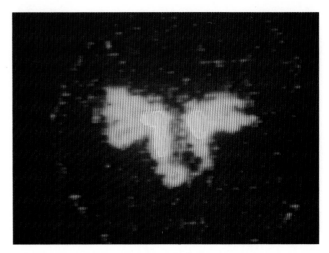

FIG. 2. Color-coded nuclear lacrimal scan shows blue as areas with weaker activity and orange as areas of more concentrated activity.

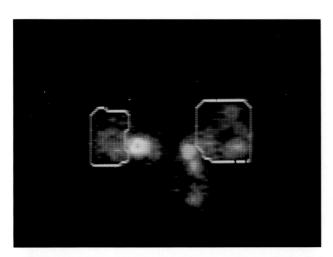

FIG. 3. Areas of interest may be drawn on the color-coded nuclear lacrimal scan and time-activity curves and T-1/2 values plotted.

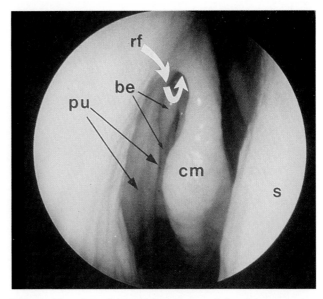

FIG. 4. View into right middle meatus. rf, frontal recess; be, bulla ethmoidalis; pu, uncinate process; cm, middle turbinate; s, septum. (Courtesy of Dr. Michael Hawke, Toronto.)

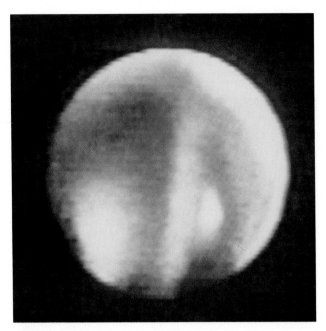

FIG. 5. Canaliculoscopy image of two canaliculi joining at common canaliculus.

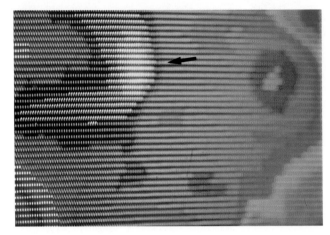

FIG. 6. Thermogram showing lacrimal sac heat radiation from dacryocystitis.

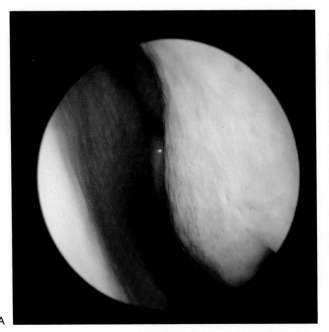

A

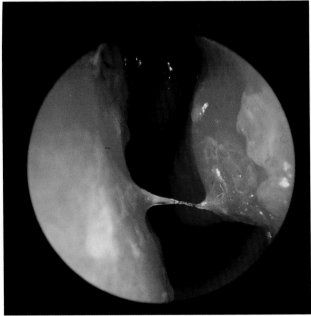

B

FIG. 7. Nasal photographs. **A:** Allergic rhinitis. **B:** Atrophic rhinitis.

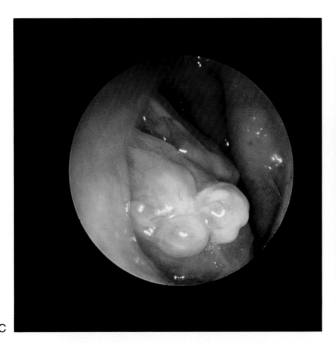

C

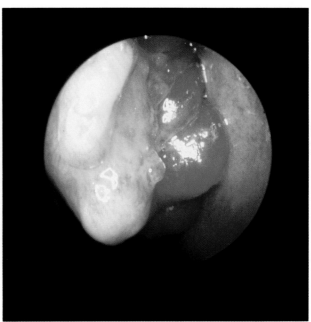

D

FIG. 7. (*Continued.*) **C:** Inverted papilloma. **D:** Reddish looking mass (*white straight arrow*) between the right middle turbinate (*curved white arrow*) and the nasal septum. Biopsy showed an esthesioneuroblastoma which is a malignant neoplasm arising from the olfactory epithelium. (Courtesy of Dr. Michael Hawke, Toronto.)

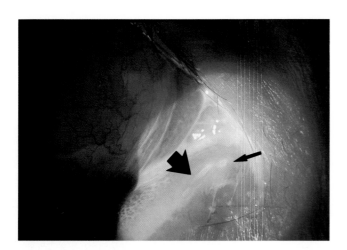

FIG. 8. Fluorescein staining of normal punctum (*large arrow*) connected to gutter in canaliculus. Accessory canalicular opening medial to gutter (*small arrow*).

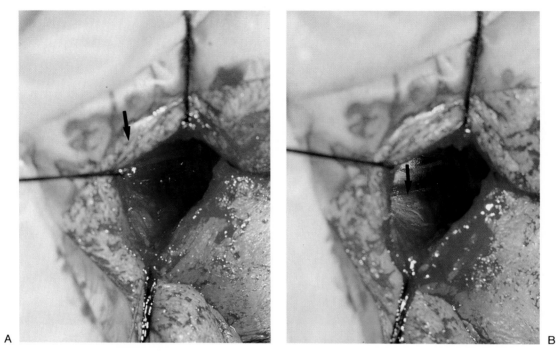

FIG. 9. Indentification of sac lumen. **A:** DCR open and sac exposed. **B:** Healon injected into sac and sac distented.

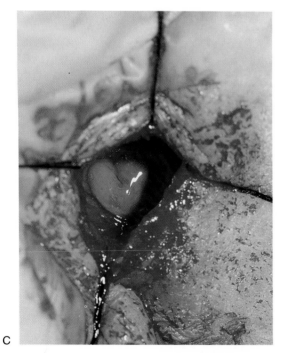

FIG. 9. (*Continued.*) **C:** Sac incised. Healon in lumen liberated.

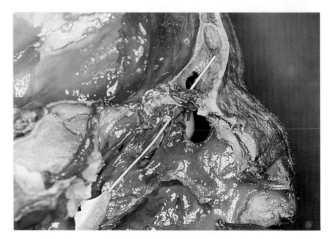

FIG. 10. Relationship of nasofrontal duct (probe) to DCR opening.

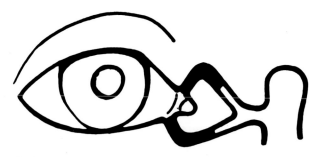

FIG. 9. Lateral obstruction of the upper and lower proximal canaliculi. Marsupialization of the medial residual canaliculi yields a low success rate and Jones' tube procedure is usually indicated. (From Hurwitz, ref. 43, with permission.)

this indeed is the procedure we use. Tubes made from other materials do not drain as well.

It is our feeling that because a Jones tube is a permanent prosthesis, one should try if possible to reconstruct the lacrimal system to permanently create a patent system. It would seem that this would be more advisable than leaving in place a life-long prosthesis such as a Lester Jones' tube, which may result in problems in the short term or the long term (27).

We have attempted to marsupialize patent canaliculi medial to the obstruction (Fig. 9) but have not had much success.

TREATMENT ALTERNATIVES: DISTAL OBSTRUCTION

Bicanalicular Intubation

The passage of bicanalicular tubes employing the method of Crawford (28) will allow for a total intubation of the system with a loop of the tube at the inner canthus and the free ends tied to each other within the nose. It would be necessary in a canalicular obstruction for one to probe the canalicular obstruction and then put in Silastic tubes to prevent reclosure. It would seem that this procedure would be more successful in a patient in whom the canalicular obstruction was intracanalicular as opposed to pericanalicular. Certainly it would seem that if a surgeon is to attempt bicanalicular intubation for an obstruction of the common canaliculus or individual canaliculi, that should the tubes not be able to be passed, the surgeon should be prepared to perform an open canaliculodacryocystorhinostomy operation.

We have managed a few patients with bilateral canalicular obstruction in whom the obstructions were between 5 and 9 mm from the punctum with bicanalicular intubation. Our success rate has been approximately 40% to 50% in these difficult cases. In these situations, we offer the patient the option of bicanalicular intuba-

tion, but we feel bias toward open surgery because our success rate ultimately has been higher.

Canalicular Surgery Similar to the Canaliculodacryocystorhinostomy But Without Opening Into the Nose (29)

The canaliculodacryocystostomy can be performed without opening into the nose and it is felt that this may simplify the procedure somewhat, especially because the sac-duct anastomosis (which sometimes may fail) does not have to be performed. However, we feel that once the sac has been opened laterally, one can probably effect better drainage through a larger DCR opening than through the smaller natural opening of the sac down into the nasolacrimal duct. Intubation of the system with a bicanalicular tube, especially with a larger sleeve around it in these situations where the sac is usually normal size, will help to decrease the possibility of a sac-nasal mucosal closure (30).

Thermal Membranectomies (Laser, Radiosurgery)

Transcanalicular-Yag thermal ablation may be performed on a canalicular membrane and followed by silicone intubation. Although this is still in the experimental stages (31), it would seem that the use of the laser to ablate soft tissue in this situation as opposed to destroying bone in the "laser DCR operation" would be a better potential application for the laser and may hold some promise in treating patients with these difficult obstructions.

As well, an insulated needle on the Ellman surgitron (32) can be used in a similar fashion to the transcanalicular laser in performing thermal membranectomies. These patients would have to be treated with silicone tubes probably for 3 to 6 months as stents. We have performed this procedure in three patients with canalicular obstructions, with obstructions in each canaliculus, between 4 and 6 mm from the punctum. In two of these

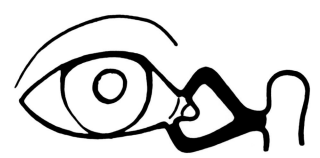

FIG. 10. Total upper and lower canalicular obstruction necessitating Jones' tube insertion. (From Hurwitz, ref. 43, with permission.)

patients we have had long-term patency, and in the other patient there was obstruction shortly after the tube was removed.

Balloon Catheter Dilatation

The concept of dilating a stricture with a balloon catheter is indeed an intriguing one. We would think that just as laser thermal ablation of a soft tissue membrane would be a better use for the laser than attempting to do a full DCR with bone ablation with the laser, so it would also seem to make more sense if a balloon catheter is to be used, to use it to dilate a soft tissue obstruction in a canaliculus where there is no bony structure around it, as opposed to attempting to dilate a nasolacrimal duct obstruction. We are now looking at using the balloon catheter in soft tissue obstructions in the canaliculus, and in failed DCRs as has been described by Becker et al. (33).

TREATMENT ALTERNATIVES: PROXIMAL OBSTRUCTION

Bicanalicular Intubation

If it is possible to probe the obstruction, silicone tubes may be inserted in a bicanalicular fashion.

Thermal Membranectomy

The Yag laser in a transcanalicular fashion, or an Ellman surgitron using radiosurgery techniques, may be used to perforate the membrane and then silicone tube may be used for 3 to 6 months afterward as a stent.

Balloon Dilatation

If the system can be probed, then dilation with a balloon catheter, followed by a 3- to 6-month period of a silicone stent, might play a role in preventing reclosure of the system.

Drainage Tubes

Tubes can be used to drain the inner canthus into the nasolacrimal duct without doing a DCR. Silicone rubber tubes have been devised that sit at the inner canthus and drain directly into the duct (34). However, we prefer, if we are to use a permanent artificial device, to be able to visualize both the ocular and the nasal end of the tube for assessment, and to be able to remove the tube easily (such as one would be able to do with a Jones tube). Therefore, we have not used these tubes.

External Conjunctivorhinostomy

Murube has devised tubes that sit at the inner canthus and pass subcutaneously down into the nose under the inferior turbinate without going into the lacrimal system at all (35). We have not used these tubes and we understand that there can be problems with blockage and displacement of the tubes, and they are not being used as often as they once were (36).

Lacorhinostomy (37)

The conjunctival sac may be drained directly into the nose or may be drained into the lacrimal sac and thereby into the nose. We have not performed this operation and we have always felt that it would be necessary to insert a Jones bypass tube to drain tears via a capillary tube into the nose.

Draining the Conjunctiva into the Antrum (38)

We have drained the conjunctival cul-de-sac down into the maxillary antrum on two occasions, but we have also done antrorhinostomies to allow drainage from the antrum into the nose. One of these procedures remains patent but the other obstructed and was treated ultimately with a Jones tube. We have not found much use for this procedure in our practice.

Vein Grafts

Veins taken from the back of the hand or the foot have been used to line the space between the conjunctival sac and the nose (39). However, we have felt that even though an open system may be present between the conjunctiva and the nose, the lacrimal pump has been circumvented. It is our feeling that it is therefore possible to get better drainage through the patent system by placing a capillary tube such as a Jones tube.

Skin and Mucosa Grafts (40)

Just as with vein grafts, there may be a patent opening from the conjunctiva into the nose, but it has been our feeling that tearing would be improved by inserting a capillary tube (Jones) that would increase the drainage from the conjunctiva into the nose.

SUPPURATIVE CANALICULAR OBSTRUCTION

The patient with a chronic unilateral follicular conjunctivitis should be assessed for having an etiology of

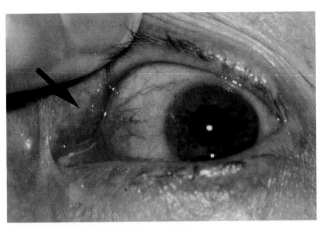

FIG. 11. Patient with upper canaliculitis, pouting punctum, and swelling of canaliculus. (From Demant and Hurwitz, ref. 41, with permission.)

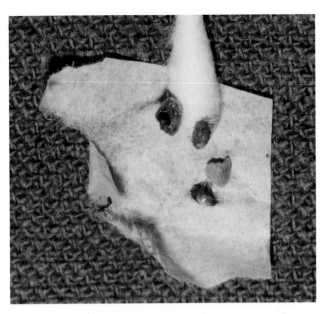

FIG. 13. Sulfur granules from canaliculitis seen on applicator.

canaliculitis. The patient typically presents with a pouting punctum, with discharge coming from the punctum (Figs. 11 and 12). This is even more obvious on expression of the punctum when one milks the canaliculus laterally. There is often point tenderness overlying the canaliculus with a swelling. The affliction may involve one or both canaliculi but is much more commonly unilateral and isolated to one canaliculus. The patient will complain of epiphora but more often will complain of a discharging pussy eye. Only rarely is there an underlying dacryocystitis, and the patient with canaliculitis will not have discharge through each punctum when one presses on the lacrimal sac, unless there is indeed an underlying dacryocystitis.

Etiology

Canalicular obstruction that is suppurative (canaliculitis) is usually caused by actinomycetes (41). In the early literature this was called "streptothrix." *Actinomycetes israeli* is an anaerobic, gram-positive branching filamentous bacterium. It is a normal inhabitant of the human mouth. The infections are characterized by sinus tracks that may suppurate, and often form scarring. The exudate from the sinus tracks contain "sulfur granules" (Fig. 13). These are gram-positive organisms that tend to coalesce and are seen best on Gram stain. Other forms of fungi have been described to cause this condition, such as *Fusobacterium neucleatum* (42). *Aspergillus fumigatus,* nocardia, and other fungi have been described as causes of canalicular obstruction and unilateral kerato-

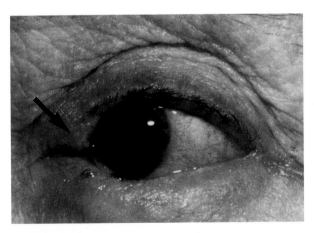

FIG. 12. Patient with upper canaliculitis and secondary irritation causing a spastic entropion. (From Demant and Hurwitz, ref. 41, with permission.)

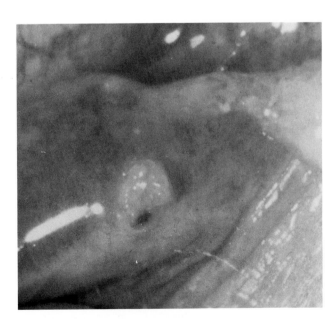

FIG. 14. Patient with canaliculitis and discharge from punctum.

conjunctivitis. Mycotic infections due to sporotrichosis aspergillus, candidiasis, and rhinosporidiosis have also been described.

What is common to all the etiologic agents is that there are saccular dilatations of the involved canaliculus. These may be seen on dacryocystography. The recurring infection causes increased dilatation of the canalicular saccules that predisposes to areas of stagnation and further organism contamination and growth. Secondary overgrowth of bacteria is often observed.

In the early stages there is often a chronic persistent conjunctivitis that may last for a long time. The diagnosis becomes more obvious when one sees the prominent pouting punctum. Once frank infection develops within the saccules of the dilated canaliculi, there is much discharge and the diagnosis becomes more obvious. Syringing of the tear duct may surprisingly reveal patency of the irrigated fluid to the nose. This suggests that the fibrosis process within the canaliculus has not developed to such an extent as to completely occlude the canaliculus. In

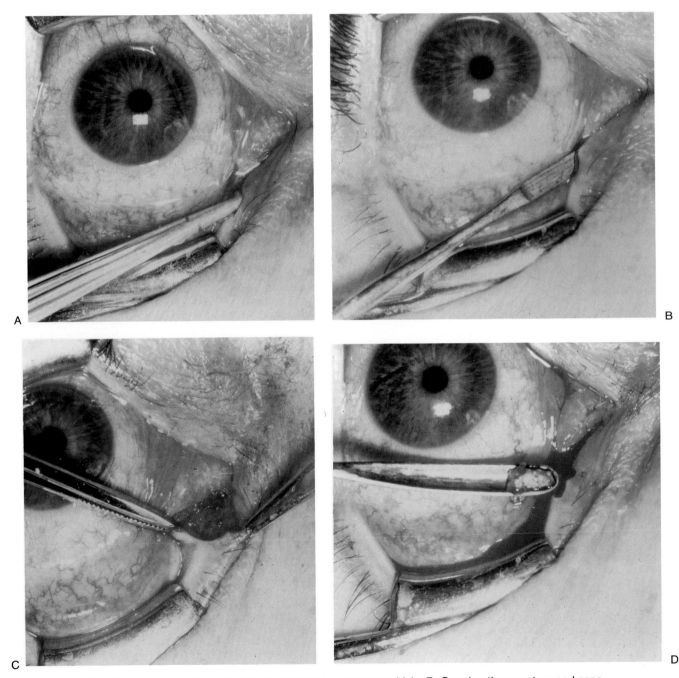

FIG. 15. Treatment of canaliculitis. **A:** Dilating the punctum widely. **B:** Opening the punctum and canaliculus with a canaliculotomy knife. **C:** Exposing widely dilated punctum. **D:** Curetting the stones. (Courtesy of Mr. Richard Welham.)

fact, it is the exception that the canaliculus becomes totally obstructed. On passing of the cannula, one will feel a grittiness as one strikes the sulfur granules that have coalesced into stones within the canaliculus. Diagnosis is verified by expressing stones through the punctum when one grasps the canaliculus with two cotton swabs and milks toward the punctum.

TREATMENT OF SUPPURATIVE CANALICULAR OBSTRUCTION (CANALICULITIS)

Medical Treatment

The mechanical milking of stones and debris out of the canaliculus through the punctum often decreases the symptoms, but is usually not curative.

Actinomyces is usually sensitive to chloramphenicol. This may be used in the form of topical eyedrops and/or ointments. The systemic use of oral penicillin is also helpful. However, there are time limitations for the use of topical chloramphenicol and also systemic penicillin.

Surgical Treatment

Canaliculotomy (Figs. 14 and 15) is the procedure of choice (41). The canaliculus is opened up (approximately 5 mm) and the canaliculus and its saccules curetted. Antibiotics may be injected into the canaliculus. Silver nitrate or iodine can be used in the rare recurrence, should it occur.

The punctal slit will gradually reduce to a normal-sized punctum in a year in most patients.

REFERENCES

1. Dawson CR. Lids, conjunctiva and lacrimal apparatus: eye infections with chlamydia. *Arch Ophthalmol* 1987;93:854.
2. Sandford-Smith JH. Herpes Simplex canalicular obstruction. *Br J Ophthalmol* 1970;54:465.
3. Valieve-Vialeix V, Robain A, Chaput C. Obliterations canaliculaires: etiologie diagnostic, traitement. *Ann Ocul* (Paris) 1961;194:259.
4. Bouzas A. Canalicular inflammation; in ophthalmic cases of Herpes Zoster and Herpes Simplex. *Am J Ophthalmol* 1965;60:713.
5. Bouzas A. Canalicular inflammation. *Br J Ophthalmol* 1973;57: . 849.
6. Jones LT. Conjunctivodacryocystorhinostomy. *Am J Ophthalmol* 1965;59:773.
7. Werb A. In: Rycroft B, ed. *Corneal plastic surgery.* Pergamon Press: London, 1969.
8. Putterman AM. Reconstruction of the absent lacrimal puncta. *Ophthal Surg* 1979;10:30.
9. Hurwitz JJ, Archer KF. Canaliculodacryocystorhinostomy. In: Linberg JV, ed. *Lacrimal surgery.* New York: Churchill Livingstone; 1988.
10. Hurwitz JJ, Howcroft MJ. Use of Lester Jones tubes: a review of 40 cases. *Can J Ophthalmol* 1981;16:176.
11. Veirs ER, Brindley GO. Management of canalicular obstruction. *Adv Ophthal Plast Reconstruct Surg* 1984;3:165.
12. Barishak R, Romano A, Stein R. Obstruction of lacrimal sac caused by topical epinepherine. *Ophthalmologica* 1969;159:373.
13. Auran JD, Hornblass A, Rose ND. Stevens Johnson's syndrome with associated nasolacrimal duct obstruction treated with dacryocystorhinostomy and Crawford silicone tube intubation. *Ophthal Plast Reconstruct Surg* 1990;6:60.
14. Fraunfelder FT, Meyer SM. Ocular toxicity of antineoplastic agents. *Ophthalmology* 1983;90:1.
15. Lovato AA, Char DH, Castro JR, Kroll SM. The effect of silicone nasolacrimal intubation on epiphora after helium ion radiation on corneal melanomas *Am J Ophthalmol* 1989;108:431.
16. Coll NB, Welham RAN. Epiphora after radiation of medial canthal tumours. *Am J Ophthalmol* 1981;92:842.
17. Glatt HJ, Chan AC. Lacrimal obstruction after medial maxillectomy *Ophthal Surg* 1991;22:757.
18. Desmet MD, Buffam SD, Fairey RN, Voss NJS. Prevention of radiation induced stenosis of the nasolacrimal duct. *Can J Ophthalmol* 1990;25:145.
19. Williams R, Ilsar M, Welham RAN. Lacrimal canalicular papillomatosis. *Br J Ophthalmol* 1985;69:464.
20. Garrett AB, Dufresne RG, Ratz JL, Berlin AJ. Basal cell carcinoma originating in the lacrimal canaliculus. *Ophthal Surg* 1993;24:197.
21. Fasanella RM. Common canaliculus or internal common punctum problems with lacrimal sac problems. In: Yamaguchi M, ed. *Recent advances on the lacrimal system.* Japan: Asahi Evening News. 1979;97.
22. Hisatomi C. Preservation of lacrimal drainage after punctum excision. *Orbit* 1990;9:241.
23. Hurwitz JJ. The slit canaliculus. *Ophthal Surg* 1982;13:572.
24. Viers ER. *Lacrimal disorders, diagnosis and treatment.* St. Louis: CV Mosby; 1979;68.
25. Nik NA, Hurwitz JJ, Chin-Sang H. The mechanism of tear flow after DCR and Jones tube surgery. *Arch Ophthalmol* 1984;102:1643.
26. Rutherford S, Hurwitz JJ. A computerized programme for the assessment and documentation of lacrimal patients. *Ophthalmology* 1986;93:14.
27. Rose GE, Welham RAN. Jones' lacrimal canalicular bypass tubes: twenty-five years' experience. *Eye* 1991;5:13.
28. Crawford JS. Intubation of obstruction in the lacrimal system. *Can J Ophthalmol* 1977;12:289.
29. Busse H, Meyer P, Rustenberg HW, Kroll P. Canaliculodacryocystotomy. *Orbit* 1985;4:69.
30. Archer KF, Hurwitz JJ. An alternative method of canalicular stent tube placement in lacrimal drainage surgery. *Ophthal Surg* 1988;19:510.
31. Silkiss RZ. Nd:Yag Nasolacrimal duct recanalization. *Ophthal Surg* 1993;24:772.
32. Hurwitz JJ, Johnson D, Howarth D, Molgat Y. Experimental treatment of eyelashes with high-frequency radio-wave electrosurgery. *Can J Ophthalmol* 1993;28:62.
33. Becker BB, Berry FD. Balloon catheter dilatation in lacrimal surgery. *Ophthal Surg* 1989;20:193.
34. Carroll JM, Beyer CK. Conjunctivodacryocystorhinostomy using silicone rubber lacrimal tubes. *Arch Ophthalmol* 1973;89:113.
35. Murube Del Castillo J. External conjunctivorhinostomy. In: Smith BC, et al. eds. *Ophthalmic Plastic and Reconstructive Surgery*, vol 2. St. Louis, Washington, Toronto: CV Mosby; 1987.
36. Murube del Castillo J. *Personal communications.*
37. Moulie HB. Lacodacryocistorrinostomia en un solo tiempo. *Arch Oftalmol Buenos Aires* 1944;19:466.
38. Bennet JE. Dacryoantrorhinostomy. *Arch Ophthalmol* 1959;62:248.
39. Paufique L, Duran D. Traitment chirurgical du Larmoiement canaliculaire; reflection du canulicule par une greffe veineuse. *Ann Oculist* Paris 1969;202:22.
40. Rycroft BW. Surgery of external rhinostomy operations. *Br J Ophthalmol* 1951;35:328.
41. Demant E, Hurwitz JJ. Canaliculitis—a review of 12 cases. *Can J Ophthalmol* 1980;25:73.
42. Weinberg RJ, Sartoris MJ, Berger GF, Novek JF. Fusobacterium in presumed actinomyces canalicultis. *Am J Ophthalmol* 1977;84:371.
43. Hurwitz JJ. Treatment of canalicular obstructions. *Canad J Ophthal* 1982;17:13.

CHAPTER 24

Diseases of the Punctum

Jeffrey Jay Hurwitz

The punctum lies medial to the most medial of the meibomian gland orifices. The punctum has a papilla, which is a nodular excrescence on the lid margin. The lid margin has a rectangular formation lateral to the punctum and a more triangular formation medial to the punctum. The punctum has a fibrous ring around it that may undergo cicatrization either due to noxious stimuli or potentially as part of the aging process. Epithelium of the skin comes up to the surface of the punctum anteriorly to join the stratified squamous mucosa within the punctum. Similarly, on the posterior aspect of the punctum, the conjunctiva comes up and becomes contiguous with the mucosa from within the punctum. Therefore, the punctum may be subject to diseases that affect both the conjunctiva and the mucosa within the punctum, and also those afflictions of the skin.

STENOSIS OF THE PUNCTUM

Congenital Malformation

Congenital stenosis of the punctum usually is primary due to a congenital malformation (Fig. 1). Two forms of congenital punctal atresia exist:

1. one in which there is imperforation of the punctal opening. In this situation a punctal papilla exists and one may simply, with a #25 needle tip, perforate the punctum and then dilate the punctum to achieve patency. In these situations, there is a papilla that is present and the rest of the canalicular system is normal.
2. absence of the punctum and papilla. In this situation there is no papilla, and the more distal canalicular system is usually obliterated. The eyelid margin medial

J. J. Hurwitz: Oculoplastics Program, Mount Sinai Hospital; and Department of Ophthalmology, University of Toronto Faculty of Medicine, Toronto, Ontario M5S 1A8, Canada.

to where the punctum should be is usually shortened and flat, and this usually suggests that no canalicular tissue medial to the punctum exists (1).

Obstructions Due to Medications

Those medications such as idoxuridine, phospholine iodide, and chemotherapeutic agents such as 5-fluorouracil may cause punctal as well as canalicular obstructions. These have been dealt with in the section under Canalicular Obstructions.

Cicatrizing Diseases of the Conjunctiva

Diseases such as Stevens-Johnson syndrome and ocular pemphigoid may cause punctal obliteration as well as canalicular obstruction. Severe lime burns may cause punctal obstruction as well.

Infections

As was mentioned under Canalicular Obstruction, viruses, bacteria, and certain fungi may occlude the punctum as well as the canaliculus.

Dermatologic Diseases That May Affect the Skin on the Anterior Surface of the Punctum Up to and Including the Mucocutaneous Junction (Fig. 2)

Diseases such as dermatitis, acne rosacea, psoriasis, and any disease that may cause inflammation of the skin may cause keratinization and closure of the punctum. However, more often these conditions cause eversion of the punctum and secondary closure. These conditions are discussed more fully in the section Eyelid Malposition.

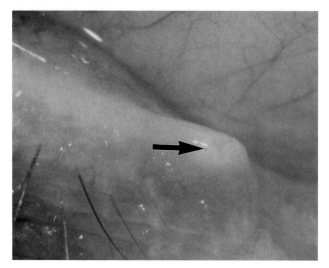

FIG. 1. Patient with congenital absence of lower punctum.

Tumors of the Punctum

Tumors may arise from the conjunctiva involving the wall of the punctum (2). Papillomas may also grow from within the system and involve the mucosa of the lining of the punctum (3) (Fig. 3). These lesions are probably best treated before they grow to a large size. They may be treated by excision and possibly followed up with cryotherapy. The cryotherapy can be a double freeze-thaw cycle to −30°C for 25 seconds.

Nevi around the puncta are extremely common and do not have to be treated (Fig. 4). If there is any change in the color, distribution of the pigment, or any history of growth, the lesion should be biopsied away from the

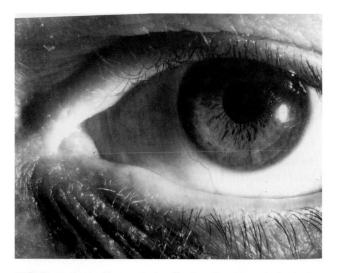

FIG. 2. Patient with psoriasis affecting the skin anterior to the punctum. There is a secondary punctal eversion that has gone on to a stenosis.

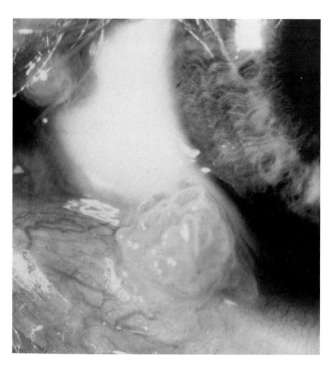

FIG. 3. Papillomatosis involving the puncta. (Courtesy of Mr. R.A.N. Welham.)

mouth of the punctum so as not to damage the opening of the punctum and interfere with tear drainage. It is unusual to have a malignant melanoma in this area, but they do exist (Fig. 4B). If malignancy is detected on biopsy, a large excision with margins should be performed.

Skin tumors such as basal cell carcinomas certainly may arise from the skin of the punctum. These should be biopsied and then treated with excision and frozen section control. We prefer not to use radiation in the treatment of basal cell carcinomas in the area of the lacrimal canaliculi.

Small cysts arising from the sweat glands and glands of Moll are extremely common. If one does not want to interfere with the integrity of the punctum or canaliculus, one can merely do a small incision and drainage with the end of a #25 needle, open up the contents of the cyst, and curette them. We do not use any cautery in the base of the cyst for fear of potentially damaging the integrity of the punctum and/or canaliculus.

Iatrogenic Damage

The punctum may be damaged from surgery or potentially from repeated dilatations. Prevention is the best management. As well, cautery or thermal damage such as that caused by electrolysis or diathermy for removal of lashes may cause punctal damage. Cryotherapy is another potential iatrogenic cause of punctum and canalic-

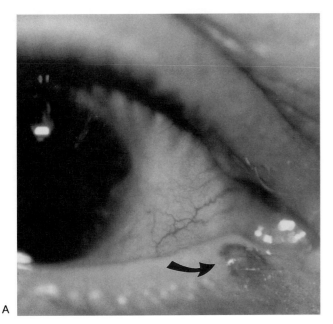 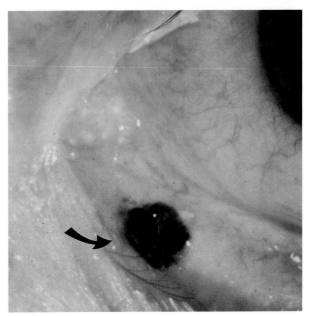

FIG. 4. A: Nevus around the punctum. There is no punctal stenosis and there has been no growth of this lesion for more than 20 years. No treatment is indicated. **B:** Patient with pigmented lesion around punctum. This is a biopsy-proven malignant melanoma. Compare this with the nevus in A.

ular obstruction. The punctum and canaliculi are generally felt to be resistant to damage from freezing at those temperatures that are needed for ablation of the lashes. It has been stated that the punctum and canaliculus probably are not injured until temperatures exceed −70°C (4).

Secondary Punctal Obstruction

Most punctal obstructions are probably due to primary eversion of the punctum where the punctum has been drawn out of the lacrimal lake. The punctum probably needs fluids going through it to keep it open. The fluids also help to prevent keratinization of the walls of the punctum. Certainly when punctal stenosis begins, and symptoms of epiphora commence, the patient will begin to wipe the tears from the eyelid. Unfortunately, this is usually done in a downward and/or horizontal direction, which indeed increases the cicatricial and atonic factors that cause ectropion, leading to further punctal eversion and stenosis. As well, the lysozymes of the tears cause changes in the skin. The excessive tear spillage complicated by the wiping will lead to an acute or chronic dermatitis. These dermatitides may become complicated by secondary bacterial superinfection or allergic contact sensitization. In fact, the chronic tear spillage occasionally may give rise to a mild form of acute eczema, which is called infectious eczematoid dermatitis. This tends to exacerbate the condition (5).

MANAGEMENT OF PUNCTAL STENOSIS

Dilating the Punctum

Incomplete punctal stenosis may be treated by dilating the punctum. We prefer to instill some steroid antibiotic drops twice a day for 3 days following the dilatation as long as one can be sure that the stenosis is not due to herpes simplex. We feel that with repeated dilatations, the fibrous ring around the punctum may be inflamed, which may ultimately lead to a permanent occlusion of the punctum. Therefore, we prefer to dilate the punctum only twice before doing a definitive punctal enlarging procedure.

Controversy has existed as to whether a one-snip, two-snip, or three-snip procedure is the best way of enlargening the punctum. In a one-snip procedure, a single cut along the posterior wall of the punctum on the conjunctival surface toward the ampulla is made. This can be done with a small Vannas scissors and usually just with tetracaine anesthesia. A two-snip procedure utilizes the incision of the one-snip, but a second incision is made from the area of the ampulla horizontal to the lid margin in a medial fashion. This allows more of a funnel to develop along the vertical limb of the canaliculus and on to the horizontal limb (6). Jones and Wobig (6) prefer the two-snip procedure over the three-snip procedure because they feel that compared to the three-snip procedure, where the two arms of the triangle are extended to a full triangle which is excised, the integrity of the ampulla is better maintained with a two-snip procedure. In fact, rather than an incision along the posterior wall, a trough may be produced to open completely the back of the vertical limb of canaliculus, ampulla, and horizontal canaliculus into the lacrimal lake (7).

We prefer to use a Holth punch, which has a 2-mm inner blade and 3-mm outer blade (Fig. 5). Under local anesthesia with 1% xylocaine with epinephrine injected around the punctum, the punctum is widely dilated (Fig. 6), and the punch is inserted into the lower punctum (Fig. 7). When one reaches the ampulla, one elevates the punch slightly and the jaws are closed so that the posterior wall is taken off the punctum and vertical canaliculus without getting into the ampulla and interfering with the important ampullary function in tear drainage. We use a mild steroid antibiotic drop for 3 days after this procedure (if herpes simplex is not present). No suturing is necessary nor is patching. There is negligible bleeding that stops quickly.

Complete Obstruction of the Punctum

Membrane Occlusion

If a punctal papilla exists, at the slit lamp a #25 needle may be used to perforate the membrane and then the

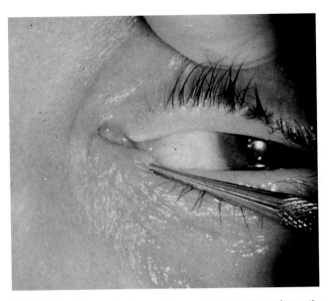

FIG. 6. In the posterior wall punctectomy procedure, the punctum is dilated widely.

punctum dilated with a punctal dilator. This almost always produces long-lasting patency and relief of symptoms.

Complete Occlusion: No Punctum Present

The position of the punctum can sometimes be seen by a small dimple just medial to the last meibomian gland orifice; one may try to insert a #30 needle vertically into the eyelid and then follow with a dilatation. Occasionally even if no papilla seems present, one may be able

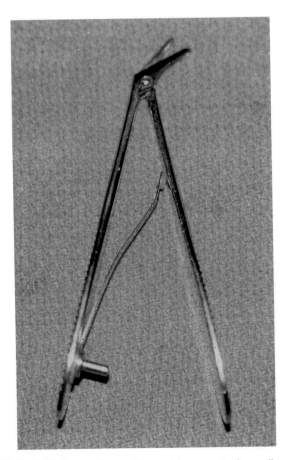

FIG. 5. A Holth punch used for making a posterior wall punctectomy to permanently enlarge a punctum (a form of a three-snip procedure).

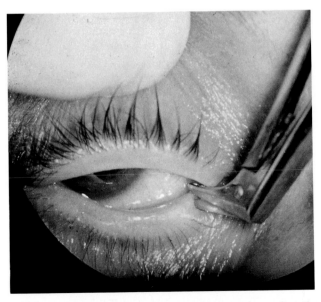

FIG. 7. In the posterior punctectomy procedure after the punctum is widely dilated, the smaller inner blade of the Holth punch is inserted and a punch taken off the back wall of the vertical limb of the canaliculus.

to achieve some patency if indeed the rest of the canalicular system is present. As stated above, more often than not, even with cut-downs of the canaliculus, the distal canaliculus is absent and usually one has to resort to a Lester Jones bypass tube. If one is able to successfully dilate through the punctum, it must be remembered that these patients tend to reobstruct. Therefore, if the procedure is repeated, we prefer to use a monocanalicular stent tube (Eagle vision) and leave the stent in place hopefully for 6 weeks. These stents are like punctal plugs and tend to grasp on to the punctum. However, if there is any mobility of the stent, we prefer to use an 8-0 polypropylene suture, which is placed through the plug onto the edge of the punctum.

Secondary Punctal Obstruction

The secondary punctal obstructions are usually secondary to eversion of the punctum with a medial ectropion. We treat these patients with a bland ointment and have them massage the lid in an upward direction to try and get the punctum back into the lacrimal lake. If there is a lot of dermatitis we use a steroid eye ointment for a short period of time. The punctum is dilated widely. Usually if the lid can be reposited so that punctum is in the lacrimal lake, tears will flow through the punctum that has been dilated. Procedures that can reposit the punctum into the lake will be discussed in the section under Eyelid Malposition.

Occasionally the upper lid may droop down so low that the upper lid obstructs the lacrimal punctum and causes obstruction of the punctum (8). This temporary cause can be treated by ptosis surgery.

Occasionally the conjunctiva may become redundant and folds may rest in front of the punctum so that tears may not get into the punctum (9). Although one can excise the redundant conjunctiva, we are concerned that there is the possibility of causing some restriction of motility of the eye because of conjunctival scarring. We prefer to use a bipolar diathermy and place the redundant conjunctiva within the arms of the instrument and then shrink the tissue with cauterization. Fluorescein dropped on the lid should be able to be seen to enter the punctum after this procedure, thereby suggesting a cure.

SLIT PUNCTUM AND CANALICULUS (FIG. 8)

A punctal slit can be congenital or acquired. The acquired slit is usually iatrogenic because of a three-snip or

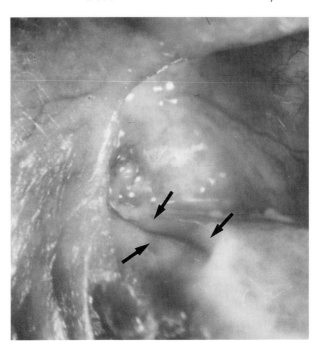

FIG. 8. A slit canaliculus secondary to a Crawford tube insertion with a DCR. The DCR is patent. There is no epiphora.

because of a canalicular tube. Treatment is usually not necessary.

REFERENCES

1. Welham RAN, Hughes SM. The results of paediatric lacrimal surgery. In: Bosniak SL, Smith BC, eds. *Advances in ophthalmic plastic and reconstructive surgery, vol 3, lacrimal system.* New York: Pergamon Press; 1984.
2. Miller DM, Brodell RT, Levine MR. The conjunctival wart: report of a case and review of treatment options. *Ophthal Surg* 1994;25: 545.
3. Karcioglu ZA, Caldwell DR, Reed HT. Papillomas of lacrimal drainage system: a clinical pathological study. *Ophthal Surg* 1984;15:670.
4. Wingfield DL, Fraunfelder FT. Possible complications secondary to cryosurgery. *Ophthal Surg* 1979;10:47.
5. Novick NL. Cutaneous complications of epiphora. In: Bosniak SL, Smith BC, eds. *Advances in ophthalmic plastic and reconstructive surgery.* Pergamon Press; 1984.
6. Jones LT, Wobig J. *Surgery of the eyelids and lacrimal system.* Birmingham, AL: Aesculapius; 1976.
7. Mindlin AM, Nesi SA. Punctoplasty an alternative technique—the trough procedure. In: Bosniak SL, Smith BC, eds. *Advances in ophthalmic plastic and reconstructive surgery*, vol 3. New York: Pergamon Press; 1984.
8. Glatt H. Epiphora caused by blepharoptosis. *Am J Ophthalmol* 1991;110:649.
9. Liu D. Conjunctivochalasis a cause of tearing and its management. *Ophthal Plast Reconstruct Surg* 1986;2:25.

CHAPTER 25

Eyelid Malpositions

Jeffrey Jay Hurwitz and Cary Hurwitz

Lower eyelid malpositions may produce tearing in two ways:

1. Ectropion. A medial ectropion will cause eversion of the punctum leading to secondary punctal stenosis and epiphora. Eyelid laxity with weak orbicularis function and an elongated lower eyelid will lead to a "lacrimal pump dysfunction" (1), and this may lead to tearing with or without frank ectropion.
2. Irritation of the eye due to trichiasis and lashes hitting on the conjunctiva and/or cornea due to trichiasis, distichiasis, or frank entropion.

A. Ectropion

Medial Ectropion

The punctum may be dragged out of the lacrimal lake (Fig. 1) for a number of reasons:

1. *Atonic changes in the lid:* A minimal eversion of the medial eyelid will often lead to secondary stenosis of the punctum and this will cause the patient to wipe the eyelid and pull the punctum away from the lacrimal lake. This will be complicated by dermatitis and lid changes as mentioned in the previous chapter.
2. *Eyelid inflammation:* Inflammations of the skin such as dermatitis, rosacea, psoriasis, etc. will cause a vertical cicatricial contracture and pull the eyelid away from the globe (Fig. 2).
3. *Mechanical:* Tumors of the cheek and lower lid will pull the lid away from the globe. This also occurs with an atonic lower face and facial palsy.
4. *Iatrogenic:* Surgery in the lower lid (especially cosmetic blepharoplasty) may cause a vertical contracture in the skin of the lower lid. This may occur when an excessive amount of skin has been removed at the time of blepharoplasty. However, it may also be due to scarring between the capsulopalpebral fascia and the septum, or indeed between the capusolopalpebral fascia, septum, and periosteum. It may also occur because of hemorrhage and/or infection in the lid.

Management of Medial Ectropion

Why does punctal eversion cause tearing? It would seem that the epiphora is due to two main causes: (a) there is no flow through the lower punctum and canaliculus, and (b) probably more importantly, the lids on closure do not meet. Therefore, with the lower punctum being everted, there is also no flow through the upper punctum because of the loss of the suctioning effect. If the surgeon is to put the lower lid back into the proper position, epiphora might decrease even if the lower punctum is not open because the suctioning effect may be increased through the upper canaliculus and indeed the upper canaliculus may carry the tears. It is important that the surgeon should also check the integrity of the upper punctum and canaliculus when the lower everted punctum is being put back in position. If the upper canaliculus is found to be closed, the patient may still be rendered tear-free if the lower punctum and eyelid is fixed. However, it is advisable to open up the upper can-

J. J. Hurwitz: Oculoplastics Program, Mount Sinai Hospital; and Department of Ophthalmology, University of Toronto Faculty of Medicine, Toronto, Ontario M5S 1A8, Canada.

C. Hurwitz: Mount Sinai Hospital, Toronto, Ontario, M5G 1X5, Canada.

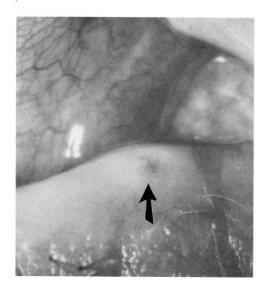

FIG. 1. Medial ectropion with secondary punctal stenosis.

aliculus as well, in the off chance that the lower punctum and canalicular dilatation and repositioning does not work.

Nonsurgical Management.. The patients must be taught to massage their lids in an upward direction and to wipe their eyes in an upward direction to try and offset the tendency toward ectropion. This alone may reposit the punctum in the lacrimal lake and if tears are going through the punctum, the punctum will usually stay open and symptoms of tearing will be less. In approximately 50% of patients with punctal eversion and epiphora, we have found that massage helps the patients significantly so that they will not request surgery at a later date. If dermatitis changes occur in the skin, it is useful to use a steroid ointment with the massage for a short period of time. However, the patients must be reminded that they must not use steroids over the long term because the skin may thin somewhat, and there are of course the risks of cataracts and glaucoma.

Retropunctal cautery may be useful in treating punctal eversion (Fig. 3). A double row of cautery is placed under the punctum on the conjunctival surface. We prefer to use the Ellman surgitron single needle, which has little lateral heat spread. Presumably scarring will occur between the two vertical rows of cautery and cause the punctum to invert. It is important that the cautery must extend lateral to the punctum as well. This will perhaps also allow for some horizontal shortening. It is also important that the tip of the cautery must be placed through the conjunctiva to the subconjunctival tissues to allow enough fibrosis to invert the punctum. The maximum effect is to be expected in 6 weeks (2).

Surgical Management of Punctal Eversion (see Fig. 9). We prefer to take a tarsal conjunctival spindle from inside the punctum. A drop of tetracaine is placed on the conjunctiva surface and then 2% xylocaine with epinephrine is injected using a #30 needle under the conjunctiva. The anesthetic is flattened with a cotton applicator. A diamond-shaped spindle is taken below and on each side of the punctum inferior to the canaliculus. The resected part measures approximately 5 mm in width and 10 mm in length. The resection should begin approximately 4 mm inferior to the punctum and the long axis should be kept horizontal. We do not insert a lacrimal probe while we are doing this, but it certainly does no harm. We suture the defect using two or three 6-0 plain gut sutures with the knots deep within the tissues

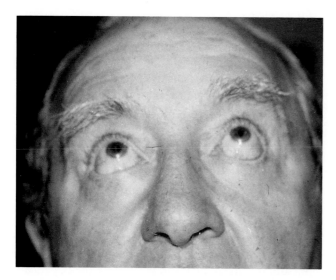

FIG. 2. Patient with cicatricial lower lid ectropion accentuated by opening of the mouth, looking up and putting the skin on the stretch.

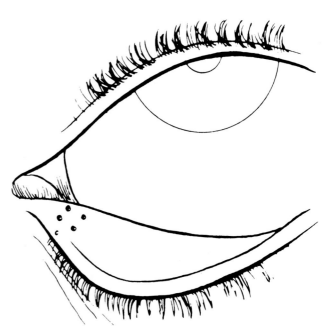

FIG. 3. Double row of retropunctal cautery to treat a punctal eversion.

so that no knots will irritate the cornea. The larger the incision vertically, the more inversion to be expected (3). The sutures may be taken in a mattress through the whole of the lid and tied externally. We prefer not to take the sutures through the lid for fear of violating the anterior lamella and producing a cicatricial change in the anterior lamella, which may evert the punctum.

If there exists with the punctal eversion a laxity of the medial canthal tendon as well, one may perform a medial canthal tendon plication, as well as a punctal inversion. There are many modifications of the procedure such as the "lazy T" operation that Byron Smith described (4), a direct operation on Horner's muscle (5), and a conjunctival approach whereby horizontal sutures are placed to fixate the punctum horizontally, and vertical sutures are placed to fixate the punctum vertically (6).

MANAGEMENT OF EYELID LAXITY (LACRIMAL PUMP DYSFUNCTION)

In this situation, the orbicularis muscle may become lax, the lateral canthal tendon and often the medial canthal tendon will become lax and stretch, and perhaps the tarsus may undergo changes where it may become lengthened. All these conditions tend to decrease the apposition of the eyelid to the globe and decrease the pumping function of the lids to move the tears from the lateral canthus to the medial canthal lacrimal lake. The same cicatricial changes that may develop from the irritation of the tears on the skin, worsened by wiping the lid in a downward direction, will exacerbate the condition.

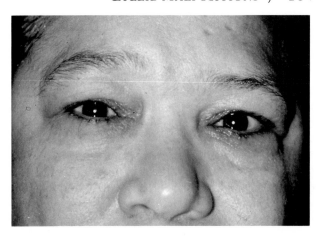

FIG. 5. Patient with tearing and facial palsy on the left side. (From Hurwitz et al., ref. 11, with permission.)

As well, horizontal wiping of the lid tends to stretch out the orbicularis even more and perhaps decreases pumping function. There is clinically a poor snap-back of the lid onto the globe when the lid is horizontally distracted from the globe (Fig. 4). As well, if the patient is asked to look in an upward direction and the lid is pulled inferiorly, the lid does not snap back against the globe. These changes suggest a lax lid and a potential lacrimal pump dysfunction. These changes may be corroborated if necessary with lacrimal scintillography (7). Patients with suspected eyelid laxity must be checked closely for signs of facial nerve paresis. Examination of the mouth and forehead will give clues to a facial palsy and/or aberrant regeneration of the facial nerve. The management of this condition will be discussed in Chapter 26 (Figs. 5 and 6).

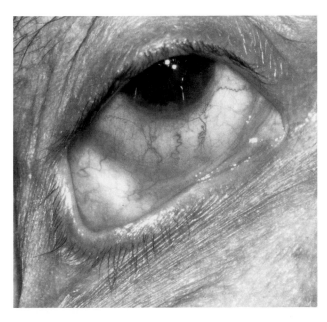

FIG. 4. Demonstrating the test for eyelid laxity in a patient with ectropion and tearing due to lacrimal pump dysfunction. (From Hurwitz et al., ref. 11, with permission.)

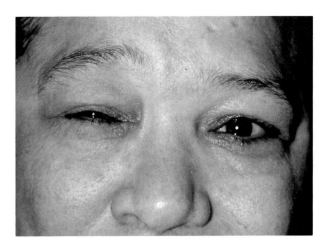

FIG. 6. Patient in Fig. 5; when this patient closes the eyes, there is incomplete closure of the left eye and aberrant regeneration of the facial nerve. Notice the exaggerated movement on the right side of the face. (From Hurwitz et al., ref. 11, with permission.)

Treatment of Eyelid Laxity

Lateral Canthal Tendon Tightening

If the punctum is situated in the lacrimal lake and there is definite eyelid laxity, one must make sure that if the lateral canthal tendon is tightened, that the punctum will not be distracted laterally out of the lacrimal lake. In most cases of lacrimal pump dysfunction with eyelid laxity and not frank ectropion, the medial canthal tendon is not significantly lax. If the medial canthal tendon is lax, frank ectropion usually develops. Pathologic studies that we have performed on tarsal tissue have shown that there is some change in the stromal matrix of the collagen fibrils with disorientation, and that indeed some tarsal lengthening can occur. However, more significantly, the lateral canthal tendon stretches. Some surgeons have addressed the lateral canthal tendon laxity by tightening up the lateral canthal tendon (8,9). However, we prefer to resect a full thickness triangle of lid laterally, encompassing both the lateral canthal tendon and some of the tarsus. This is referred to as to the Bick procedure (10). However, in 1966 when Bick described the procedure, because there was not the selection of sutures that we have available today, some of the resected eyelids would open up and there would be significant complications from this procedure. We have modified this operation, and we have found the results to be gratifying (11). This procedure has the advantage of resecting some orbicularis muscle with the concept that by shortening the muscle one would increase the strength of contraction of the muscle, and therefore aid in alleviating the "lacrimal pump dysfunction."

Modified Bick Procedure (Fig. 7)

Two percent xylocaine with epinephrine is injected into the lower lid laterally. A full thickness is resected. Hemostasis is secured with bipolar cautery. A 3-0 Dexon (Davis and Geck) suture is used to anchor the cut edge of tarsus to the lateral orbital tubercle located 2 mm inside the lateral orbital rim. This fixates the tarsus directly to the periosteum inside the lateral orbital rim to give good lid-globe apposition. We feel that it is not necessary to dissect out a piece of tarsus to give good fixation. Occasionally there may be a slight granuloma from the suture, but this has not been a problem in our hands. We also feel that a nonabsorbable suture is not necessary because the 3-0 Dexon seems to stay in place long enough to allow the healing process to occur; it is rare for the lid to open up following the surgery because of suture absorption. Then a 5-0 Dexon suture is placed at the lateral canthus with the knot tied laterally in the soft tissues between the upper and lower lids. The suture enters 2 mm inside the upper and lower lids at the gray line and is tied

to recreate an angle. A 5-0 Dexon suture is then used to reapproximate the pretarsal orbicularis and a 5-0 Dexon suture is used to tighten the preseptal orbicularis. These muscle-tightening sutures presumably help to shorten the muscle and increase pump function. The skin is sutured with 4-0 silk or nylon. The sutures are removed in 1 week. Postoperatively, some antibiotic ointment is placed on the sutures and the scarring usually blends in with the lateral canthal angle lines within 6 to 12 weeks. It is most important that the patients preoperatively are told that they must never wipe their eyes in a downward or sideways direction because if they were in this habit, they may increase the tendency to ectropion and lid laxity postoperatively.

Potential Complications

1. *Opening up of the wound.* We have found in the few cases in which the lid does open up, that it is not necessary to resuture the lid. In fact, resuturing seems to cause more trauma and tissue necrosis. We treat these patients with antibiotic ointments into the defect and an eye shield at night. Usually within a few weeks the defect will close and in fact the lid pump function will improve.

2. *Granuloma formation of the suture.* Pyogenic granulomas may occur around the sutures. The sutures may be snipped away no earlier than 3 weeks postoperatively and usually the pyogenic granulomas can be snipped away at the same time if this is a problem. The pyogenic granulomas bleed, but we have not had to cauterize one and we treat this with pressure for a few minutes after the excision.

3. *Unsightly scar.* It is unusual to have an unsightly scar from this procedure if one places the upper arm of the triangle in line with the natural flow of the upper lid laterally.

4. *Operation unsuccessful.* We inform patients that at least 50% of the patients in whom we are doing this procedure to treat a lacrimal pump dysfunction will be significantly improved of their tearing. We tell them as well that there will be some patients who will notice only a small improvement and some who will indeed have little improvement. In fact, some of the patients who have had little or no improvement from the procedure still seem to have some eyelid laxity postoperatively and either a repeat Bick procedure was performed or some medial canthal tendon tightening was performed as well.

Medial Canthal Tendon Tightening

If laxity of the medial canthal tendon exists, one prefers to perform the medial canthal procedure first and then determine on the table whether a lateral canthal tightening has to be done at the same time, or to wait for some months postoperatively and perhaps perform a

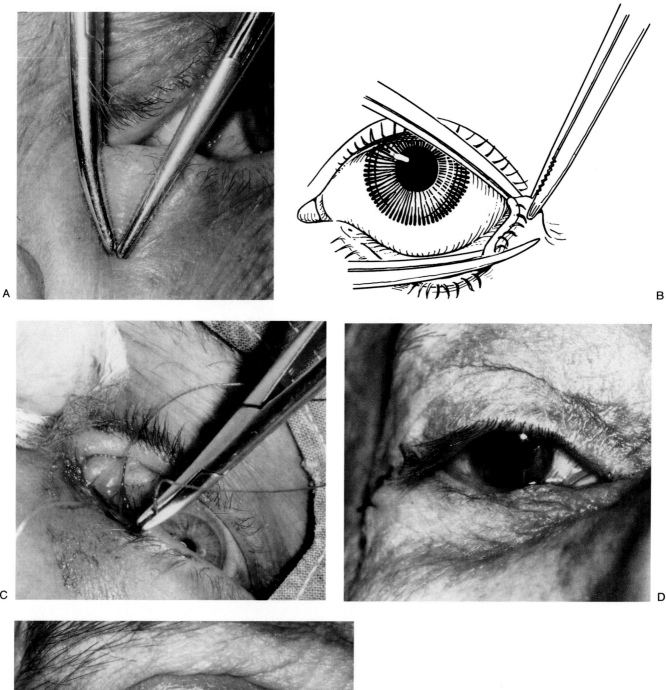

A

B

C

D

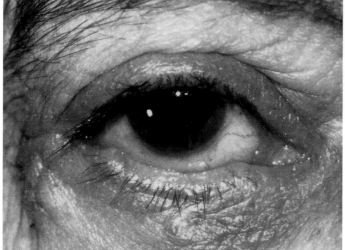

E

FIG. 7. A: Lacrimal pump tightening (Bick procedure). Artery forceps are placed on the lid in a triangular fashion to outline the lid to be excised. B: The full thickness triangle is excised laterally. C: A 3-0 Dexon suture is used to tighten the cut edge of the tarsus to the lateral orbital tubercle. The angle of the lid is then recreated using a 5-0 Dexon suture. D: After the orbicularis is sutured with 5-0 Dexon sutures to tighten the muscle, the skin is sutured using 4-0 black silk. Good apposition between the lid and the globe is observable. E: The patient 1 month after surgery. The scar has faded. (From Hurwitz et al., ref. 11, with permission.)

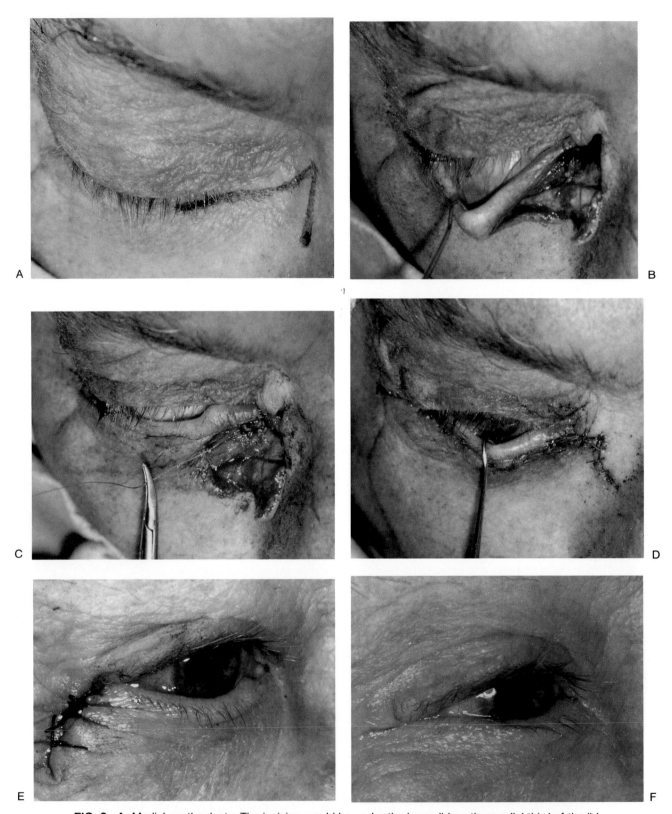

FIG. 8. A: Medial canthoplasty. The incision would be under the lower lid on the medial third of the lid and then down along the side of the nose. **B:** An incision is made to open up the flap, based inferolaterally. The laxity of the lid can be seen. **C:** After the suture has been placed from the medial tarsus burrowing subcutaneously through the orbicularis to the anterior limb of the medial canthal tendon, and then burrowing back to the tarsus where it is tied, the lid can be seen to be tighter. **D:** After the extra skin has been excised and skin sutured, the tightness of the lid can be seen. **E:** Another patient with a medial canthoplasty and a lateral Bick procedure. **F:** The patient in E 1 month after the sutures have been removed. The scars are fading nicely.

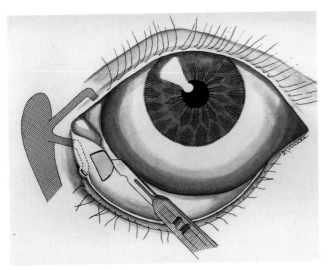

FIG. 9. The diamond-shaped excision beneath the punctum to invert the punctum. We prefer to use 6-0 plain gut sutures, but we prefer to bury the knots deep within the subconjunctival tissues rather than leaving the knots exposed. (Courtesy Drs. S. Tucker and J. Hurwitz, Toronto, Ontario, Canada.)

lateral canthal tendon tightening at a later date. One must ensure that any procedure done to tighten the lid horizontally is performed medial to the punctum. Ideally, the posterior limb of the medial canthal tendon should be tightened, but this indeed may be difficult for fear of damaging the lacrimal system. We might attempt this only in conjunction with a dacryocystorhinostomy (DCR) but indeed we have abandoned this procedure for another procedure that we feel in our hands gives a better success rate. We have also attempted to incise the periosteum medially and reflect it laterally to use the periosteum as flaps (12). However, we have found that the periosteum is often extremely dehiscent medially, and we

have had difficulty making flaps. As well, we have preferred not to resect the canaliculus and do a canalicular repair or perform a canaliculostomy for a medial ectropion, even if a facial nerve palsy is the cause of the ectropion (13).

Technique (Fig. 8)

Two percent xylocaine with epinephrine is injected under the skin of the lower lid and the side of the nose. This procedure is performed under local anesthesia and one may occasionally use some intravenous sedation. An incision is made starting in the medial one third of the lower lid in the crease and proceeding superonasally to the side of the nose. Then the incision is directed vertically in an inferior direction as one would for a DCR. The triangular skin flap is dissected inferiorly. A 5-0 Dexon (Davis and Geck) suture on a CE 23 needle is used and the suture starts along the tarsal plate inferior to the punctum and canaliculus. Two deep bites are taken of the subcutaneous tissues along the inferior aspect of the medial canthal tendon and orbicularis as the needle moves in a superomedial direction. Then another bite is taken at the anterior lacrimal crest whereby the needle is turned inferolaterally and passed toward the tarsus, with two deep bites being taken again in the deeper tissues and then another final bite in the tarsus. This forms a mattress suture and, when the suture is tied, the punctum may be seen to move medially. Because of the deeper bites, the punctum is not pulled anteriorly and out of the lacrimal lake but slides along the surface of the lacrimal lake to stay in position. This suture then can be tied and the skin flap redraped. Often some of the superior and/or nasal aspect of the skin flap needs to be excised. A deep 5-0 Dexon suture is placed under the flap to the

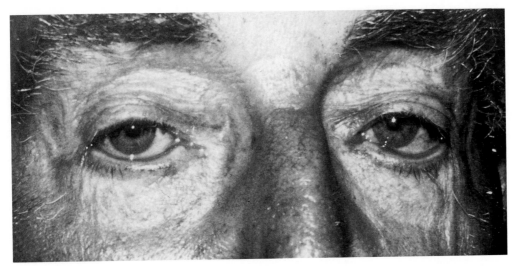

FIG. 10. Patient with cicatricial changes in the lower lid with punctal eversion. (From Hurwitz et al., ref. 11, with permission.)

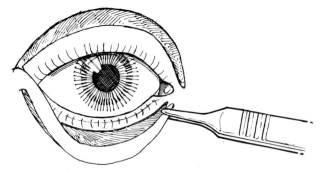

FIG. 11. Rotational flap from upper lid to lower in a cicatricial ectropion with flap based laterally. (From Hurwitz et al., ref. 11, with permission.)

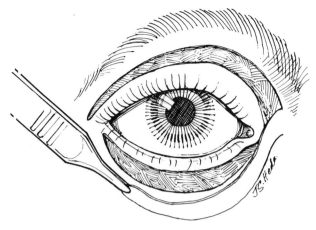

FIG. 12. Rotational flap from upper lid to lower lid in patient with cicatricial ectropion with flap based medially. (From Hurwitz et al., ref. 11, with permission.)

deeper tissue to prevent an anterior migration of the flap or webbing, and allow the recess of the medial canthus to be maintained. The skin is sutured with 6-0 nylon sutures. Then the lateral canthus can be assessed to see if a lid tightening is also needed. We have found this procedure to be helpful in repositing the punctum in the lacrimal lake. If the punctum is also vertically migrated anteriorly out of the lacrimal lake, the diamond wedge excision that has been previously described can be performed as well (Fig. 9).

Cicatricial Changes in the Lower Lid

To improve lid-globe apposition if there are cicatricial changes in the lower lid, massage over a period of time will often help. If it does not, and the skin is tight, then surgery can be performed on the skin. We have found that the usual cause of tautness of the skin vertically is following surgery (such as blepharoplasty or excessive re-

moval of xanthelasma) or dermatitic skin changes. (Fig. 10). Surgery is best performed under local anesthesia so the patient can be asked to open and close the eyes and the lid-globe apposition can be best achieved. A subciliary incision is made, and the skin is dissected from the muscle inferiorly toward the orbital rim. Then with the patient opening his mouth and looking upward, the amount of skin deficit can be ascertained. It is often found at this time that there is still some contraction and it may be necessary to do some deeper dissection to relieve some scarring at the level of the capsulopalpebral fascia. It is often found that once the skin is released, the lid indeed is horizontally lax and we need to perform a modified Bick procedure at the same time. Skin can be rotated from the upper lid laterally (14) (Fig. 11) or medially (15) (Figs. 12 and 13). However, if there is not

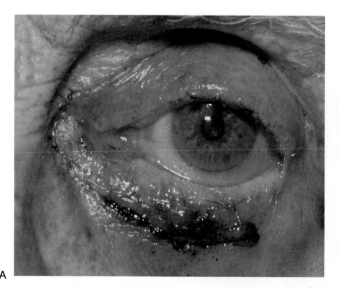

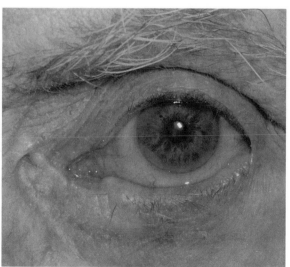

FIG. 13. A: Patient having had upper lid rotation flap based medially in a condition of cicatricial lower lid ectropion 1 week after the surgery when sutures are removed. **B:** Same patient 6 weeks after sutures are removed. The flap has taken well and is only barely visible. (From Hurwitz et al., ref. 11, with permission.)

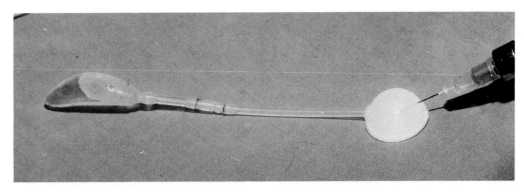

FIG. 14. Specially made tissue expander with reservoir (Heyer-Schulte). The cigar-shaped expander fits in a pocket between the skin and orbicularis muscle to stretch the skin. Saline is injected into the reservoir to blow up the balloon. (From Hurwitz, ref. 19, with permission.)

enough excess skin in the upper lid we prefer to use a retroauricullar skin graft. The skin can be harvested from behind the ear. We prefer to inject 2% xylocaine with epinephrine behind the ear and take approximately one half of the graft from the ear itself and one half of the graft from the scalp. This graft can be taken as thick or thin as desired, but in a skin deficiency the graft should be very thin. We close the donor site with deep 3-0 Dexon and supeficially with running 5-0 Dexon sutures. The graft can be trimmed and put into place. We prefer to hold the graft in place for a few days with a tight pressure bandage. It is also important to put deep sutures between the undersurface of the graft and the orbicularis to hold the graft in place. We often place a double-armed Dexon suture through the conjunctiva coming out at the lower border of tarsus and tied over the anterior surface of the graft to hold the graft tightly against the eyelid. We treat the patient with hot compresses for 2 weeks following this procedure. It is unusual to have a graft failure.

If possible, we prefer to use flaps from the upper lid to the lower lid because the flaps do tend to give some elevation of the lower lid either at the lateral canthus if the flap is based laterally, or more importantly at the medial canthus with punctal elevation if the flap is based medially. However, for large defects the skin of the upper lid is not as thick as the retroauricular skin and we prefer to use a retroauricular graft. In the lower lid with its rich vascular supply, failure of the grafts is rare and there is no real need (other than mechanical) to use an upper lid flap rather than a graft.

Tissue Expansion

If one does not want to operate on the lids one can insert a tissue expander at the lateral canthus into the lower lid subcutaneous pocket (Fig. 14). This can expand the eyelid skin if left in place for approximately 6 weeks (16). However, we prefer if possible a skin flap or graft to

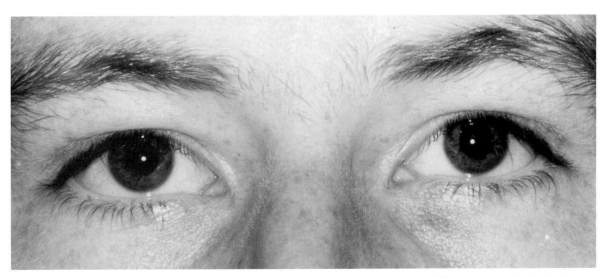

FIG. 15. Patient with tearing of both eyes due to anteriorly placed puncta with respect to the lacrimal lake (Centurion syndrome). Note the prominent bridge of the nose and a short interpalpebral distance.

treat the lower lid ectropion rather than using the specially designed tissue expanders.

Lid Surgery in Conjunction with DCR

Many patients with blocked tear ducts who need lacrimal surgery are also found to have eyelid malposition presumably due to the prolonged wiping of the eyes. There is no reason why a lid procedure cannot be done at the same time as a DCR, CDCR, or Jones tube procedure (17).

Punctal Malposition with Respect to the Lacrimal Lake (Centurion Syndrome)

Certain patients are born with a congenital defect whereby the punctum is anterior to the lacrimal lake (Fig. 15). These patients may have abnormalities of their nasal bridges (18), and we have found some of our patients to have a short interpalpebral distance. Sullivan et al. were able to help some of these patients by lysing the anterior limb of the medial canthal tendon to allow the punctum to migrate posteriorly into the lacrimal lake. A posterior wall punctectomy with a Holth punch may also be attempted.

REFERENCES

1. Doane MG. Blinking and tear drainage. In: Bosniak SL, Smith BC, eds. *Advances in Ophthalmic Plastic and Reconstructive Surgery*, vol 3. New York: Pergamon Press; 1984.
2. Jones BR. Cautery to treat epiphora from punctal eversion. *Trans Ophthal Soc UK* 1973;93:597.
3. Jones LT, Wobig JL. Surgery of the eyelids and lacrimal system. Birmingham AL: Aesculapius; 1976.
4. Smith B. "Lazy T" operation for the correcton of ectropion. *Arch Ophthalmol* 1976;90:1149.
5. Ritleng T. Medial canthoplasty for recurrent lacrimal ectropions. *Orbit* 1998;8:43.
6. Hurwitz JJ, Tucker S. Posterior horizontal and vertical tightening to treat combined punctal ectropion with medial canthal tendon and laxity. *Ophthal Surg* 1990;21:721.
7. Doucet TW, Hurwitz JJ, Chin-Sang H. Lacrimal scintillography: advances and functional applications. *Surv Ophthalmol* 1982;27: 105.
8. Tenzel RR, Buffam FC, Miller GR. The use of "lateral canthal sling" in ectropion repair. *Can J Ophthalmol* 1977;12:199.
9. Anderson RL, Gordy DD. The tarsal strip procedure. *Arch Ophthalmol* 1979;97:2192.
10. Bick MW. Surgical management of orbital tarsal disparity. *Arch Ophthalmol* 1966;75:386.
11. Hurwitz JJ, Mishkin SK, Rodgers KJA. Modification of Bick's procedure for treatment of eyelid laxity. *Can J Ophthalmol* 1987;22:262.
12. Edelstein JP, Dryden RM. Medial palpebral tendon repair for medial ectropion of the lower lid. *Ophthal Plast Reconstruct Surg* 1990;6:27.
13. McCord CD. Canalicular resection and reconstruction by canaliculostomy. *Ophthal Surg* 1980;11:440.
14. Hurwitz JJ, Lichter M, Rodgers J. Cicatricial ectropion due to essential skin shrinkage: treatment with rotational upper lid pedicle flaps. *Can J Ophthalmol* 1983;18:269.
15. Anderson RL, Hatt MU, Dixon R. Medial ectropion a new technique. *Arch Ophthalmol* 1979;97:521.
16. Victor WH, Hurwitz JJ. Cicatricial ectropion following blepharoplasty: treatment by tissue expansion. *Can J Ophthalmol* 1984;19: 317.
17. Hurwitz JJ. Investigation and treatment of epiphora due to lid laxity. *Trans Ophthal Soc UK* 1978;98:69.
18. Sullivan TJ, Welham RAN, Collin JRO. Centurion syndrome Idiopathic anterior displacement of the medial canthus. *Ophthalmology* 1993;100:328.

B. Tearing Due to Trichiasis and Entropion

Lashes may irritate the cornea and thereby the trigeminal nerve to cause increased tearing. Whereas the abnormal lashes do not of themselves cause a lacrimal obstruction, the lashes must be treated to help with the patient's symptoms.

Trichiasis

Abnormal lashes are often the result of chronic eyelid inflammation, or cicatrizing diseases. The lashes tend to grow from their normal roots but in a misdirected fashion.

Treatment of Trichiasis

Epilation

Repeated epilation may be performed but this is often a nuisance for the patient. Many of these patients are quite presbyopic and it is difficult for them or their spouses to pull the lashes.

Hyfercation

Burning of the lash with diathermy whereby the root of the follicle is excised is an effective way of removing the offending eyelash. We prefer to use the Ellman surgitron, which produces the least amount of lateral heat spread because of the nature of its high frequency radio waves (1). This minimizes lid damage. However, there is some question as to whether cicatrizing conditions such as ocular pemphigoid can be exacerbated by any form of cautery or diathermy.

Cryotherapy

Aberrant eyelid lashes may be removed with cryotherapy to a temperature of -20°C for 20 seconds in the lower

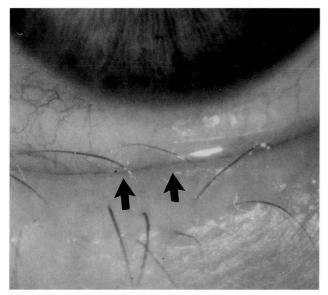

FIG. 16. Patient with congenital distichiasis. Notice the abnormal lashes coming from the meibomian gland orifices.

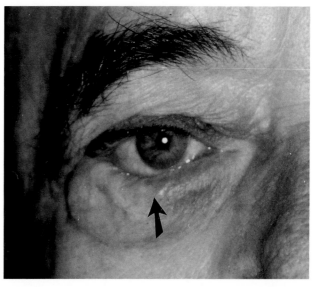

FIG. 17. Patient with entropion and trichiasis. There is lid laxity. The patient was cured with a modified Bick procedure.

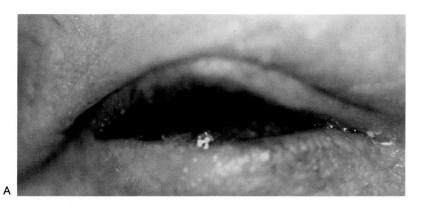

A

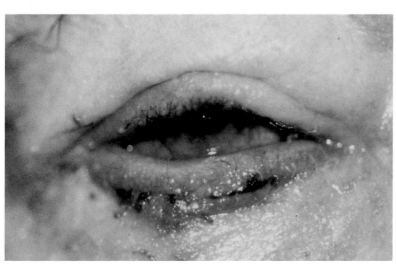

B

FIG. 18. A: Patient with mild right-sided entropion and ocular pemphigoid. **B:** Following a "marginal roll" procedure the lid is in excellent position and there is no longer any entropion.

lid and 25 seconds in the upper lid to destroy the aberrant lashes (2). Cryotherapy works well in removing the aberrant lashes, but there are a number of side effects that can occur. The most common side effect is depigmentation of the skin, which is especially a problem in black patients. There may also be change of the junction of the mucous membrane and the skin, which may lead to chronic inflammation and/or to keratitis from the skin rubbing on the cornea (3). There is also the possibility of reactivating herpes zoster and ocular pemphigoid (4). Eyelid damage and necrosis may occur either due to the cryoprobe or perhaps from overtreatment. Pre-existing lid notches may be exacerbated as well (4).

Argon Laser Ablation

Lashes may be removed using the Argon laser, but we prefer electrolysis because it is much more readily available and more cost effective.

Surgical Excision

If the abnormal lashes occur in a clump, a lid resection can be performed to remove part of the lid harboring the abnormal lashes.

Mucous Membrane Grafting

The eyelid margin with the offending lashes may be removed and the mucous membrane may be grafted from the conjunctiva in either eye or from the mouth. We have seldom seen a situation where this procedure needed to be done.

Distichiasis

When abnormal lashes come from the meibomian gland orifices such as in congenital distichiasis (Fig. 16) or in acquired distichiasis due to conditions such as sta-

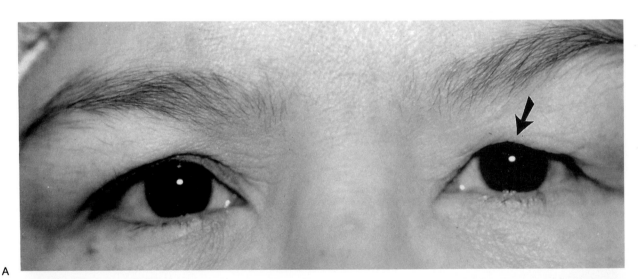

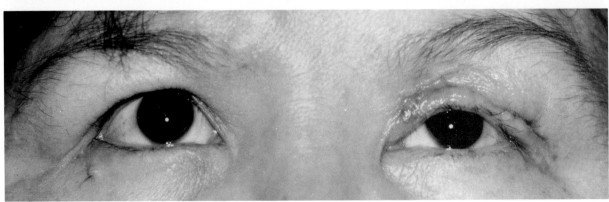

FIG. 19. A: Patient with mild upper lid entropion with some overhanging skin secondary to trauma. **B:** Patient with the entropion and trichiasis cured following a small "marginal roll" procedure.

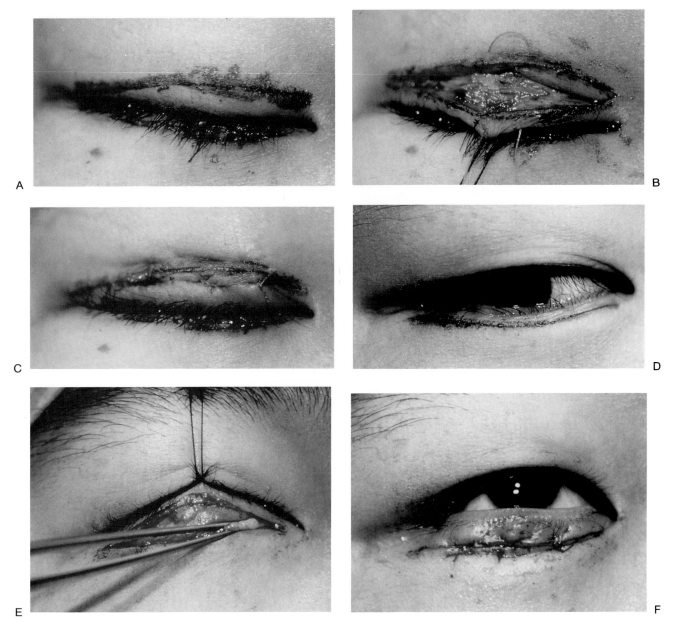

FIG. 20. The "margainal roll" procedure (epiblepharon procedure). **A:** Skin incision marked out. Upper lid. **B:** Skin incision; muscle exposure. **C:** Suturing of skin higher up on tarsus on upper lid to evert upper lid margin. **D:** Marking out skin for procedure on lower lid. **E:** Shrinkage of fat with bipolar diathermy after strip of muscle excised. **F:** The lower lid following shrinkage of fat with bipolar diathermy and inserting sutures through skin edges lower down on tarsus to evert margin slightly to rotate lashes from the globe.

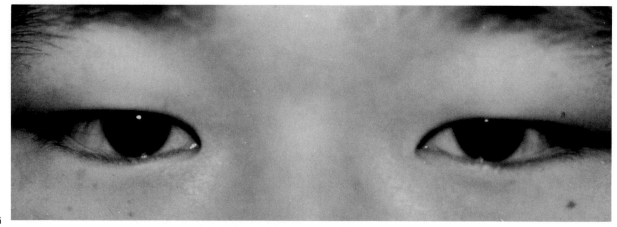

G

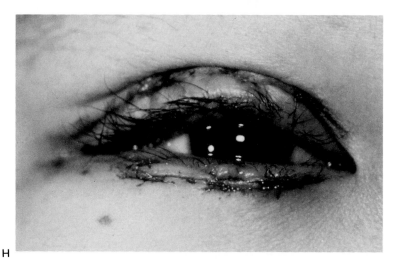

H

FIG. 20. (Continued.) **G:** Preoperative appearance of patient with epiblepharon, lash irritation, and tearing. **H:** Postoperative appearance of upper and lower marginal rolls (epiblepharon procedure).

phylococcoblepharoconjunctivitis, ocular pemphigoid, burns, or Stevens-Johnson syndrome. The treatment is more difficult. We prefer to split the gray line, insert an insulating device between the anterior and posterior lamella, and to cryotherapy the posterior lamella (5).

Corneal Irritation from Eyelashes

The lashes from the lower lid may rub against the floppy upper eyelid in a floppy eyelid syndrome (6). This is seen more frequently when the lid everts. If the upper lid does not evert, the lower lid lashes can rub on the conjunctiva of the upper lid ("eyelid imbrication") (7). A lid resection performed laterally in the upper lid is all that is usually necessary.

Entropion Due to Horizontal Lid Laxity (Fig. 17)

We prefer to tighten the lid by doing a full thickness pentagonal excision of the eyelid laterally (modified Bick procedure) (8). The insertion of sutures to tighten the or-

bicularis laterally fixates the lower border of tarsus, preventing it from everting.

Trichiasis with Early Entropion (Cicatricial)

We prefer in these patients to perform a small anterior lamella surgical procedure. We call this the "margainal roll" (Figs. 18–20).

A small skin-muscle resection is performed along the length of the eyelid. A 5-0 Dexon suture is placed through the proximal skin edge and picks up tarsus more distally, before it passes through the other skin edge. Tying the suture everts the lid margin. This is effective in more than 75% of cases. If it recurs, the operation can easily be repeated.

Increased eversion is achieved by:

1. taking the proximal incision closer to the lid margin
2. taking the tarsal bites farther away from the lid margin
3. cutting through the tarsus (tarsotomy) (9).

This procedure seems to be especially useful in patients with ocular pemphigoid where there is a fear of exacerbating the condition by violating the conjunctiva.

REFERENCES

1. Hurwitz JJ, Johnson D, Howarth D, Molgat Y. Experimental treatment of lashes with high-frequency radio wave electrosurgery. *Can J Ophthalmol* 1993;28:62.
2. Johnson RLC, Collin JRO. Treatment of trichiasis with lid cryoprobe. *Br J Ophthalmol* 1985;69:267.
3. Kavelec CC, Ragbeer M, Harvey JT. Conjunctivalization of lid skin following cryotherapy for trichiasis. *Can J Ophthalmol* 1994;29: 143.
4. Wood JR, Anderson RL. Complications of cryosurgery. *Arch Ophthalmol* 1981;99:460.
5. Anderson RL, Harvey JT. Lid splitting and posterior lamella cryosurgery for congenital and acquired distichiasis. *Arch Ophthalmol* 1981;99:631.
6. Culbertson WW, Ostler HB. The floppy eyelid syndrome. *Am J Ophthalmol* 1981;92:568.
7. Karesh JW, Nirankari VS, Hameroff SB. Eyelid imbrication an unrecognized cause of chronic ocular irritation. *Ophthalmology* 1993;100:883.
8. Hurwitz JJ, Mishkin SK, Rodgers KJA. Modification of Bick's procedure for treatment of eyelid laxity. *Can J Ophthalmol* 1987;22: 262.
9. Kersten RC, Kleiner FP, Kulwin DR. Tarsotomy for the treatment of cicatricial entropion with trichiasis. *Arch Ophthalmol* 1992;110: 714.

CHAPTER 26

Facial Paralysis

Paul LaPierre and Jeffrey J. Hurwitz

ANATOMY OF THE FACIAL NERVE

The facial nerve is a mixed nerve originating in the pons (Fig. 1). It contains approximately 7000 neurons and includes motor, sensory, and parasympathetic fibers, all of which originate or end in various nuclei in the lower third of the pons. These nuclei are the motor nucleus, the superior salivary nucleus (responsible for the innervation of the sublingual salivary, lacrimal, some palatine, pharyngeal, and nasal mucosal glands), and the sensory nucleus.

Upon exiting from the pons, the seventh nerve is composed of two branches: a large motor root and a smaller sensory root (nerve of Wrisberg). The latter nerve branch contains special sensory fibers of taste and parasympathetic secretory fibers (which eventually provide innervation to the lacrimal gland). The corticobulbar fibers reaching the motor nuclei of the lower part of the face are entirely crossed, whereas those connecting with the upper part of the face are both crossed and uncrossed. This difference in the corticobulbar fibers supplying the upper and lower face explains the sparing of the forehead (upper face) movements in supranuclear lesions of the seventh nerve.

The seventh nerve joins the acoustic nerve (8th cranial nerve) upon its exit from the pons. Together they enter a bony canal, the internal auditory canal, whereupon the eighth nerve abandons the facial nerve as the facial nerve continues on in the fallopian canal. The fallopian canal is approximately 33 mm long. During its passage, the seventh nerve is firmly encased in a rigid structure and thus most susceptible to injury from any sort of swelling

(i.e., edema in idiopathic palsy), especially at the labyrinth section. Here not only is the nerve at its smallest diameter (0.68 mm), but the blood supply to the nerve at this point is unique—this is the only segment of the facial nerve that has no anastomosing arterial arcades (1). During its passage through the fallopian canal, the seventh nerve gives off four branches: (a) greater petrosal nerve, (b) lesser superficial petrosal nerve, (c) stapedius muscle nerve, and (d) chorda tympani nerve. The nerve exits the skull at the stylomastoid foramen to enter into the parotid gland. Before entering the gland it gives a further two branches: (a) posterior auricular nerve and (b) a branch supplying the posterior belly of the digastric muscle.

In the parotid gland, the nerve divides into two main trunks: (a) upper temporofacial division and (b) lower cervicofacial division. Each of these gives various branches and interconnections with each other in a plexiform manner.

The greater petrosal nerve leaves the geniculate ganglion and joins the deep petrosal nerve to form the nerve of the pterygoid canal—Vidian's nerve. The Vidian nerve enters the sphenopalatine ganglion and joins with postganglionic fibers and ultimately gives branches that innervate the lacrimal gland. Thus, any process that severs the nerve proximal to the geniculate ganglion may, during regeneration (if aberrant), affect the way the lacrimal gland functions. Such is the case in "crocodile tearing."

FACIAL NERVE TESTING

There exists two principal modes of testing seventh nerve function: topognostic and electrical. The former are more historical and falling out of favor, whereas the latter are growing in popularity and usefulness.

P. LaPierre: Oculoplastics Program, Mount Sinai Hospital, Toronto, Ontario M5G 1X5, Canada.

J. J. Hurwitz: Oculoplastics Program, Mount Sinai Hospital; and Department of Ophthalmology, University of Toronto Faculty of Medicine, Toronto, Ontario M5S 1A8, Canada.

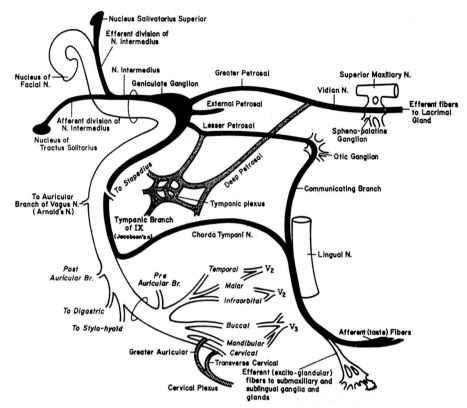

FIG. 1. Anatomical communications of the seventh cranial nerve. (Modified from May, ref. 40, with permission.)

Topognostic Testing

Topognostic testing relies on the fact that lesions below the point at which a particular branch leaves the facial nerve trunk will spare the function subserved by that branch. Tschiassny (2) popularized these tests in the early 1950s (Fig. 2).

The various tests include lacrimal function (i.e., Schirmer's test), the stapedius reflex, taste, salivary flow, salivary pH, hearing, and balance tests.

In complete focal lesions, topognostic tests can be reliable; however, the most common facial nerve injury, Bell's palsy, is usually a mixed lesion with varying degrees of conduction block and degeneration changes, making topognostic tests of little value in the diagnosis and prognostication of this illness.

In general, these tests are inappropriate to prognosticate or are cumbersome to perform and thus are not used clinically to any great extent. In comparison, electrical tests, most notably the electroneurography (ENOG), are easier to perform, interpret, are readily available, and have proved more useful in the prognostication of various nerve injuries.

Electrical Testing

Testing the electrical response of the nerve after activation by either mechanical, voluntary, or electrical stimulation is the basis for evaluation of nerve conduc-

tivity and thus nerve integrity. These tests are useful in prognostication following nerve trauma as well as intraoperative monitoring of the nerve function during surgical dissection in proximity to nerve fascicles. The various tests include nerve excitability test, maximum stimulation test, ENOG, and electromyography (EMG). They are usually of no value in establishing an etiology per se. Each test has its own limitations and purposes. None of these tests, except electromyography, are of great value if the response to electrical stimulation is lost completely.

Nerve Excitability Test

Introduced by Laumans and Jonkes in 1963 (3), the nerve excitability test (NET) remains one of the simplest and best known. A stimulating electrode is placed at the stylomastoid foramen along with a return electrode on the forearm. Electrical pulses are delivered at steadily increasing currents until a facial twitch is barely noticeable. The lowest amount of current required to produce a twitch is called the "threshold of excitation." This procedure is performed on both the affected side and the normal side. The results are then compared and the difference in thresholds is noted. A difference of 3.5 mA or more is considered a reliable indicator of degeneration. It is important to remember that a lag of 3 to 4 days after complete axonal degeneration is required before loss of electrical excitability will be demonstrated.

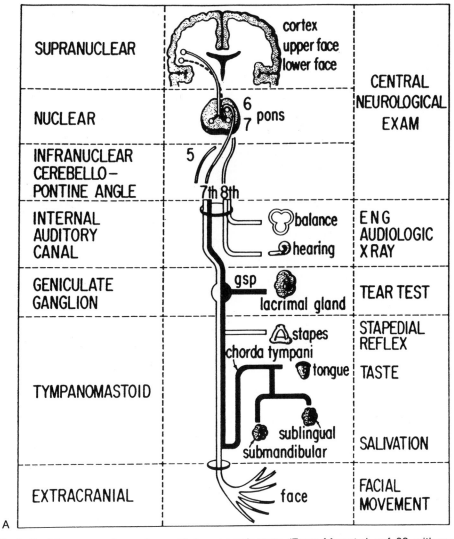

FIG. 2. A: Facial nerve anatomy along with topognostic tests. (From May et al., ref. 39, with permission.)

Proponents of this test suggest daily testing until complete loss of response is found. The limitations of this test are that it is subjective and the patient must have a complete facial palsy with some remaining nerve conductivity in order to perform the test.

Maximum Stimulation Test

In the maximum stimulation test (MST), similar to the NET in that it involves visual (subjective) evaluation of facial movements, one does not consider the threshold for facial movements, but rather the current used to provide maximal facial muscle stimulation as judged by an observer. Again the intraobserver error as well as interobserver error can often be very high.

Electroneurography (Evoked Electromyography)

To perform ENOG, a bipolar electrode is placed at the stylomastoid foramen and is used for electrical stimulation while another pair of bipolar electrodes, placed in the nasolabial groove, records muscle response (objective endpoint). What is measured is in fact the compound muscle action potential (CMAP) as in electromyograms. The normal difference from side to side in the average person is 3%. Test-retest errors in the range of 20% have been reported in the literature and there is a certain technical ability required to master this test (4). Notwithstanding these limitations, one of the most beneficial results of this test is the ability to prognosticate in patients with Bell's palsy. Various studies have shown that amplitude reduction below 10% as measured by ENOG were correlated with a poor response (5). This test is superior to both the NET and MST as it is objective and does not require a patient to have a complete paralysis to interpret its results.

Electromyography

Needle electrodes are placed directly into muscle tissue and electrical activity is recorded. This test allows the

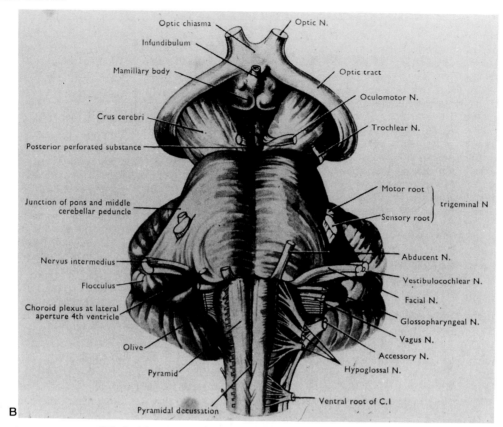

FIG. 2. (*Continued.*) **B:** Brain stem demonstrating facial nerve.

evaluation of muscle that has lost its innervation completely. Loss of excitability is no longer a limiting factor as it is in the other electrical stimulation tests. After 10 to 14 days of axonal degeneration, one can measure fibrillation potentials. Of more interest are the polyphasic re-innervation potentials that are seen 4 to 6 weeks after the onset of paralysis. These precede clinically detectable recovery and predict a fair to good outcome (6). The value of EMG lies in its ability, along with muscle biopsy, to determine the probability of success of nerve grafting many months after paralysis when no electrical activity can be recorded by any other means. Similarly, it may be useful to determine the results of nerve grafting in patients by tracking the arrival of polyphasic potentials in facial muscles.

PATHOLOGY OF NERVE INJURY

Degeneration and Regeneration

Sunderland (7,8) described five degrees of nerve injury. From his classification, it is possible to predict the chance of restoration of nerve function given its degree of injury (Table 1). Once injured, a nerve sprouts a growth cone where it was severed that puts forth fan-like protoplasmic processes that actively extend as they seek a favorable milieu in which to grow. Because of the nu-

merous protoplasmic processes of the growth cone, a regenerating axon is likely to branch and enter several tubules into a single Schwann cell, whereby a Schwann cell may be shared by many small axons. Thus, the invariable result of regeneration of the facial nerve is that an axon that previously supplied a single muscle now supplies widely separated muscle fibers causing synkinesis or associated movements. The regenerating axon grows at the rate of 1 mm per day in a thin thread-like filament less than 1 μm in diameter. Upon reaching a motor endplate in facial muscle, the nerve begins to thicken and acquire myelin when it is 1 to 2 μm thick (9). In a regenerated nerve there are many more distal branches and they tend to be of smaller caliber and nonmyelinated when compared to a normal nerve. The deficient insulation of these axons results in the mass movement and spasm of the facial muscles one encounters clinically with aberrant regeneration. The gustolacrimal reflex (crocodile tearing) is found in 6% to 30% of patients following idiopathic facial nerve paralysis (10,11). The etiology of this syndrome is felt to be due to facial nerve fibers that regenerate in the wrong direction and stray into another nerve bundle. If the sprouting fibers destined for the gustatory nerve reach the lacrimal nerve instead, an increase in lacrimal secretion occurs when taste is stimulated. Other possible etiologies of crocodile tearing include misdirected regeneration from the minor

TABLE 1. *Neuropathology and spontaneous recovery correlated with degree of facial nerve injury*

Degree of injury	Pathology of injury	EEMG response	Neurobiology of recovery	Clinical recovery begins	Spontaneous recovery— result one year post injury
1	Compression. Damming of axoplasm. No morphologic changes. (Neuropraxial)	Normal	No morphologic changes noted	1–4 weeks	Grade I Complete: without evidence of faulty regeneration
2	Compression persists, increased intraneural pressure. Loss of axons but endoneurial tubes remain intact. (Axonotmesis)	25% of normal	Axons grow into intact empty myelin tubes at a rate of 1 mm/day which accounts for longer period for recovery in 2° injuries compared to 1°. Less than complete recovery is due to some fibers with 3° injury.	1–2 months	Grade II Fair: Some noticeable difference with volitional or spontaneous movement, minimal evidence of faulty regeneration.
3	Intraneural pressure increases. Loss of myelin tubes. (Neurotmesis)	0–10% of normal	With loss of myelin tubes the new axons have an opportunity to get mixed up and split causing mouth movement with eye closure referred to as synkinesis.	2–4 months	Grade III–IV Moderate to poor: Obvious incomplete recovery to crippling deformity with moderate to marked complications of faulty regeneration.
4	Above plus disruption of perineurium. (Partial transection)	No response	In addition to problems caused by 2° and 3° injuries, now the axons are blocked by scarring which impairs regeneration.	4–18 months	Grade V Motion barely perceptible
5	Above plus disruption of epineurium. (Complete transection)	No response	Complete disruption with a scar-filled gap presents an insurmountable barrier to the regrowth of axons and neuromuscular reanastomosis.	Never	Grade VI None

From ref. 41.

petrosal nerve to the greater petrosal nerve, and cross-stimulation due to the loss of insulation of the injured nerve (12). Others (13) believe that an already present phylogenic reflex is released by the pathology affecting the nerve.

Various treatment modalities have been tried to stop tearing including blockage of postganglionic fibers with cocaine or alcohol, resection of the lesser superficial petrosal nerve, and resection of the tympanic branch of the glossopharyngeal nerve. None have proved to be absolute in their response.

ETIOLOGY OF FACIAL NERVE DYSFUNCTION

There is a long differential of seventh nerve palsy (Table 2) and one must remember that Bell's palsy, although

TABLE 2. *Etiology of facial palsy from a review of the medical literature*

Birth	*Neoplastic*
Molding	Cholesteatoma
Forceps delivery	Seventh nerve tumor
Dystrophia myotonica	Glomus jugulare tumor
Mobius syndrome (facial diplegia associated with other cranial nerve deficits)	Leukemia
Trauma	Meningioma
Basal skull fractures	Hemangioblastoma
Facial injuries	Sarcoma
Penetrating injury to middle ear	Carcinoma (invading or metastatic)
Altitude paralysis (barotrauma)	Anomalous sigmoid sinus
Scuba diving (barotrauma)	Hemangioma of tympanum
Lightning	Hydradenoma (external canal)
Neurologic	Facial nerve tumor (cylindroma)
Opercular syndrome (cortical lesion in facial motor area)	Schwannoma
Millard-Gubler syndrome (abducens palsy with contralateral hemiplegia due to lesion in base of pons involving corticospinal tract)	Teratoma
	Hand-Schüller-Christian disease
	Fibrous dysplasia
Infection	von Recklinghausen disease
External otitis	*Toxic*
Otitis media	Thalidomide (Michlke syndrome, cranial nerves VI, VII with congenital malformed external ears and deafness)
Mastoiditis	Tetanus
Chicken pox	Diphtheria
Herpes zoster cephalicus (Ramsey-Hunt syndrome)	Carbon monoxide
Encephalitis	*Iatrogenic*
Poliomyelitis (Type I)	Mandibular block anesthesia
Mumps	Antitetanus serum
Mononucleosis	Vaccine treatment for rabies
Leprosy	Post immunization
Influenza	Parotid surgery
Coxsackie virus	Mastoid surgery
Malaria	Post tonsillectomy and adenoidectomy
Syphilis	Iontophoresis (local anesthesia)
Scleroma	Embolization
Tuberculosis	Dental
Botulism	*Idiopathic*
Acute hemorrhagic conjunctivitis (enterovirus 70)	Bell's, familial
Cnathostomiasis	Melkersson-Rosenthal syndrome (recurrent alternating facial palsy, furrowed tongue, faciolabial edema)
Mucormycosis	Hereditary hypertrophic neuropathy (Charcol-Marie Tooth disease, Dejerine Sottas disease)
Lyme disease	Autoimmune syndrome
Metabolic	Temporal arteritis
Diabetes mellitus	Thrombotic thrombocytopenic purpura
Hyperthyroidism	Periarteritis nodosa
Pregnancy	Landry-Cuillan-Barré syndrome (ascending paralysis)
Hypertension	Multiple sclerosis
Acute porphyria	Myasthenia gravis
	Sarcoidosis (Heerfordt syndrome-uveoparotid fever)
	Osteopetrosis

From ref. 41.

the most common by far, is a diagnosis of exclusion. The five most common causes of seventh nerve palsy are: a) Bell's palsy, b) herpes zoster cephalicus, c) trauma, d) tumor, and e) infection. These five account for more than 90% of all cases (Table 3) (14).

The onset of facial palsy is not diagnostic in itself whether complete, incomplete, sudden, or delayed, but it may have prognostic implications. Excellent recovery will most likely occur in cases of incomplete palsy that do not progress to complete palsy.

Approximately 50% of patients with Bell's palsy present with a sudden complete facial paralysis. However, 40% of patients with confirmed tumors involving the facial nerve also present with sudden and complete facial paralysis. Bilateral simultaneous palsy is usually due to Guillain-Barre Syndromé (15), whereas the differential includes idiopathic palsy (Bell's), leukemia, bulbar palsy, sarcoidosis, skull fracture, mobious syndrome, and myotonic dystrophy.

Recurrent palsy has been noted to occur with a) idiopathic palsy, b) Melkersson-Rosenthal syndrome, and c) tumors. With recurrent ipsilateral palsy frequently due to Bell's—81% of cases (15)—a tumor must be ruled out as a cause of recurrence as 17% of patients with ipsilateral recurrence will harbor a malignancy.

If, on the other hand, the patient experiences a recurrence on the opposite side, one can be confident that the patient has idiopathic Bell's palsy, although other very rare disorders may be responsible (i.e., Melkersson-Rosenthal syndrome).

Any and all patients with slowly progressive facial paralysis do not have Bell's palsy and must be evaluated to rule out a malignancy. The differential diagnosis in this scenario includes a) primary neuromas of the facial nerve, b) metastasis from squamous cell carcinomas, c) melanomas of the face and scalp, and d) distant metastases from kidney, breast, lung, and prostate (16). Progressive palsy may also occur from other primary temporal bone and cerebellopontine angle lesions as well as from carotid artery aneurysms (17,18).

Bell's Palsy

Bell's palsy infers acute peripheral facial palsy of unknown cause. This disorder is self-limiting, nonprogressive, non–life-threatening, and spontaneously remitting. It is neither preventable nor curable. The lifetime incidence is between 15 and 40 per 100,000 population. A higher percentage of patients are over 65 and under 13 (19–21). Typically it involves the tympanomastoid portion of the facial nerve (Fig. 3).

Taverner (22) outlined the diagnostic criteria for Bell's palsy:

1. paralysis or paresis of all muscle groups on one side of the face
2. sudden onset
3. absence of signs of central nervous system disease
4. absence of signs of ear or cerebellopontine angle disease.

This entity may be bilateral but is unlikely to be so. It may recur in 12% of patients (4% ipsilateral to the first involvement and 8% contralateral) (15,23). Outcome prognostication is obtained from electrical investigation.

Various etiologies have been advanced for this entity: viral, microvascular, ischemic, and autoimmune; however, none has been proved conclusively. Currently, a viral pathogen is the most common accepted etiologic factor.

Peitersen (24) examined the natural history of more than 1,000 patients with Bell's palsy and found a satisfactory recovery rate in 84% of patients within 15 years of onset. Of the remaining 16%, only 4% had sequelae that were crippling. Peitersen argued that when earlier recovery is noted, better the prognosis for a satisfactory and speedy recovery. He found that recovery proceeded within 3 weeks of onset of paralysis in 85% of patients.

Numerous authors have shown that the prognosis is satisfactory in up to 80% of patients without any treatment. Using the ENOG, if the response rate remains above 10% during the first 14 days following onset of paralysis, more than 80% of patients will have a satisfactory recovery, whereas only 50% will have a satisfactory outcome if the activity falls below 10% (5).

Although reported by some to promote a more rapid and complete recovery, a large randomized double-blind trial has not been done to prove that corticosteroids alter the final outcome of facial paralysis. However, the use of steroids may be indicated for reasons other than the facial paralysis itself. Some authors (19) found that prednisone dramatically relieved the pain of Bell's palsy.

Currently, no other medical modality has been shown

TABLE 3. *Causes of facial nerve disorders in 1575 patients over 20 years old by one clinician*

Cause	Patients
	No. (%)
Bell's plasy	895 (57%)
Herpes zoster cephalicus	117 (7%)
Trauma	268 (17%)
Tumor	91 (6%)
Infection	70 (4%)
Birth (congenital and acquired)	48 (3%)
Hemifacial spasm	28 (2%)
Central nervous system (axial) disease	18 (1%)
Other	30 (2%)
Questionable	10 (1%)
TOTAL	1575 (100%)

From ref. 41.

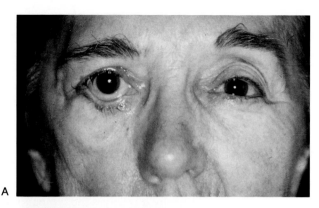

FIG. 3. A: This woman demonstrates the common presentation of patients with seventh nerve paralysis. **B:** Close-up of eye. **C:** When she attempts to close her eyes, there is no closure, plus we see aberrant regeneration is present in the facial musculature.

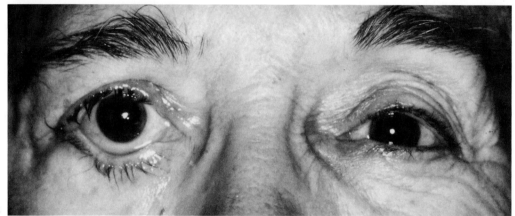

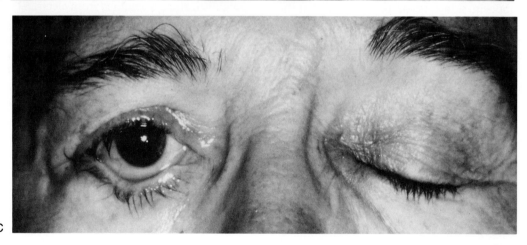

to improve on the natural course of idiopathic facial nerve palsy and surgical therapy remains even more controversial in Bell's palsy.

Trauma

Trauma may be iatrogenic, surgical, or accidental. Trauma causing temporal bone fractures is the most common cause of accidental trauma to the facial nerve. This is especially true of transverse temporal bone fractures. When paralysis occurs several days after the traumatic event, it can be assumed that the nerve has not been transected and that satisfactory spontaneous recovery will most likely occur without surgical intervention. If, on the other hand, there exists evidence that the nerve has been transected, surgery is indicated to repair the fracture and explore and decompress the nerve with or without subsequent nerve grafting. Success in restoring function is guarded.

Tumors

Tumors represent approximately 5% of cases of facial palsy, with more than half these cases being acoustic neuromas (Schwannomas) located in the cerebellopontine angle or internal auditory canal. Surprisingly, acoustic neuromas rarely cause facial paralysis even though the nerve is thinned and stretched considerably over the surface of a large neuroma (Fig. 4). Other lesions to consider are meningiomas, angiomas, and arteriovenous malformations.

Malignant tumors may also affect the facial nerve. According to May (15), the two most common are adenoid cystic and mucoepidermoid carcinomas at the level of the parotid gland. During tumor removal, the surgeon must consider not only resection of the tumor but facial reanimation as well. In most benign tumors, the functional, cosmetic, and emotional consequences of complete tumor removal outweigh the benefits of partial resection with preservation of nerve function.

Clinical Assessment

Trauma, infection, or tumor are the usual causes of paralysis and are usually ascertained by clinical history and examination. If the examination fails to reveal any positive findings, the nerve palsy is most likely viral in origin. Recovery from this type of lesion is excellent and close monitoring over the next 2 to 3 weeks is important to exclude any other cause of paralysis.

The time and degree of recovery are determined by assessing:

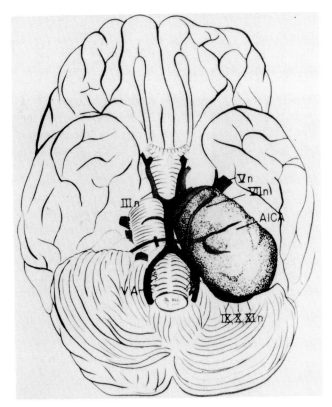

FIG. 4. Common location of acoustic neuroma with stretched seventh cranial nerve overlying tumor.

1. the completeness of the palsy (subjectively)
2. the response to electrical tests (MST or ENOG).

Almost every patient with idiopathic palsy or acute facial palsy due to trauma or infection, who retains some facial movement beyond 14 days after onset, will have a satisfactory recovery from this disorder (Sunderland group I or II recovery). After an initial evaluation within 14 days of onset, the patient is given a return appointment in 3 to 4 weeks and instructed to monitor his nerve function at home. Specifically, he is told to return if he notices any worsening of his palsy or if complete paralysis ensues. If the patient with persistent incomplete palsy does not begin to recover within 6 weeks or the paresis worsens, a tumor should be suspected and the patient should undergo appropriate investigations such as a computed tomography scan.

Patients who have complete paralysis at the onset can be evaluated initially with MST or ENOG to determine the likelihood of recovery. Early partial recovery of facial function, within the first 3 weeks, is a reliable indication that recovery will be satisfactory. The patient is evaluated electrically daily during the first 14 days; if electrical activity remains above 10% of normal then significant recovery is expected in 80% of cases (5).

Once the prognosis has been established, patients are asked to return at 3, 6, and 12 months for evaluation of facial function employing the system established by House and Brackmann (25). During this time, medical treatment is implemented and necessary precautions must be taken to prevent possible sequelae of facial nerve paralysis.

Medical treatment includes warm compress, heat, massage, facial muscles exercises, and lubrication drops if the cornea appears exposed. No pharmacologic treatment, including steroids, have proved to be efficacious in the treatment of patients with facial nerve paralysis.

One must not forget to address the psychological factors that accompany the facial disfigurement brought on by the facial nerve paralysis. Appropriate counseling and/or referral should be provided as necessary.

Ocular Assessment

The facial nerve supplies innervation to the orbicularis muscle via the upper temporofacial division of the nerve. It is essential to verify its integrity during examination. Other important considerations include a) an intact and adequate Bell's phenomenon to protect the cornea, b) normal corneal sensation, c) adequate tear production, and d) any degree of lagophthalmos. It is also important to detect any predisposing ocular condition that may be aggravated by a lack of normal lid function and/or tear film instability.

Tearing is an extremely frequent symptom that may be attributed to hypersecretion following corneal irritation or secondarily to malfunction of the tear pump (poor lid position and/or function).

With no drainage through the patent system due to a pump paralysis, there may be a chronic stagnation within the lacrimal passages, which may lead to an obstruction. Therefore, a nasolacrimal obstruction must be ruled out by syringing. Lacrimal pump dysfunction with or without punctal eversion is the usual cause of tearing. Mild pump dysfunction may exist in an apparently fully recovered case with only the presence of aberrant regeneration being the telltale sign. A nuclear lacrimal scan can be used to demonstrate decreased flow from the palpebral aperture and from the sac.

During subsequent visits, the integrity of the cornea is closely monitored to detect any dehydration. Various nonsurgical modalities may be tried to prevent this. The most useful include daily lubricants (ideally nonpreserved) as well as lubricating ointment at night. Other therapies include a thin sheet of cellophane taped over the eye to trap moisture, a moist chamber placed over the eye, or simply taping the lids shut. Patients should be instructed to wipe and massage the eyelids in an upward direction in an attempt to improve lid-globe apposition.

When these measures fail to protect the cornea sufficiently, we must consider one of the surgical options.

SURGICAL MANAGEMENT IN THE REPAIR OF SEVENTH NERVE DAMAGE

Many variables must be considered when deciding on the appropriate management of any patient:

1. *Ocular assessment (including corneal assessment):* corneal anesthesia and/or corneal breakdown suggest more radical measures such as tarsorrhaphies are in order (26).
2. *Time elapsed since injury:* a temporary tarsorrhaphy may be performed in the early phases; a permanent procedure is advisable in long-standing disorders.
3. *Age:* the older patient often requires a lid-lengthening procedure as well as a tarsorrhaphy
4. *Current lid position (i.e., ectropion, retraction)*
5. *Etiology of facial paralysis (i.e., tumor vs. trauma):* if spontaneous improvement may be expected
6. *Diabetes or other nutritional/metabolic/vascular disorders*

In addition, if dynamic repair is considered:

1. presence of partial regeneration
2. previous attempts at surgical repair
3. proximal and distal nerve integrity
4. nerve donor site consequences
5. viability of facial muscles (EMG findings).

There are two fundamental ways of viewing surgical repair of the seventh nerve: functional and cosmetic.

Functional repair may be divided further into dynamic repair where restoration of kinetic function is attempted and second, static repair where one attempts to protect the eye. Cosmetic procedures relate to improving the esthetic component of facial paralysis that causes significant psychological sequelae to many patients.

Functional Repair

1. *Static:*
   tarsorrhaphy: medial and/or lateral
   lower lid tightening procedure
   upper lid lengthening
   gold weights
   lid spring
2. *dynamic (reanimation):*
   nerve transplantation
   muscle transposition/free graft
   Arion sling
   electrodes (27)
     glasses
     implantable

Cosmetic Repair (upper face)

1. Ectropion repair
2. brow elevation
3. blepharoplasty

Static Repair

Tarsorrhaphy (Acute)

Once corneal exposure is established, a simple yet effective mode of treatment is a tarsorrhaphy, which may be critically placed to provide the maximum amount of benefit. We prefer a "double adhesion" tarsorrhaphy. The gray line is split and the eyelids are separated into anterior and posterior halves. The posterior lamellae are sutured with interrupted 5-0 Dexon (Davis and Geck) sutures. The anterior lamellae are sutured with a 4-0 silk suture over eyelid bolsters. This provides a "permanent tarsorrhaphy" that can be easily opened if desired, without affecting the eyelashes (Fig. 5). A lateral tarsorrhaphy is usually adequate but may need to be augmented by a medial tarsorrhaphy in order to decrease exposure (Fig. 6). If the eyelid is also lax or if ectropion is present, a lateral lid-tightening procedure should be done in conjunction with a tarsorrhaphy (28) (Fig. 7).

Lateral Lid Tightening

If ectropion exists with any amount of lid laxity, one may perform a lateral lid-tightening procedure such as a

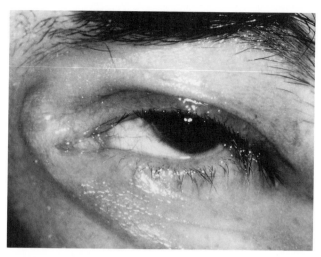

FIG. 5. Lateral double-adhesion tarsorrhaphy in a patient with facial palsy.

modified Bick (29) procedure. A medial canthoplasty is often indicated with lax medial canthal tendons. Older patients with facial nerve palsy often have lagophthalmos due to lower lid ectropion, whereas in younger patients upper lid retraction from unopposed action of the superior rectus and levator complex often produces lagophthalmos. Given this fact, lower lid–tightening procedures seem more useful in the older patients whereas the younger patients often do quite well with lengthening of the upper lid (Fig. 7).

Upper Lid Lengthening

Upper lid lengthening is most often used in younger patients who present with upper lid retraction from unopposed levator and Muller's muscle action. A simple conjunctivo-Mullerectomy is effective in lowering the retracted upper lid. Under local anesthesia, a conjunctival approach is used, as one would for a lid-lengthening procedure in Graves' disease. Two percent xylocaine with epinephrine (1:10,000) is injected beneath the conjunctiva. The conjunctiva is incised and Muller's muscle and/or the levator aponeurosis is recessed. The amount of recession is assessed by the lid position with the patient opening the eye during surgery. The conjunctiva is sutured with a 6-0 plain gut suture.

Gold Weights

Weighting of the upper lid was first described by Sheehan and Smellie (30). Most surgeons now prefer to insert the gold weight and attach it to the tarsus. The current standard weights vary from 0.6 to 1.6 g in 0.2-g increments. There exist several weight configurations, each varying in thickness and/or width. Most commonly they tend to be 1 mm thick, with a width of 5 mm and the length variable according to the total weight. This procedure is ideally performed under neurolept or local anesthesia. An appropriate gold weight may be selected before surgery and taped to the upper lid to provide a presurgical evaluation of the amount of lid ptosis produced. Under local anesthetic, the incision is placed in the patient's natural lid crease. A skin muscle flap is then dissected down to 2 to 3 mm from the lash line. The weight is placed between the tarsus and the orbicularis and sutured using nonabsorbable material (i.e., 5-0 Ticron) to the tarsus. The incision is closed using a running nylon suture.

Some patients may experience extrusion of the weight, especially those with thin skin and diminished pretarsal orbicularis muscle. Usually this is first noticeable at the lateral corner of the weight. Should this arise, the weight should be removed and reimplantation postponed until all tissues have completely healed.

Although they provide only static passive movement,

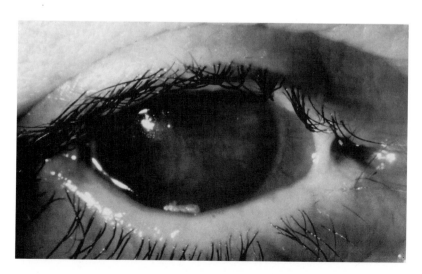

FIG. 6. This patient underwent both a lateral and medial tarsorrhaphy to protect his cornea following seventh nerve paralysis. The medial pillar could be enlarged with another suture.

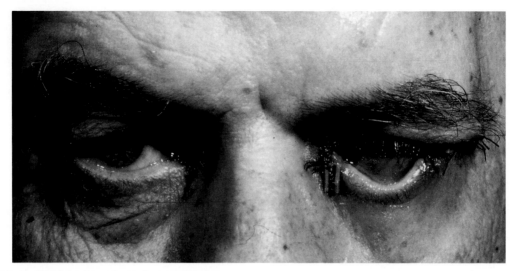

FIG. 7. Patient referred with facial palsy and worsening corneal exposure. Lateral and medial tarsorrhaphy performed without taking into account the severe lid laxity. One can clearly see the amount of lid bowing centrally with poor lid-globe apposition and increased corneal exposure. The tarsorrhaphies were taken down and a lid-tightening procedure with a small lateral tarsorrhaphy was performed.

most patients are quite happy with the surgical results. The extrusion and infection rate for these implants are very low (31).

Lid Spring

Lid springs were first introduced by Morel-Fatio in 1964 (32). The spring consists of two limbs of 30-mm stainless steel wire with a coil at the center resembling a safety pin. Unlike gold weights, it has a closing effect regardless of the position of the patient. It also provides a faster blink and therefore better and more frequent coverage of the cornea (33). Among its disadvantages are a higher extrusion rate and need for frequent readjustments. Most surgeons now use 0.010″ nonmagnetic stainless steel orthodontic wire to fashion a spring that is inserted under local anesthesia. The purpose is to close the lid with the spring and have the levator and Muller's muscle open the eye (34).

Dynamic Repair

Facial Nerve Grafting and Muscle Transposition

In most instances, the techniques used for facial reanimation depend on the status of the proximal limb of the facial nerve. For example, tumor ablation with facial nerve resection requires immediate nerve reconstruction with a nerve graft, whereas facial palsy following resection of a cerebellopontine neuroma will often regress without any further surgical intervention if the nerve was not inadvertently transected during surgery. Hence, no one modality is universally appropriate for all afflictions

of facial nerve function. In general, the order of preference for reanimation is:

1. facial nerve regeneration (laissez-faire)
2. facial nerve neurorrhaphy
3. facial nerve cable graft
4. nerve transposition

Several points remain highly controversial as to when, how, and which nerve and which material should be used in the repair of the seventh nerve. In general, one should attempt to reapproximate the damaged ends fairly quickly (3–7 days) with a graft that is obtained from the sural nerve, the greater auricular nerve, the lateral cutaneous nerve of the thigh, or the cervical plexus.

If it is not possible to locate the proximal end of the severed seventh nerve, then one may consider performing a cross-over graft. The hypoglossal, spinal accessory, glossopharyngeal, or phrenic nerve have all been used for this purpose. Some surgeons advocate cross-face nerve grafting, where a nerve graft is attached to the healthy facial nerve and tunneled through skin to the distal end of the contralateral distal portion of the facial nerve to provide innervation.

Muscle Transfer and Grafts

In long-standing paralysis, where there is atrophy of the mimetic muscles, a regional muscle transfer may provide adequate movement. The transposed muscles provide a large volume of dynamic and living tissue that augments atrophic areas. The most popular muscles used for this technique are the temporalis and masseter muscles. The latter is restricted to the oral and cheek area and the temporalis is used for the orbital region as well.

Both these muscles are innervated by the trigeminal nerve and thus movement is not natural in appearance. To rectify this, some surgeons prefer to use a facial nerve graft or a cross-face graft whereas other surgeons (35–37) prefer to graft muscle from other sites (i.e., palmaris longus, extensor digitorum brevis, pectoralis minor, latissimus dorsi, etc.).

Arion Sling

The silicon palpebral sling was originally described by Arion in 1972 (38). Under local anesthesia, numerous horizontal small incisions are placed along the border of both the upper and lower lids near the lashes. A silicone rod is then placed subcutaneously surrounding the lids while both ends protrude laterally. The tension is adjusted to provide maximum movement and the ends are tied and then buried. The disadvantage of this technique is that it lasts approximately 6 months and needs to be repeated. Extrusion is frequent as well.

Electrodes

Recently, several surgeons have begun to look at electrical stimulation of the orbicularis using electrodes that are placed on the surface skin or implanted into the orbicularis. These electrodes may be used with varying amounts of success in exciting the underlying orbicularis to contract using electrical stimulation. Although experience with these techniques has been limited, the results hold promise for a more physiologic restoration of the blink response.

Cosmetic Repair

Brow Lift

A direct browplasty is often useful to lift the brow and elevate excess skin from the eyelids (Fig. 8). Local anes-thesia is injected above the brow and a wedge-shaped incision of skin, muscle, and galea is performed. The subcutaneous tissues from the edges of the excision are fixated to the periosteum in the immobile eyelid. The incision is sutured in layers. Placing the lower end of the incision in the upper row of brow hairs will minimize the appearance of any eventual scar. One must ensure that lagophthalmos is not made worse (Fig. 9).

Ectropion

A standard ectropion procedure with or without a blepharoplasty and fat excision may help lower lid cosmesis.

Blepharoplasty

Upper lid skin may be removed but care must be taken that the lagophthalmos is not worsened and the middle of the eyebrow is not pulled into the eyelid.

MANAGEMENT OF THE TEARING PATIENT WITH FACIAL NERVE DYSFUNCTION

When assessing patients who present with tearing and have facial nerve dysfunction, one must ultimately decide on the etiology of the tearing to define the appropriate management. Patients with more tearing while eating exhibit aberrant regeneration (crocodile tearing). Treatment is focused at cutting the nerve-relaying information from the parotid gland to the lacrimal gland. The procedure, where Vidian's nerve is transected (Vidian neurectomy), has in our experience a 50% success rate.

During our examination, we must assess lid function, lid laxity, punctal position, and the patency of the lacrimal outflow tract as we would do in any other patient who presents with tearing. Particular attention must be

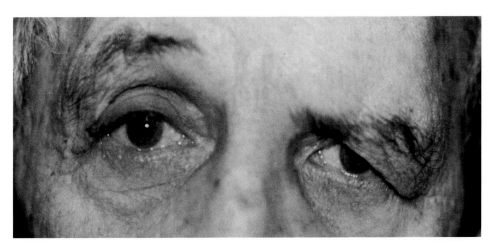

FIG. 8. This patient developed severe brow ptosis following seventh nerve paralysis.

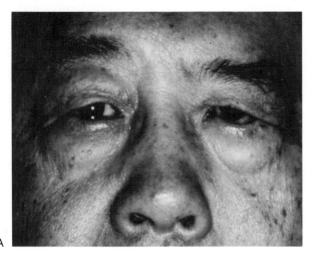 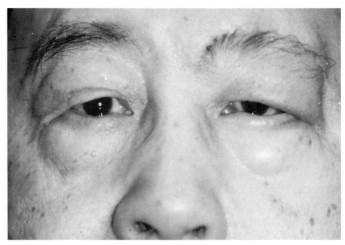

A

B

FIG. 9. A: Patient with brow ptosis before surgical correction. **B:** Same patient postbrowplasty.

paid to a) the cornea—is there any evidence of exposure?, b) the lid pump—how well is it functioning?, c) nasolacrimal duct function—is there any blockage or stagnation in the sac?

The management of these patients will be determined by our clinical findings. Simple lubrication may be the only required form of treatment for patients presenting with exposure, whereas one may contemplate lid tightening, either lateral or medial, in patients with pump abnormalities, and lacrimal drainage surgery may be considered in patients with lacrimal obstruction. Finally, reanimation of the lids may be offered to a certain subgroup of patients who present with pump abnormalities.

The insertion of Jones tubes does not usually significantly reduce symptomatology in these patients as the tube is dependent on adequate pump function for drainage of tears. The role of capillarity of the tube helps somewhat in tear drainage, but the relief of epiphora depends on the level of orbicularis dysfunction.

REFERENCES

1. Blunt MJ. The possible role of vascular changes in the etiology of Bell's palsy. *J Laryngol* 1956;70:701.
2. Tschiassny K. Eight syndromes of facial paralysis and their significance in locating lesions. *Ann Otol Rhinol Laringol* 1953;62:677.
3. Laumans EP, Jonkes LBW. On the prognosis of peripheral facial paralysis of endotemporal origin. *Ann Otorhinolaryngol* 1963;72:621.
4. Fisch U. Maximal nerve excitability testing vs. electroneurography. *Arch Otolaryngol* 1980;106:352.
5. May M, Blumenthal F, Klein S. Acute Bell's palsy: prognostic value of evoked electromyography, maximal stimulation, and other electrical tests. *Am J Otolaryngol* 1983;5:1–7.
6. Esslen E. *The acute facial palsies: investigations on the localization and pathogenesis of meato-labyrinthine facial palsies.* Berlin: Springer; 1976.
7. Sunderland S. *Some anatomical and pathophysiological data relevant to facial nerve surgery.* New York: Aesculapius; 1977.
8. Sunderland S. *Nerve and nerve injuries,* 2nd ed. London: Churchill Livingstone; 1978.
9. Aitken JT. Growth of nerve implants in voluntary muscle. *J Anat* 1950;84:38.
10. Taverner D. The prognosis and treatment of spontaneous facial palsy. *Proc R Soc Med* 1959;52:1077.
11. Tumarkin IA. Some aspects of the problem of facial paralysis. *Proc R Soc Med* 1936;29:1685.
12. Fisch U. Lacrimation. In: Fisch U, ed. *Facial nerve surgery.* New York: Aesculapius; 1977.
13. Sadjadpour K. Postfacial palsy caused by artificial synapse?, *Neurology* 1976;26:292.
14. May M. *The facial nerve.* New York: Thieme-Stratton Inc; 1986.
15. May M. Facial nerve paralysis. In: Paparella MM, Shumrick DA, Meyerhoff W, et al., eds. *Otolaryngology,* 3rd ed. Philadelphia: WB Saunders; 1991.
16. Muhlbauer WD, Segeth H, Viessman H. Restoration of lid function in facial palsy with permanent magnets. *Chirmaxilofac Plast* 1973;1:295.
17. Brandt TW, Jenkins HA, Coker NJ. Facial paralysis as the initial presentation of an internal carotid artery aneurysm. *Arch Otolaryngo Head Neck Surg* 1986;112:198.
18. Gruber H, et al. Prostate cancer presenting as facial paralysis. *Otolaryngol Head Neck Surg* 1989;100:333.
19. Adour KK, et al. The true nature of Bell's palsy: analysis of 1000 consecutive patients. *Laryngoscope* 1978;88:787.
20. Hadar T, et al. Specific IgG and IgA antibodies to herpes simplex virus and varicella zoster virus in acute peripheral facial palsy patients. *J Med Virol* 1983;12:237.
21. Katusic SK, et al. Incidence, clinical features, and prognosis in Bell's palsy. Rochester, Minnesota 1968–1982. *Ann Neurol* 1986;20:622.
22. Taverner D. Bell's palsy. *Brain* 1955;78:209.
23. May M. Chapter 14. In: Paparella MM, Shumrick DA, Meyerhoff W, Gluckman JL, eds. *Facial nerve paralysis in otolaryngology,* 3rd ed. Philadelphia: WB Saunders, 1991;1097.
24. Peitersen E. The natural history of Bell's palsy, *Am J Otol* 1982;4:107.
25. House JW, Brackmann DE. Facial nerve grading system. *Otolaryngol Head Neck Surg* 1985;93:146.
26. Collin JRO. Ophthalmic management of seventh nerve palsy. *Aust N Z J Ophthalmol* 1990;18:267.
27. Cowen D, Oestricher J, Kavalec C. ASOPRS, Presented at November 1994 meeting.
28. Rosenstock T, Hurwitz JJ, Nedzelski J, Tator C. Ocular complication following excision of cerebellopontine angle tumors. *Can J Ophthalmol* 1986;21:134.

29. Hurwitz JJ, Rodgers KJA, Mishkin S. Modification of Bick's procedure for treatment of eyelid laxity. *Can J Ophthalmol* 1987;22: 262.

30. Smellie GD. Restoration of the blinking reflex in facial palsy by a simple lid loading operation. *Br J Plast Surg* 1966;19:279–283.

31. Townsend DJ. Eyelid reanimation for the treatment of paralytic lagophthalmos: historical perspectives; and current applications of the gold weight implant. *Ophthal Plast Reconstruct Surg* 1992;8: 196.

32. Morel-Fatio D, Lalardri JP. Palliative surgical treatment of facial paralysis: the palpebral spring. *Plast Reconstruct Surg* 1964;33: 446–456.

33. Sobol S, May M, Mester S. Early facial reanimation following radical parotid and temporal bone tumor resection. *Am J Surg* 1990;1660:382–386.

34. Sheehan JE. Progress in correction of facial palsy with tantalum wire and mesh. *Surgery* 1950;27:122.

35. Thompson N. A review of autogenous skeletal muscle grafts and their clinical applications. *Clin Plast Surg* 1974;1:349.

36. Hakelius L. Free muscle grafting. *Clin Plast Surg* 1979;6:301.

37. Mackinnon SE, Dellon AL. A surgical algorithm for the management of facial palsy. *Microsurgery* 1988;9:30.

38. Arion HG. Dynamic closure of the lids in paralysis of the orbicularis muscle. *Int Surg* 1972;57:48.

39. Peitersen E. The natural history of Bell's palsy. *AM J Otol* 1982;4: 107.

40. May M. *Gray's Anatomy,* 36th British edition. Philadelphia: WB Saunders; p. 1068.

41. May M. *The facial nerve.* New York: Thieme-Stratton, pp.182–183, 328.

CHAPTER 27

Lacrimal Sac Tumors

Pathology

David J.C. Howarth and Jeffrey Jay Hurwitz

The pathologist is called on to give a definitive diagnosis on tissue, as to the presence or absence of tumor, or the pathologic condition present. It is useful to understand the pathologist's approach to, and limitations in, diagnosis at the time of frozen section.

The pathologist does not operate in a "black box," so the more clinical information given to him/her, including the exact site of the lesion, the more definitive the diagnosis can be. An adequate amount of tissue is required. Crush and cautery artifact can render tissue uninterpretable.

Frozen sections should be used to determine if lesional tissue is present, if there is uncertainty as to exact localization, or to guide complete surgical excision of tumors by assessment of margins. Orientation is crucial in the assessment of margins of resection and orientation by the surgeon or by diagrammatic representation as to the position of the specimen is extremely helpful. Separately submitting margins is another useful method that can be used.

Definitive diagnosis on frozen section tissues is frequently difficult as freezing artifact distorts cytologic detail, leaving only architectural abnormalities for assessment. The diagnosis of malignancy depends on the assessment of the nuclear/cytoplasmic ratio and nuclear abnormalities. Nuclear pleomorphism, enlargement of the nucleus (with a subsequent increased nuclear/cyto-

plasmic ratio), irregular nuclear contours (angulation), hyperchromasia (intense nuclear staining possibly due to increased DNA synthesis, or chromosomal abnormalities), and nuclear molding (when one nucleus compresses another, indicating a fragile nuclear membrane and a lack of respect for normal cytoplasmic borders) are all cytologic features that help define a cell as being malignant. The cytoplasm of a cell defines the cell's histogenesis by its content. Frozen sections, because of the formation of ice crystals, cause nuclear enlargement and irregularity. This distortion does not entirely revert with thawing of the tissue, which may render the tissue nondiagnostic.

It is impossible to accurately assess lentiginous spread of a malignant melanoma because of the cytologic distortion introduced at frozen section, and the best advice to the surgeon is to excise all the pigmented lesion and if possible include nonpigmented margins as widely as possible. Diagnosis of lymphomas on frozen section slides is also not possible, and further permanent sections are mandatory to make the diagnosis. The population of cells must be destructive and (in most cases) proven to be monoclonal by immunophenotyping. Assessment of epithelial lesions is also rendered difficult on frozen section assessment, unless frankly invasive carcinoma can be identified, with individual malignant cell infiltration. Tangential cutting of tissue can render assessment of invasion difficult.

The tumors that can arise in the lacrimal sac are related to the indigent component cells therein, or may represent metastatic disease or contiguous spread (secondary) from adjacent tissues.

The broad categories into which these primary and secondary tumors fall are shown in Table 1.

D. Howarth: Departments of Pathology and Ophthalmology, Mount Sinai Hospital, and Department of Pathology, University of Toronto Faculty of Medicine, Toronto, Ontario M5S 1A8, Canada.

J. J. Hurwitz: Oculoplastics Program, Mount Sinai Hospital; and Department of Ophthalmology, University of Toronto Faculty of Medicine, Toronto, Ontario M5S 1A8, Canada.

TABLE 1. *Lacrimal sac tumors*

Epithelial tumors	Nonepithelial tumors

Squamous cell carcinoma
Adenocarcinoma
Transitional cell carcinoma
Mucoepidermoid carcinoma
Oncocytoma/oncocytic carcinoma
Adenoid cystic carcinoma
Benign mixed tumor (pleomorphic adenoma)
Although not described, a monomorphic adenoma could possibly arise from small intrinsic glands present.
	Mesenchymal (stromal)
	  Fibrous histiocytoma
	  Skeletal muscle
	    —Rhabdomyosarcoma (secondary)
	  Peripheral nerve tumors
	    —Schwannoma/neurofibroma
	  Vascular tumors
	    —Hemangioma/hemangiopericytoma/angiosarcoma
	  Adipose tissue tumors
	  Lipoma
	Although not yet described, further tumors could include malignant fibrous histiocytoma, leiomyoma/leiomyosarcoma, lipoma/liposarcoma, and osteosarcoma.
	
	Hematopoietic
	  Lymphomas, plasmacytomas, chronic lymphocytic leukemias, granulocytic sarcoma
	Although not yet described, eosinophilic granuloma is also a possibility.
	
	Neuroectoderm
	  Melanomas—primary or secondary
	Neuroendocrine
	  Metastases from small (oat) cell carcinoma
	Although not yet described, a retinoblastoma could potentially involve the lacrimal sac from contiguous spread.

The broad categorizations allow for a differential diagnostic template to be drawn up.

EPITHELIAL TUMORS

Epithelial tumors account for the bulk of lacrimal sac tumors. In general, these tumors can be grouped into papillomas, carcinomas, and adenomas.

Papillomas

Papillomas (Fig. 1) can have a squamous epithelial lining with a central fibrovascular core (squamous papilloma) or a transitional epithelial lining (transitional cell papilloma) or a mixture of both (1). These tumors and a few of the carcinomas have recently been shown to be associated occasionally with human papilloma virus (HPV types 11 and 18) infection (2). This association could help to account for local recurrence due to the continuing effects of the viral genome in residual affected cells, postexcision.

Papillomas can have exophytic, endophytic, or mixed growth patterns. Exophytic tumors tend to recur less frequently than the others (1,3). This is similar in nature to inverted papillomas of the nasal and paranasal sinuses, in which an inverted growth pattern confers the potential for recurrence, possibly with subsequent dysplastic changes and malignant transformation (4).

Varying degrees of dysplasia can arise in squamous papillomas from mild to severe to carcinoma in situ. The degree of dysplasia will correlate with recurrence and potential malignant spread (Fig. 2).

The degree of dysplasia of squamous epithelium is based on the thickness to which the atypical cells infiltrate the epithelium. *Mild dysplasia* indicates the atypical cells are present only in the lower third of the epithelium; *moderate dysplasia* denotes atypical cells extending to the middle third. *Severe dysplasia* contains atypical cells virtually throughout the full thickness of the epithelium and *carcinoma in situ* indicates full thickness atypia with complete loss of the polarity of the epithelium, as conferred by the normal maturation sequence, with flattening of the surface epithelial cells with or without keratinization. (In the mind's eye, one can turn the atypical epithelium of carcinoma in situ upside

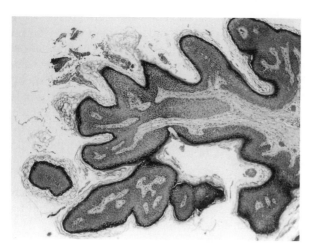

FIG. 1. Squamous papilloma. H & E ×250.

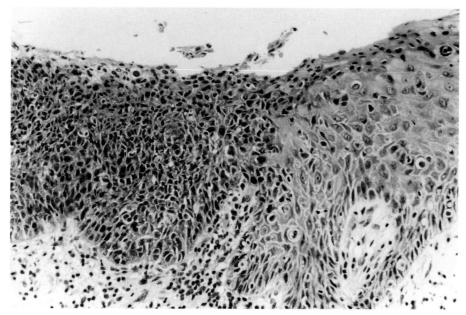

FIG. 2. Severe dysplasia of squamous epithelium. H & E ×250.

down, and not be able to note a difference, because of the complete loss of any maturation sequence at the surface).

CARCINOMAS

Squamous cell carcinomas are composed of cells that form intercellular bridges (desmosomes) recognized at a light microscopic level, and produce keratin that can be recognized at a light microscopic or electron microscopic level (intermediate or tonofilaments) or by immunohistochemical studies (keratin positivity).

Squamous cell carcinomas are graded with respect to the degree of differentiation as mild, moderate, or poorly differentiated. Most tumors will fall into a moderate category, indicating that the invasive component is readily identified as a squamous cell carcinoma, but there is a considerable amount of cytologic atypia. Well differentiated squamous cell carcinomas differ only minimally from their normal squamous counterpart. Poorly differentiated squamous cell carcinomas and poorly differentiated tumors in general reveal few clues as to their histogenesis at a light microscopic level, and therefore ancillary studies are required to determine differentiation, such as electron microscopy and immunohistochemistry.

Epithelial tumors in general share certain features such as keratin positivity [AE1, AE3, CAM 5.2, possibly epithelial membrane antigen (EMA)] by immunohistochemistry and well formed desmosomes at the electron microscopic level.

Transitional epithelium is in a transition state between pseudostratified columnar epithelium (with or without goblet cells) and stratified squamous epithelium. It is our contention that the transitional cell carcinomas be classified according to the grading system used for transitional cell carcinomas of the bladder (5). This would in all likelihood be a predictor for recurrence and malignant potential (6). The other significance of this comparison is that, perhaps, as in bladder tumors, a field effect may occur in which multiple foci of dysplastic epithelium develops, rendering complete surgical excision exceedingly difficult (7) (Fig. 3).

In the bladder, transitional cell carcinomas are classified into grades ranging from I to III (5). The classification is as follows:

Grade I: epithelium >7 cells thick; minimal cytologic atypia; slight loss of polarity
Grade II: epithelium usually >10 cells thick; moderate cytologic atypia; greater loss of polarity
Grade III: marked cytologic atypia; loss of polarity; fragmentation of superficial layers.

It is not surprising given the presence of small accessory glands that tumors similar to lacrimal and salivary gland tumors should arise in this region.

There are cases of adenocarcinomas arising primarily in the lacrimal sac that have been reported (3). An adenocarcinoma is composed of cells that produce mucin and therefore stain histochemically positive by the periodic acid-Schiff with diastase stain (PAS-D).

Mucoepidermoid carcinomas have also rarely been reported as primary tumors in the lacrimal sac (8–10). These tumors represent a hybrid degree of differentiation between squamous cell carcinomas and adenocarcinomas. In these tumors there is an intimate admixture of mucin-secreting and squamous epithelial cells. The

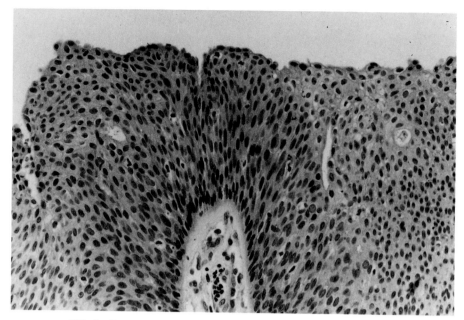

FIG. 3. Transitional epithelium lining of a papilloma. H & E ×400.

greater the proportion represented by squamous differentiation, the more malignant these tumors will be expected to behave. This method of grading these tumors means that the highest grade (3 of 3) is composed of malignant squamous cells with positivity within these cells for PAS-D (i.e., representing mucin production) (Fig. 4).

A rare adenoid cystic carcinoma has been described (11,12). This is a tumor that is derived from duct cells that form gland-like spaces into which they secrete basement membrane material. This is the opposite polarity to which these cells normally function, in that in normal circumstances, they lay down basement membrane material at their base, onto which they anchor, with their luminal surface on the opposite side forming the duct. When these tumors proliferate they often form a cystic or cribriform or "Swiss cheese" pattern, hence the name "adenoid cystic carcinoma." Adenoid cystic carcinomas have a tendency toward perineural and bony extension, making their complete excision exceedingly difficult as the tumor may extend well beyond the tumor bulk. In

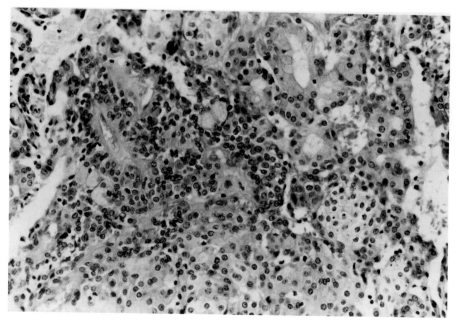

FIG. 4. Mucoepidermoid carcinoma. H & E ×400.

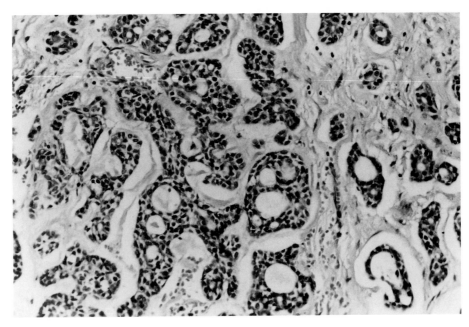

FIG. 5. Adenoid cystic carcinoma. H & E ×400.

this situation, frozen section–guided resection margins are suggested. Adenoid cystic carcinomas are usually slow-growing tumors with a propensity to local recurrence because of the aforementioned reasons. Because of their slow-growing nature, they are not particularly susceptible to radiotherapy (Fig. 5).

ADENOMAS

Oncocytic adenomas (3,13), also known as oncocytomas or oxyphilic adenomas, are benign tumors that can arise in the lacrimal sac. They are composed of cells that, stained with hematoxylin and eosin, by light microscopy have an abundant eosinophilic granular cytoplasm (oncocytes or oxyphils). By electron microscopy the cells are found to contain numerous mitochondria. These cells are felt to represent degenerative serous secretory epithelial cells that are histologically present in the walls of the lacrimal sac. These cells can undergo hyperplasia, termed "oncocytic hyperplasia." Oncocytic carcinomas have also been described, in which there is significant cytologic atypia (i.e., malignant changes). In the case of oncocytic adenomas, local excision is curative (Figs. 6 and 7).

Benign mixed tumors (pleomorphic adenomas) have been described rarely (3). These are benign, well circumscribed tumors composed of an intimate admixture of cells representing epithelial (squamous, glandular differentiation) and mesenchymal (fibrous, chondroid, and adipose) differentiation, hence the name. As in the parotid gland, these tumors may have small finger-like protuberances outside the main tumor bulk, which, if not fully excised, may result in multifocal recurrence.

It is not surprising to find rare cases of the aforementioned minor salivary/lacrimal gland tumors (mucoepidermoid carcinomas, adenoid cystic carcinomas oncocytic adenomas, and pleomorphic adenomas) in this site because of the finding of serous and mucinous secretory glands in the walls of the lacrimal sac. We would not be surprised if eventually a monomorphic adenoma were identified in the lacrimal sac. In all these tumors, as wide a local excision as possible is recommended with expectant follow-up.

NONEPITHELIAL TUMORS

There are rare case reports of nonepithelial tumors.

Mesenchymal/Stromal

Stromal tumors stain immunohistochemically positive for the intermediate filament vimentin. Stromal cells form a reticulin framework around each individual cell. This is in contrast to epithelial tumors, in which reticulin is seen around cell nests, but not between individual cells.

Fibrous histiocytomas (3,14) are benign tumors, and as the name implies, are composed of a combination of fibroblasts producing a collagenous matrix and histiocytes (macrophages). Macrophages stain immunohistochemically positive for alpha-1-antitrypsin, alpha-1-antichymotrypsin, and lysozyme, all degradative enzymes present in the cytoplasm. The tumor is cured by local excision. Its malignant counterpart is a malignant

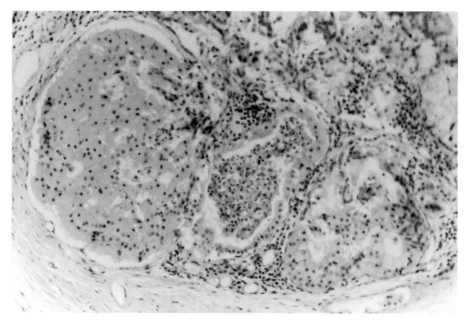

FIG. 6. Oncocytic metaplasia in serous glands in lacrimal sac wall. H & E ×250.

fibrous histiocytoma. This has not been, to our knowledge, described in the lacrimal sac.

Rhabdomyosarcoma (15), a tumor of striated muscle, arises most commonly in children. This tumor recapitulates skeletal muscle differentiation and is immunohistochemically positive for desmin (a contractile protein), myosin, and myoglobin. By electron microscopy, abortive attempts at the production of sarcomeres may

.be seen. Cases of secondary extension into the lacrimal sac have been reported.

Nerves in the vicinity of the lacrimal sac may give rise to tumors. Neurilemmomas (Schwannomas) (16) are peripheral nerve sheath tumors composed of Schwann cells that proliferate adjacent to the axonal bundles of the nerve. The cells tend to palisade and can form organoid (Verocay) bodies. Antoni A (cellular) and Antoni B

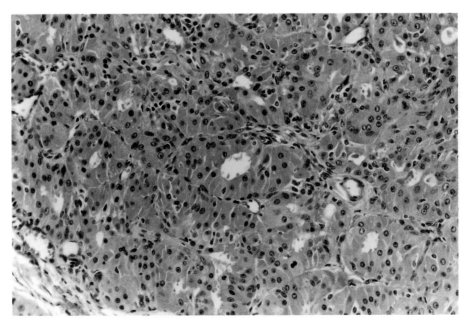

FIG. 7. Oncocytoma. H & E ×400.

(myxoid and cystic) areas are admixed. Immunohistochemically, the cells stain positively for S100 protein. By electron microscopy, mesoaxons may be formed. These are benign tumors, which do not recur after local excision.

The other type of peripheral nerve tumor that can occur in this vicinity is the neurofibroma (14). This is also a benign peripheral nerve tumor, which is composed of a combination of Schwann cells and perineural fibroblasts that proliferate to entrap axons of the nerve bundle, which then course through the tumor bulk. The tumor cells also tend to palisade, but there are no intermixed areas of cellular, myxoid, or cystic change. Neurofibromas are not encapsulated. Plexiform neurofibromas are pathognomic of von Recklinghausen's disease.

Vascular tumors can occur in the lacrimal sac. Hemangiomas represent a benign proliferation of endothelial-lined vascular channels and have been reported in the lacrimal sac. Their malignant counterpart, the angiosarcoma (17), has also been reported in this region. Tumors derived from endothelium should stain positively by immunohistochemistry with factor VIII. By electron microscopy, the tumor cells would be expected to contain Weibel-Palade bodies. Hemangiopericytomas (18–20) are vascular tumors arising from the pericyte present in close association with normal endothelium. The constituent vessels are lined by a single layer of attenuated endothelial cells, surrounded by a basal lamina. The tumor cells do not stain positively by immunohistochemistry with factor VIII. The vascular channels coursing through the tumor can be made to stand out more readily by histochemical staining with PAS-D. Histologic assessment of these tumors cannot predict biologic behavior with respect to recurrence or metastases. This tumor has been described in the lacrimal sac.

Hematopoietic

Tumors of the hematopoietic system have been reported in the lacrimal sac (14,21–23). Lymphomas could arise from the "adenoid" layer of lymphocytes in the lacrimal sac. These tumors usually display B-cell immunophenotype (L-26, MB2 positive). They are immunohistochemically positive for leukocyte common antigen, a marker useful for distinguishing them from other poorly differentiated tumors. The tumor cells are generally not patchy in distribution and destroy the tissue in which they grow. Plasmacytomas have also been described in this region, as well as "granulocytic sarcoma" (an unusual variant of myeloid malignancy) and chronic lymphocytic leukemia. If such a lesion is suspected, the tissue should be sent fresh from biopsy/excision to the pathologist for further processing. Depending on the amount of tissue, this will be divided for fixation (B5, a mercury-based fixative and formalin), snap frozen at −70°C for cell surface marker assessment, flow cytometry, and tissue culture. A frozen section may be performed to rule out a carcinoma, if possible. The patient will require further systemic work-up in all these cases.

Although not described, eosinophilic granuloma, a proliferation of Langerhans' cells (histiocytosis X), could occur. These cells contain Birbeck granules, identified by electron microscopy.

Neuroectoderm

Primary malignant melanomas have been described in the lacrimal sac (24–26). They are felt to arise from indigenous melanocytes. Melanoma cells usually have nuclei containing large "brick-red" or purple nucleoli. They may or may not produce melanin pigment (positive with Warthin-Starry histochemical stain). By electron microscopy, melanosomes and premelanosomes may be found to determine histogenesis. Immunohistochemically, these cells are positive for S100 protein and HMB-45 (a specific melanoma marker).

Neuroendocrine

Metastatic small (oat) cell carcinoma from a lung primary to the lacrimal sac region has been seen by our group. These represent neuroendocrine tumors, which are poorly differentiated. They are positive for neuron-specific enolase (NSE) and chromogranin by immunohistochemistry. By electron microscopy, scant neurosecretory granules (dense-core granules) can be identified.

REFERENCES

1. Ryan SJ, Font RL. Primary epithelial neoplasms of the lacrimal sac. *Am J Ophthalmol* 1973;76(1):73–88.
2. Madreperla SA, et al. Human papilloma virus in primary epithelial tumors of the lacrimal sac. *Ophthalmology* 1993;100(4):569–573.
3. Stefanyszyn, et al. Lacrimal sac tumors. *Ophthal Plast Reconstr Surg* 1994;10(3):169–184.
4. Anderson KK, et al. Invasive transitional cell carcinoma of the lacrimal sac arising in an inverted papilloma. *Arch Ophthalmol* 1994;112:306–308.
5. Murphy WM. Current topics in the pathology of bladder cancer. *Pathol Annu* 1983;18(1).
6. Robbins SL, Cotran RS. *Pathologic basis of disease,* 4th ed. Philadelphia: WB Saunders; 1989.
7. Paxton BR, et al. Carcinoma of lacrimal canaliculi and lacrimal sac. *Arch Ophthalmol* 1970;84:749–753.
8. Fliss DM, et al. Mucoepidermoid carcinoma of the lacrimal sac: a report of three cases with observations on the histogenesis. *Can J Ophthalmol* 1993;28(5):228–235.
9. Khan JA, et al. Mucoepidermoid carcinoma involving the lacrimal sac. *Ophthal Plast Reconstr Surg* 1988;8:153–157.
10. Blake J, et al. Lacrimal sac mucoepidermoid carcinoma. *Br J Ophthalmol* 1986;70:681–685.

11. Kincaid MC, et al. Adenoid cystic carcinoma of the lacrimal sac. *Ophthalmology* 1989;96:1655–1658.
12. Parnell JR, et al. Primary adenoid cystic carcinoma of the lacrimal sac: report of a case. *Ophthal Plast Reconstr Surg* 1994;10(2):124–129.
13. Ni C, et al. Tumors of the lacrimal sac. *Int Ophthalmol Clin* 1982;22:121–140.
14. Pe'er JJ, et al. Nonepithelial tumors of the lacrimal sac. *Am J Ophthalmol* 1994;118:650–658.
15. Baron EM, et al. Rhabdomyosarcoma manifesting as acquired nasolacrimal duct obstruction. *Am J Ophthalmol* 1993;115:239–242.
16. Sen DK, et al. Neurilemmoma of the lacrimal sac. *Eye Ear Nose Throat Monthly* 1971;50:179–180.
17. Harry J, Ashton N. The pathology of tumours of the lacrimal sac. *Trans Ophthalmol Soc UK* 1969;88:19–35.
18. Gurney N, et al. Lacrimal sac hemangiopericytoma. *Am J Ophthalmol* 1971;71:757–759.
19. Carnevali L, et al. Haemangiopericytoma of the lacrimal sac: a case report. *Br J Ophthalmol* 1988;72:782–785.
20. Roth SI, et al. Hemangiopericytoma of the lacrimal sac. *Ophthalmology* 98(6):925–997.
21. Kheterpal S, et al. Previously undiagnosed lymphoma presenting as recurrent dacryocystitis. *Arch Ophthalmol* 1994;112:519.
22. Munro S, et al. Nasolacrimal obstruction in two patients with chronic lymphocytic leukemia. *Can J Ophthal* 1994;29(3):137–140.
23. Karesh JW, et al. Dacryocystitis associated with malignant lymphoma of the lacrimal sac. *Ophthalmology* 1993;100:669–673.
24. Radnót M, et al. Examen ultrastructural d'un mélanome malin du sac lacrymal. *Ophthalmologica* 1971;163:73–89.
25. Lloyd WC, Leone CR. Malignant melanoma of the lacrimal sac. *Arch Ophthal* 1984;102(1):104–107.
26. Eide N, et al. Primary malignant melanoma of the lacrimal sac. *Acta Ophthal* 1993;71:273–276.

CHAPTER 28

Lacrimal Sac Tumors

Management

Jeffrey Jay Hurwitz

The proper management of a lacrimal sac tumor is important not only to the ultimate relief of the patient's epiphora but, more importantly, to prevent spread and metastasis, and the ultimate demise of the patient.

PRESENTATION

A lacrimal tumor may present as a mass in the lacrimal sac fossa (Fig. 1). The mass is usually hard, nonfluctuant (as opposed to the fluctuance one finds in a lacrimal sac mucocele), does not transilluminate, and is rarely tender. Symptoms of tearing may or may not be present. Blood-stained tears may occur (1). The system is often patent to syringing. A dacryocystogram often demonstrates a fixed filling defect within the sac. Surrounding bone erosion may be present. A computed tomography (CT) scan [or CT-dacryocystogram (DCG)] demonstrates the relationship to the bone and soft tissue anatomy (Fig. 2).

MANAGEMENT

There are three situations that may arise with respect to the management of lacrimal sac tumors: unsuspected sac tumor, suspected sac tumor, and known sac tumor with spread into surrounding structures.

J. J. Hurwitz: Oculoplastics Program, Mount Sinai Hospital; and Department of Ophthalmology, University of Toronto Faculty of Medicine, Toronto, Ontario M5S 1A8, Canada.

Unsuspected Sac Tumor

During a routine dacryocystorhinostomy (DCR), one might find that the sac appears hard and enlarged. If one has not opened up the sac, it is prudent to perform a biopsy under frozen section control. A small wedge incision into the sac can be performed. If it is confirmed that a tumor is present, a dacryocystectomy should be performed. The exception to this should be when there is a round cell infiltration and one cannot be sure on frozen section whether this is a lymphoma or a pseudotumor. In this scenario it is probably best not to open up into the nose, and to close the incision pending the final pathology report. If one has already opened the sac and the mucosa looks thick and suspicious, one can take a frozen section at that time and wait for the results, and manage the patient the same as if the sac had not been opened.

Suspected Sac Tumor

The patient should be told preoperatively that if a tumor is confirmed, a dacryocystectomy and not a DCR will be performed. If there is any suggestion on frozen section of a malignancy, one should not open into the nose or complete the DCR for fear of spreading cells beyond the contained site of the lacrimal sac, and into the nose and sinuses. A biopsy can be performed similar to the case of the unsuspected sac tumor. A cryoprobe is useful to seal the site of the biopsy and prevent spillage of cells. If there is any question as to the malignancy of the lesion on frozen section, we feel that one should err on the side of conservatism and perhaps come back at

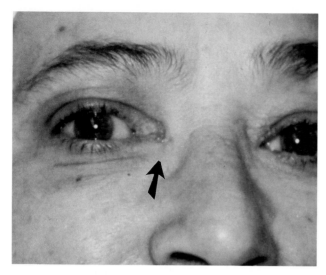

FIG. 1. Patient with firm lacrimal sac mass. The lacrimal system is patent to syringing. A sac lymphoma was found at biopsy and treated with radiotherapy. A DCR was later performed.

another sitting to complete the DCR if the lesion is benign. If a lymphoma is suspected, it is probably best not to complete the operation in the nose, or even to put in bicanalicular Silastic stents on the pretext that the patient will have radiation. The stents going through the duct into the nose may spill cells down through this passage and increase the field of radiation necessary. If a malignancy is found, a dacryocystectomy can be performed (Fig. 3).

Known Lid Tumor with Extension

We prefer before doing an en bloc excision of the site to do a frozen section to confirm that indeed there is a malignancy of the sac. We then would seal the site with the cryoprobe. The en bloc excision is performed either by the ophthalmologist alone or in conjunction with the otolaryngologist. It is difficult to get frozen section margins on the bone of the en bloc excision. This en bloc excision may involve the lateral wall of the nose and nasal mucosa, some of the ethmoids, maxillary sinus, or medial orbit, depending on the radiologic limits of the tumor. However, one often finds that the tumor is larger than one might have thought on examining the CT scan films. Depending on the soft tissue extent of the lesion, the canaliculi, puncta, and eyelids may have to be excised. The philosophy of the en bloc excision is to remove all the tumor, including some normal tissue around it. The area can be packed afterward, and reconstruction performed at a later date. It is helpful to have these patients seen by the radiotherapist preoperatively because often these patients need postoperative radiation and it is helpful if the radiotherapist has some knowledge of the patient and the disease. A prosthetics

expert will help in the ultimate rehabilitation of these patients.

DACRYOCYSTECTOMY

Indications

Dacryocystectomy is an operation to treat a lacrimal sac tumor when the sac must be excised. The operation may be done in other situations such as Wegener's granulomatosis, or in an elderly patient with a sac abscess on whom the surgeon has decided not to perform a DCR, or where at the time of DCR surgery, for one reason or another, it is not possible to perform a DCR. It must be remembered that these patients may have tearing after a dacryocystectomy, and the patients must be warned of this. They may also may be told, however, that a common canaliculorhinostomy can be performed at a later date if necessary to relieve any residual epiphora.

Surgical Technique

This procedure may be performed using a general anesthesia or a local anesthesia, but we usually do this under local anesthesia. Two percent xylocaine with epinephrine can be injected around the sac and a parainfraorbital nerve block can be given. For maximum anesthesia, an infratrochlear nerve block may also be given, but this is not mandatory.

A skin incision is made on the side of the nose as per a DCR. The section is carried down to bone and the sac is mobilized laterally from the lacrimal fossa with the plane of cleavage between the periosteum overlying the sac and the bone. It is important for the surgeon not to open the bone of the lacrimal fossa for fear of spreading any tumor cells toward the nasal mucosa. The sac must then be amputated from its connection with the common canaliculus laterally, and with the nasolacrimal canal inferiorly. We find it useful to use a cryoprobe to fixate the sac and lift it out of its fossa so the amputation can then be performed. With the dacryocystectomy, especially if a tumor is present, it is useful to freeze the whole of the sac; this seems to decrease the potential for spillage of cells in the area. A Stevens scissors can be used to amputate the sac at the common canaliculus. This allows one to lift the sac with the cryoprobe superiorly. Then the Stevens scissors can be placed at the superior aspect of the nasolacrimal canal, and as the sac is lifted it can be amputated from the nasolacrimal duct. One then can use an artery forceps within the membranous lacrimal duct to remove the mucosal lining. We do not use any bone punches to remove any of the bone of the nasolacrimal canal. Bleeding is usually negligible, but if it is a problem one can use Surgicel pieces in the surgical site to stop the bleeding. The subcutaneous tissue can be sutured with interrupted absorbable sutures and the skin with interrupted nonab-

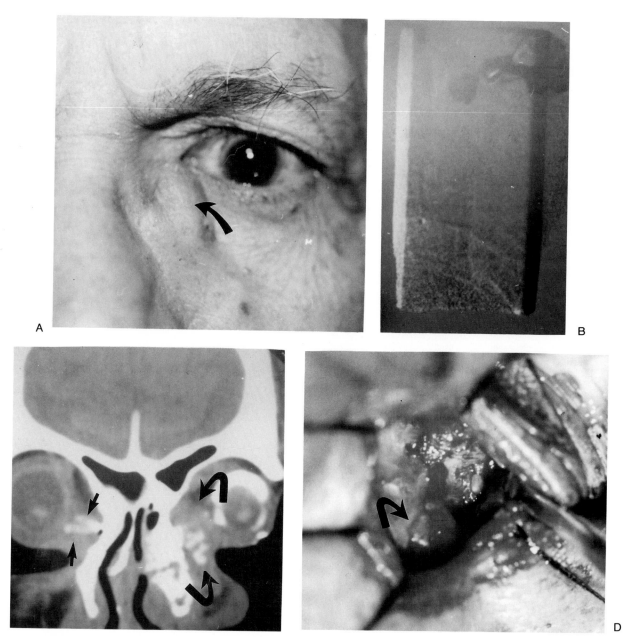

FIG. 2. A: Patient with firm left sac mass. System is not patent to syringing. **B:** DCG shows sac enlargement and obstructed sac. **C:** CT-DCG shows right-side normal (*arrows*) and left-sided mass (*curved arrows*). **D:** An epithelial tumor was found at dacryocystectomy.

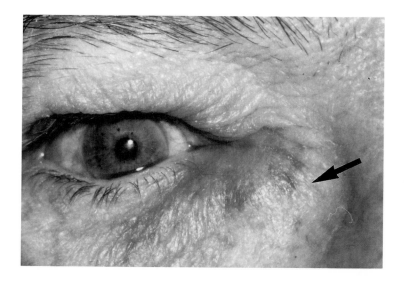

FIG. 3. A 75-year-old man with hard mass in lacrimal sac. The system was partially patent to syringing. A transitional papilloma was found, treated by dacryocystectomy (not DCR). Tearing was not a problem postoperatively, so no later surgery was necessary.

sorbable sutures. We prefer to use 5-0 Dexon (Davis and Geck) for the subcutaneous layer and 6-0 nylon sutures for the skin. A pressure dressing can be placed on the side of the nose for 24 hours.

Postoperative Management

The patients may be discharged immediately after a short recovery, or the next day if necessary. The sutures are removed afterward. The decision as to follow-up radiotherapy depends on the final pathology report, and the potential for possible spread beyond surgical site, as suggested on CT scan.

REFERENCE

1. Flanagan JC, Mauriello JA. Management of lacrimal sac tumors. *Adv Ophthal Plast Reconstruct Surg* 1984;3:399.

CHAPTER 29

Management of Nasal and Sinus Disease

Jeremy L. Freeman, Per G. Liavaag, and Jeffrey Jay Hurwitz

The lacrimal surgeon should understand diseases of the nose and paranasal sinuses that may result in increased tear formation or epiphora. Knowledge of the management of these problems is necessary because the lacrimal system may be affected either pre- or postoperatively.

CONGENITAL ANOMALIES OF THE NOSE AND SINUSES

Choanal Atresia

Choanal atresia is a failure of canalization of the nasal cavity and most often occurs in the posterior aspect of the nose, i.e., posterior choana. The atresia may be membranous or bony, complete or incomplete, and bilateral or unilateral. Infants with bilateral choanal atresia will have symptoms in the neonatal period. Neonates are obligate nasal breathers, and thus with obstruction, ventilatory problems will develop. The child will also experience feeding difficulties as he is not able to suck because of the inability to breathe at the same time as feeding. The initial treatment is to secure the infant's airway. Thereafter, one should confirm the diagnosis by passing a catheter through the nose to the oropharynx; if this is unable to be done an atresia is suspected. Plain x-ray, taken while installing contrast solution into the nose, may make the diagnosis; computed tomography (CT) may also be useful.

Early surgery, to establish an airway, is the treatment

for bilateral choanal atresia. Most atresias may be incised or punctured and then dilated transnasally; however, some of the bony types should be managed through a transpalatal approach.

In unilateral atresia the symptoms are more subtle and less dramatic and may actually present in adulthood as nasal airway obstruction, necessitating transpalatal management.

Encephalocoele/Meningocoele

Encephalocoele or meningocoele is a result of developmental entrapment of neural and/or dural tissue within the nasal cavity or over the nose. This condition is probably caused by failed closure of the frontal/ethmoidal/orbital complex. It is treated surgically for functional or cosmetic problems. This problem must be differentiated from a dacryocystocele (amniotocele).

Dermoid Cyst

Dermoids are developmental anomalies with the haphazard arrangement of one or more tissues, forming a mass on the nose or in the nasal cavity. In the former type the patient presents with a subcutaneous, cystic tumor in the midline, between the glabella and the nasal tip. Dermoids may involve the intracranial cavity, simultaneously with the nose and sinuses. The important differential diagnosis is encephalocele, and this possibility must be excluded before surgery is contemplated to avoid intracranial complication. Further, a lacrimal sac mucocele, although usually beneath the medial canthal tendon, is in the differential.

Hypoplasia and Aplasia of Sinuses

Aplasia, and more often hypoplasia, of one or more of the sinuses may occur because of failure of canalization

J. L. Freeman: Head and Neck Program, Mount Sinai Hospital, and Department of Otolaryngology, University of Toronto Faculty of Medicine, Toronto, Ontario M5S 1A8, Canada.

P. G. Liavaag: Department of Otolaryngology, Mount Sinai Hospital, Toronto, Ontario M5G 1X5, Canada.

J. J. Hurwitz: Oculoplastics Program, Mount Sinai Hospital; and Department of Ophthalmology, University of Toronto Faculty of Medicine, Toronto, Ontario M5S 1A8 Canada.

of the bones of the facial skeleton housing the sinuses. Most often the frontal sinus is affected. This condition has no clinical significance, apart from the necessity to recognize it radiographically and not confuse it with an inflammatory process; no treatment is indicated.

ACQUIRED NASAL AND SINUS DISEASE

Inflammatory Disease

Awareness of inflammatory diseases that may affect the nose and sinuses is important to the lacrimal surgeon. Because of the proximity of these anatomical areas, these problems should be diagnosed and treated before any surgery is performed on the lacrimal system.

Noninfectious Disease

Rhinitis

Allergic Rhinitis. Allergic rhinitis is a nasal inflammatory disorder initiated by a mast cell/IgE-mediated hypersensitivity reaction to allergens. It is estimated that 10% to 15% of the population has allergic rhinitis. The disease usually starts before 30 years of age. The symptoms are episodic sneezing, itching, watery nasal discharge, and nasal congestion. Other associated symptoms are itching of the palate and the eyes. The symptoms may be seasonal as in allergy to grass, flowers, and trees or may be perennial, as in allergy to house dust, mites, and molds. Examination usually reveals pale bluish nasal mucosa with stigmata of inflammation (i.e., edema, clear discharge) (see Colorplate 7A following page 142).

The treatment of allergic rhinitis is avoidance of known allergens as far as possible, local application of steroids intranasally (steroid aerosol spray), and antihistamine medication if there are systemic symptoms. Turbinate reduction surgery may be performed if the turbinates are enlarged (see below).

Nonallergic Rhinitis. Nonallergic rhinitis is a heterogeneous group of disorders. "Vasomotoric rhinitis" is a term used for a condition with symptoms similar to allergic rhinitis, where there is no history of allergy and no cause of allergy can be found by skin tests or other provocative tests. The cause of this problem is likely a triggering event such as some foods or changes in weather that stimulate increased parasympathetic outflow to the nose, resulting in discharge and engorgement. The treatment is the same as for allergic rhinitis.

Nasal obstruction may also be caused by drugs, particularly some antihypertensive agents and psychosedatives, because of their interference with the autonomic nerve system.

During pregnancy, many women may experience periods of nasal congestion as a result of hormonal changes. The nasal mucosa may be congested and inflamed and again the treatment is the same as for allergic rhinitis.

Rhinitis medicamentosa is a condition in patients who have chronically applied topical decongestants. Used over a long period of time, this medication can cause a "rebound" congestion of the nasal mucosa. The treatment consists of convincing the patient to cease the use of nasal spray combined with the use of nasal steroid spray to reduce mucosal inflammation or turbinate reduction surgery (see below).

Turbinate Reduction Surgery. Turbinate surgery is indicated when enlargement of the turbinates is a contributing factor to the patient's congestion and medical therapy has failed. The procedure may be done in a variety of manners, usually under local anesthesia. To reduce the size of submucosal tissue, electrocautery may be used by inserting the electrode submucosally into the inferior turbinate. The electrical current produced destroys the submucosal tissue, causing reduction in size of the turbinate.

Cryosurgery, probably the most widely used outpatient modality for mechanical turbinate reduction, is performed to reduce the size of the turbinate by applying a liquid nitrogen cryoprobe, which is placed on the turbinate surface for approximately 1 minute. This actually destroys the hypertrophic turbinate tissue.

Infracturing and lateral movement of the inferior (and middle) turbinate can also be performed to improve the nasal airway. This can, if necessary, be combined with surgical resection of the turbinate bone. Care should be taken with turbinate resection because of the possibility of nasal hemorrhage as an early or late complication. With removal of the whole inferior turbinate there exists the risk of atrophic rhinitis, so this should be done as a last resort when the patient has been tried on conservative and less radical surgical regimens.

Nasal Polyposis

Nasal polyps are pedunculated outgrowths of edematous mucosa that appear as smooth, soft, glistening masses. They can be translucent, white, yellowish, or pink. The polyps can be simple or multiple and most often arise in the ethmoid region or from the superior or middle turbinates. A special subgroup of polyps is the antrochoanal polyp, arising in the antrum, spreading through the natural ostium, and presenting in the choana.

Allergy is a prime etiologic factor in the development of nasal polyps. Asthma is not uncommon in polyposis patients, as well as intolerance to acetylsalicylic acid (ASA). Polyposis may occur in mucoviscidosis (cystic fibrosis).

The most common symptoms of polyposis are obstruction, rhinorrhea, and hyposmia. Examination reveals soft, whitish, or hemorrhagic grape-like masses emanating from nasal mucosa (Fig. 1).

The treatment of polyposis is surgical removal of the polyps, but recurrences are common. If this is the case, the patient may be given local steroid treatment postoperatively to help prevent recurrence. Systemic steroid administration is effective against polyps if they are small, but this modality of therapy carries with it the inherent risks of the medication, which are not minimal.

Infectious Disease

Some infectious disease of the nose and sinuses may stimulate the first division of the trigeminal nerve. The afferent fibers via a reflex arc in turn stimulate the lacrimal gland to secrete tears. Therefore, resolution of the nasal problem may decrease this hypersecretion and ameliorate the symptom of epiphora.

Nasal

Acute Viral Infective Rhinitis. The common cold is an acute rhinitis, caused by various viruses, the rhinovirus being the most common. The viruses are transmitted in an air-borne fashion, with an incubation time of 1 to 3 days. The well known symptoms are obstruction, discharge, sneezing, and fever.

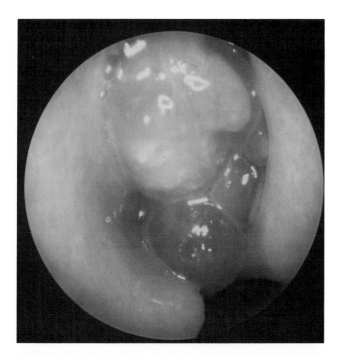

FIG. 1. The appearance of allergic nasal polyps emanating from the lateral wall of the nose. (Courtesy of Dr. Michael Hawke, Toronto.)

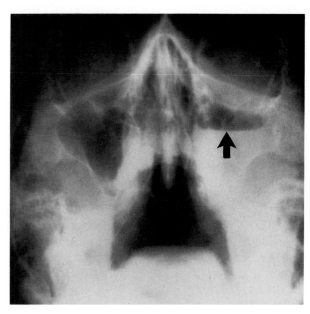

FIG. 2. Plain Water's view of the maxillary antra showing an air-fluid level in the left antrum (*arrow*).

There is no specific treatment for a common cold, but palliation includes rest, heat, analgesics, antipyretics, and local vasoconstrictors.

Sinus

Acute Bacterial Sinusitis. Acute sinusitis is most common in the maxillary sinus, followed by the ethmoid and the frontal sinus. During an upper respiratory infection the mucosa swells and obstructs the natural ostium. A sinus without drainage will be secondarily infected. Sinusitis may also be caused by foreign body, barotrauma, or dental disease. Severe deviation of the septum may predispose to maxillary sinusitis because of ostial blockage. The most common bacteria associated with sinusitis are pneumococci, streptococci, and haemophilus influenza. The symptoms include pain, nasal obstruction, and purulent discharge. Physical examination shows congested mucosa and possibly pus in the meatus. Plain x-rays of the sinuses show opacification, mucosal thickening, or an air-fluid level (Fig. 2). Transillumination, an examination method not in much use, shows decreased light transmission on the affected side because of fluid accumulation and/or thickened mucosa.

Initial therapy of acute sinusitis consists of analgesics, decongestants, and antibiotics; antral lavage is reserved for refractory disease.

Sinus Lavage. Antral lavage, which is a drainage of an empyema of the antrum, is an office procedure performed in patients who have failed to improve on medication. The procedure is most often done by puncturing the lateral wall of the nose through the inferior meatus.

The exact site for puncture is the middle meatus approximately 2 cm posterior along the nasal floor. A trocar is directed upward/laterally, toward a point between the ear lobe and the lateral canthus and then punched through the medial wall of the sinus. The stiletto is withdrawn and the cannula is pushed to the posterior wall and then withdrawn one cm. Lukewarm saline is then irrigated into the sinus, until the effluent is clear. The puncture is done without identifying the lacrimal duct since damage to the duct is a remote complication. However, if this is a consideration, the antrum can also be punctured through the canine fossa.

Trephination of the frontal sinus, for refractory frontal sinusitis, is performed through an incision at the inferomedial margin of the eyebrow. The bony opening can be made with a rotating burr. After irrigation, a temporary silicone tube is placed in the frontal sinus, for repeated irrigation.

The ethmoid sinus can be drained in the acute stage either through an intranasal, transantral (via a Caldwell-Luc), or medial canthal direct approach, which is described below. The sphenoid sinus is drained directly through the nose or via an external transethmoid approach.

Chronic Sinusitis

In chronic sinusitis there are irreversible changes to the mucosa, which discharges and becomes hypertrophic and/or polypoid. The symptoms are nasal obstruction, purulent discharge, abnormalities of smell, and pain in the head and face. On anterior rhinoscopy one may see reddened, inflamed mucosa and pus in the area of the ostium of the affected sinus. Rarely, ethmoidal sinusitis may produce a fistula draining through the skin in the medial canthal area. This must be differentiated from a lacrimal fistula. The radiographic images are much like those found in acute sinusitis. Most of these patients have failed conservative treatment with antibiotics and surgery should be considered to relieve symptoms.

For chronic ethmoiditis an exenteration of the ethmoid cells is done. Currently intranasal ethmoidectomy is done as part of functional endoscopic sinus surgery (FESS); by using this method the integrity of the nasolacrimal duct should be maintained because the procedure is done with direct visualization. (see Chapter 17).

External ethmoidectomy has been replaced by FESS and is not done as often as in the past. The external operation is performed through an incision between the medial canthus of the eye and the nasal dorsum. An approach along the medial orbital wall (the lamina papyracia) allows access to the ethmoid sinus air cells. An exenteration of the ethmoid cells is then performed, working partly through the incision and partly through the nose.

Surgery for chronic maxillary sinusitis is most often done as a FESS procedure transnasally. The well known Caldwell-Luc operation, opening of the sinus through the canine fossa, still has its place, but for widespread, chronic infective disease, infection of dental origin, or diagnosis of malignancy. It is also possible to exenterate the ethmoid sinuses through a transmaxillary Caldwell-Luc approach.

The aim of surgical treatment for chronic frontal sinusitis is to establish adequate drainage of the sinus. To effect this, an external frontoethmoidectomy may be done. An incision is made on the inferior margin of the eyebrow, extending inferiorly between the medial canthus and the nasal dorsum. The ethmoid sinus is approached as mentioned above. The floor of the frontal sinus is removed and a continuous passage is established between the frontal sinus, the ethmoid, and the nasal cavity. A plastic tube is left for several months in this "new" frontoethmoidal opening. Stenosis of the new duct is relatively common, however, resulting in recurrent disease.

Drainage may also be performed through an osteoplastic frontal sinusotomy approach. This procedure is performed through a coronal skin incision posterior to the hairline. An appropriate "template" of the frontal sinus is made from a nonmagnified plain anteroposterior film of the skull and is used as a guide to drilling out the outline of the frontal bone incision. The anterior wall of the sinus and the periosteum are elevated as a combined osteoplastic flap and the sinus is entered. If both frontal ostia are involved, the floor of the sinuses is removed and drainage is effected into the nose. If there is a normal ostium on the contralateral side to the disease, the abnormal sinus is drained into the normal. A Silastic stent is used for 2 months in the "new" ostium.

Complications of Sinusitis
Orbital complications. The ethmoid sinus' close proximity to the orbit and the extremely thin lamina papyracia between the orbit and this sinus makes it possible for infection to spread from the ethmoid cell to the orbit both directly and through the venous system. Such spread initially causes inflammatory edema of the upper eyelid because of obstruction of the venous drainage. The next step of orbital involvement is cellulitis, a diffuse inflammation of the orbital contents resulting in proptosis and chemosis (Fig. 3). A subperiosteal abscess may then develop, typically localized medially in the orbit. The globe may in these cases be displaced laterally and downward, and extraocular movements are impaired. If the infection spreads through periorbita, an orbital abscess develops with ophthalmoplegia, severe proptosis, and impairment of visual acuity. The next step in progression of a fulminant infection is spread through the orbital venous complex to the cavernous sinus, resulting in thrombosis or thrombophlebitis, characterized by

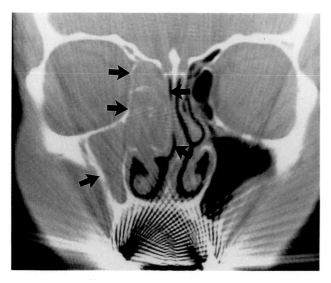

FIG. 3. CT of a patient with right pansinusitis.

pain in the face, chemosis, proptosis, visual impairment, and ophthalmoplegia—usually the patient is septic and systemically severely ill. The early stage of orbital involvement is treated with intravenous antibiotics only. If there is no resolution and CT scans show signs of subperiosteal abscess formation, drainage is necessary, through an external ethmoidectomy approach. In any medial orbital abscess, it should be determined whether the primary focus of infection is within the ethmoid sinus or the lacrimal system. Simple lacrimal duct syringing may answer this question.

Intracranial complications. Meningitis may develop from sinusitis, particularly from disease in the frontal and sphenoid sinuses. The infection spreads either directly or hematogenously. Epidural, subdural, and brain abscess may develop, as well as thrombosis of the sagittal or cavernous sinus. Appropriate antibiotics are administered and drainage is performed if necessary.

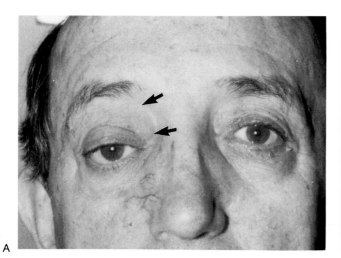

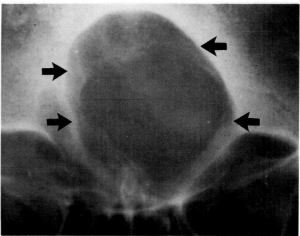

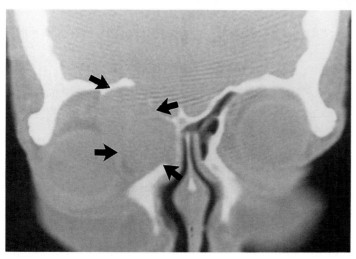

FIG. 4. A: Patient with a frontal sinus mucocele. Note the proptosis of the right eye and the mass in the superomedial aspect of the orbit (*arrow*). **B:** CT of patient with a mucocele of the frontal sinus. **C:** Plain film of another patient with a frontal mucocele. Notice the expansion of the sinus and the loss of the "scalloped border".

Osteomyelitis. Osteomyelitis may occur as a complication to sinusitis, particularly in frontal sinusitis. The most common bacteria are staphylococci and streptococci. If the frontal sinus is involved, the patient experiences frontal pain and inflammation or cellulitis of the forehead skin. If the bone is infected a severe forehead swelling may develop (Pott's puffy tumor). The diagnosis of osteomyelitis is confirmed by CT and radionuclide imaging. Treatment consists of prolonged use of high-dose antibiotics. The efficacy of hyperbaric oxygen is controversial. Surgical drainage may be required to remove necrotic bone.

Mucocele. Sinus ostial obstruction, due to sinusitis, may cause mucocele formation. Mucocele is a cystic swelling of the whole sinus and most often occurs in the frontal or frontoethmoidal sinuses, but may also occur uncommonly in the maxillary and sphenoidal sinus. In the frontal sinus, over time, with growth and pressure necrosis the mucocele may erode the thin bone in the floor of the frontal sinus and arise as a painless swelling at the medial canthus area. Displacement of the globe downward and laterally with proptosis may occur. A frontal mucocele may also extend intracranially with resultant intracranial complications as mentioned above. The mucocele may also grow anteriorly, eroding the anterior face of the frontal sinus and appear as a subcutaneous forehead mass. Plain x-rays and CT examination confirm the diagnosis (Fig. 4). Frontal sinus mucocele is treated surgically, either by external frontoethmoidectomy and drainage to the nose or through a frontal osteoplastic approach as mentioned above. An ethmoid mucocele is managed through a transfacial-medial canthal approach as mentioned above. Sphenoid mucocele is managed through a transnasal or transethmoid approach.

Fungal Infection of the Sinuses

Fungal infections of the sinuses occur, particularly in diabetics, debilitated, and immunosuppressed patients. Aspergillosis and mucormycosis are the most common mycotic infections, most often involving the maxillary sinus. The disease may be highly invasive, with rapid, aggressive behavior. Treatment consists of excision of the infected necrotic tissue and administration of systemic antifungal medication.

Allergic fungal sinusitis is an entity of diseases, where the pathogenesis is a hypersensitivity reaction in the spinal tissue, induced by the intraluminal fungus. Treatment is the same as mentioned above.

Atrophic Rhinitis

Atrophic rhinitis is a disease characterized by progressive atrophy of the nasal mucosa and turbinates, dryness, crusts, and offensive odor from the nose (ozena) (see Colorplate 7B following page 142). Although there is an enlargement of the airway, the patient feels congested. The etiology of this disease is unclear although bacteria, such as *Klebsiella ozaenae,* have been linked to it. Most likely the bacteria are present secondary to tissue changes and do not cause the disease per se. Other factors that have been regarded as causative factors are endocrine imbalance, nutritional factors, and intranasal destruction (i.e., aggressive surgical removal of anatomical structures) after previous surgery.

Treatment includes nasal irrigation with isotonic saline solution as well as surgical procedures with the aim of reducing the airway and increasing nasal surface area. Surgical closure of the nostrils, as well as bone grafting to the submucosa, have been attempted to treat this disease, but with limited success.

TUMORS OF THE NOSE AND SINUSES

Benign Tumors

Epithelial Tumors

Epithelial tumors may arise from "covering" tissue or glandular tissue. Papillomas may be fungiform, inverted, or cylindrical. They should be removed completely, preferably with a margin of normal tissue around.

Inverted papillomas commonly arise from the lateral wall of the nasal cavity, but may emanate from almost anywhere in the nose or sinuses. Histologically, the epithelial tumor grows in an inverted fashion instead of growing outward, as in fungiform papillomas. Clinically, the tumor appears as a whitish grape-like mass often not unlike nasal polyps. There is a high tendency to local recurrence without aggressive resection. This tumor can also undergo malignant transformation or be associated with concomitant malignancy, but this is quite uncommon. The imaging work-up should include CT and/or magnetic resonance imaging (MRI).

Inverted papillomas should be treated aggressively and be removed by lateral rhinotomy, medial maxillectomy, and ethmoidectomy if necessary. An alternative to lateral rhinotomy is an approach via a facial degloving approach performed through a transgingival incision. The lacrimal system may be involved with tumor or injured during surgery. Lacrimal intubation is useful if the system is compromised but intact. Otherwise, a dacryocystorhinostomy (DCR) with intubation affords the best chance for a patent system postoperatively (see Colorplate 7C following page 142). Uncommonly, benign salivary gland tumors can arise in the nose or sinuses and these are managed by local resection. Mucous retention cysts occur commonly and may be left untreated if asymptomatic, provided that they are differentiated from malignant disease.

Nonepithelial tumors

Most nonepithelial tumors are derived from mesenchymal cells. They are classified according to their tissue of origin, e.g., chondroma, hemangioma, osteoma, etc. Symptoms are consistent with the presence of a mass or, as in the case of hemangioma or angiofibroma, bleeding. The diagnostic work-up includes plain films, CT, MRI, and in the case of vascular lesions, angiography. The latter may be used in conjunction with embolization as a preoperative measure to reduce bleeding. Generally, benign mesenchymally derived lesions are removed using standard nasal or sinus approaches as described above.

Malignant Tumors

Epithelial Tumors

Squamous cell carcinomas comprise 80% to 90% of the malignant tumors in the nose and paranasal sinuses and most often arise in the ethmoidal/antral region. Workers exposed to nickel or chromate have an increased incidence of this type of cancer. Squamous cell carcinomas may also arise in the skin in the nasal vestibule. These are high grade tumors that invade locally and metastasize to regional lymph nodes and to distant sites. Malignant salivary gland tumors occur in the nasal cavity and sinuses. A high incidence of adenocarcinomas are seen in woodworkers.

Malignant Melanoma

Primary malignant melanoma can arise from the intranasal mucous membrane and can be melanotic or amelanotic. This aggressive tumor has an unpredictable, but usually a lethal, outcome.

Esthesioneuroblastoma (see Colorplate 7B)

Esthesioneuroblastoma (olfactory neuroblastoma) is a malignant, neurectodermal tumor arising from the olfactory neurosensory epithelium in the upper vault of the nasal cavity and cribriform plate area. The tumor is polypoidal and extremely vascular. This is a slow-growing lesion that invades locally and may metastasize late to regional or distant lymph nodes. The lacrimal system may be involved early in these patients and tearing may be one of the presenting symptoms. A CT-dacryocystogram (CT-DCG) will be helpful if this tumor is suspected.

Nonepithelial Tumors

Malignant nonepithelial tumors are generally derived from mesenchymal tissue. As with benign tumors, they are classified according to the tissue of origin, e.g., chondrosarcoma, angiosarcoma, osteosarcoma, etc. Sarcomas of the nose and sinus are high grade tumors, but do not usually metastasize.

Symptoms

The most common symptoms of all malignant tumors are nasal obstruction and epistaxis. Because of the large air spaces in the sinuses, these tumors do not give early symptoms and therefore often present at an advanced stage. Late disease is characterized by pain, dental symptoms (tooth loosening), and growth through the palate or into the skin. With greater growth, the tumor may also give orbital and/or lacrimal symptoms. With even further invasion, the base of skull is affected with subsequent cranial neuropathy.

Signs

On examination, malignant tumors in general appear as fungiform, hemorrhagic, destructive masses. Often there is loss of normal bony architecture. There may be evidence of the mass invading local sites such as the oral cavity, skin of the face, or orbit. At times neurologic signs may be present because of base of skull involvement. The neck may reveal regional metastatic disease.

Plain films, CT, and MRI are helpful in diagnosis and mapping the extent of the tumor.

Treatment

In general, malignant tumors of the nose and sinuses are treated with radiation or surgery as single modality treatment or a combination of the two as a planned combined effort.

The surgical approach to tumors of the maxilla is the en bloc resection of the maxilla through a transfacial access. This is performed through a Weber-Ferguson incision (infraorbital, lateral rhinotomy, and lip split). The en bloc resection is done in such a way that the tumor is encompassed by the bony margins of the extirpation. Bone "cuts" are performed with saws or drills through the hard palate, lacrimal bone, floor of orbit, zygoma, and pterygoid plates. Intraoperatively, the patient is fitted with a dental obturator to close the large oroantral fistula created; this is converted into a permanent prosthesis later.

Where the tumor abuts or actually invades the anterior skull base (e.g., esthesioneuroblastoma) a combined intra- and extracranial removal (craniofacial resection) of the tumor is done. This is performed through a frontal craniotomy done by a neurosurgical team and a transfacial approach done by the head and neck team. This formidable procedure has of late been beneficial with minimal morbidity to many patients who have heretofore been relegated to death from their disease.

TRAUMA OF THE NOSE AND SINUSES

Simple Fractures

Nasal Bone Fracture

The nasal bones may be fractured by direct blunt or penetrating trauma. The nasal bones may sustain a simple or comminuted fracture. The alignment of the bones may be in an undisplaced position or in a displaced one, resulting in an external nasal cosmetic deformity. Concomitant fracture of the septum may accompany any nasal fracture. The end result of the latter can be airway obstruction due to septal deviation. The immediate evaluation of a nasal fracture focuses on the cosmetic appearance and the status of the septum. Radiographs may be helpful in diagnosing a fracture, although the clinical appearance and the patient's perception of a change is of primary importance. The presence of a hematoma of the septum must be ruled out—if present, drainage should be done immediately to avoid infection of the hematoma and possible necrosis of cartilage with nasal collapse.

Patients with nasal fractures may have tearing due to mucosal irritation and secondary afferent stimulation of the lacrimal gland. However, trauma sufficient to fracture the nose may also fracture the bony housing of the nasolacrimal canal leading to tearing due to lacrimal obstruction necessitating lacrimal surgery in addition to nasal surgery for correction.

The treatment of displaced nasal fracture is closed reduction, which can be accomplished by a combination of manual and instrument manipulation of the nasal bones to the desired position. A repositioning of the septum, if it is significantly deviated, can be done at the time of closed reduction or at a later date. If the nasal bones do not realign to the proper position, an open reduction is indicated. This is done by introducing an osteotome through intranasal incisions to free the nasal bones so that they may be molded to the correct position. If the nasal bones have healed in an incorrect position (fusion is usually solid by about 14 days), osteotomies may have to be done to free the bones for repositioning.

If the injury is caused by a violent telescoping force from anterior, a comminuted fracture of the nasoethmoidal complex may occur. The radix of the nose is displaced backward and the nasoethmoid structures are spread laterally into the orbits. The patient presents with a flattening of the nasal root and widening of the intercanthal distance. These patients are best operated by an open approach through a bilateral medial canthal (ethmoidectomy-type) incision. The fractured fragments of bone are carefully reduced and either wired or plated together. It is important that the medial canthal tendon be repaired and reattached to avoid permanent telecanthus.

Septum Deviation

Septum displacement/deviation may be caused by pressure during intrauterine life, parturition, or nasal trauma later in life. There may be concomitant deviation of the external nasal skeleton or not—external deformity occurs if the deviation involves the supporting aspect of the septum (i.e., that portion of the cartilage anterior to a line from the radix to the anterior nasal spine). The dominant symptom caused by significant septal deviation is nasal obstruction, especially on the side to which the septum deviates. The deviation is easily noticed on anterior rhinoscopy (Fig. 5). If there is indication for surgical treatment, a repositioning or septoplasty is performed through an intranasal approach. This is performed through a submucus approach, wherein the cartilaginous and bony obstructive components of the septum are repositioned.

Occasionally, a deviated septum compromises the technical aspect of a DCR, so that in order to have enough room for the rhinostomy, a septoplasty is mandated.

Blow-Out Fracture of the Orbit

The "pure" blow-out fracture is an isolated fracture of one of the walls of the orbit, usually the floor, caused by either a sudden implosive impact on the globe resulting

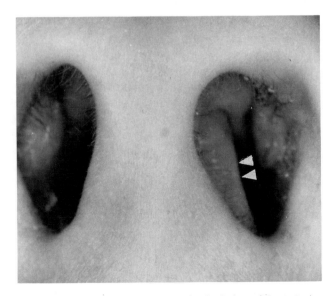

FIG. 5. The external appearance of a deviation of the anterior (caudal) aspect of the septum.

in an increase in intraorbital pressure or by a buckling force to the orbital rim. If the bone fragments are displaced, this occurs downward into the maxillary antrum; at the same time the periorbital fat may herniate into the antrum and become entrapped, causing restriction of extraocular movement commonly in the upward direction leading to diplopia. In this situation, the treatment consists of exploring the orbital floor through a subciliary or transconjunctival approach. The herniated fat is reduced and the bone fragments are replaced and wired if possible for fixation. If there is a defect in the floor, autogenous bone, nasal septum or artificial sheets may be used to reconstruct the orbital floor. Fractures involving significant herniation of orbital contents may have to be treated to avoid permanent diplopia and enophthalmous—the latter is caused by lipodystrophy of the herniated fat.

Fracture of the Zygomaticomaxillary Compound

Because of its prominent location, the zygomaticomaxillary compound is subjected to injury by direct blows to the cheek. Usually there is a disruption of the zygomaticofrontal suture and fractures of the anterior and lateral wall of the maxilla, the floor of the orbit, and the zygomatic arch; this is the so-called tripod fracture. These fractures may have the features of a "blow-out" fracture in addition to the cosmetic deformity of flattening of the malar area due to depression or rotation of the zygoma. There is characteristically sensory loss in the area innervated by the infraorbital nerve. The fracture is reduced for cosmetic and/or functional reasons. This is usually accomplished through an approach such as for "blow-out" fractures in addition to an approach to the frontozygomatic suture through the eyebrow in order to establish two-point fixation with miniplates or wires.

Frontal Sinus Fractures

These fractures are the result of direct force on the forehead and may involve the anterior or posterior wall or both. The indication for intervention is a cosmetic deformity or involvement of the anterior cranial fossa (e.g., dural tear with cerebrospinal fluid leak). The optimal approach is via an osteoplastic sinusotomy access. The necessary work can be carried out through the sinus after removal of the anterior wall. Bone fragments are either plated or wired.

Complex Facial Fractures Involving the Sinuses and Nose

Severe facial trauma usually as a result of motor vehicle accidents or gunshot wounds may cause multiple facial fractures. These are classified as Le Fort types, and there are three basic types.

Le Fort I fractures involve the lower facial skeleton with separation of the upper alveolar structure from the maxilla proper. Le Fort II fractures traverse the nasal bones, orbital floor, and lateral maxillary walls. Le Fort III fractures occur through the orbital roof, nasal bones, and frontozygomatic sutures (craniofacial separation). These injuries often occur in combination and are best managed with open reduction and appropriate plating or wiring techniques. Le Fort II fractures typically involve the lacrimal system.

GRANULOMATOUS DISEASE OF THE NOSE

Wegener's Granulomatosis

Wegener's granulomatosis can be systemic or localized and primarily affects the upper airway, lungs, and kidneys. Histologically, the disease is characterized by necrotizing granulomas and vasculitis. Patients present with nasal congestion, discharge, and eventually crusting. The nasal findings can be negligible in the beginning, but later, widespread ulcerations and septal destruction may occur with the development of systemic symptoms such as fatigue, malaise, and weight loss. Some patients have orbital and/or otologic manifestations.

In the early stages, the diagnosis is difficult because the histologic picture is not always clear cut. Diagnosis has been easier since the anticytoplasmatic autoantibody (ANCA) test was developed. The disease is treated with chemotherapy.

Lacrimal obstruction may occur with Wegener's and repair is possible using modified techniques (see Chapters 22 and 36).

Sarcoidosis

Sarcoidosis is a systemic disease that may also involve the nose. Histologically, it is characterized by noncaseating granulomata. Both the external and internal nose can be involved, with the latter more commonly involved. On intranasal examination, one may see a hyperemic, swollen mucosa or papules. Tearing may be a problem, due to secondary hypersecretion from nasal irritation or primary lacrimal obstruction. The major differential diagnosis is tuberculosis.

Serum angiotensin-converting enzyme (SACE) test has made the diagnosis easier to make, but histologic confirmation is mandatory.

Treatment is systemic steroids. Many times, however, it is necessary to establish a nasal airway for the comfort of the patient and this can be effected by turbinate-reducing surgery.

Tuberculosis

Tuberculosis localized to the nasal cavity or to the sinuses is rare and is most often secondary to disease in the lungs. Usually the cartilaginous part of the septum is involved, and septal perforation may occur. The symptoms are discharge, obstruction, and eventually pain. The diagnosis is made by bacteriologic examination and the patients are treated with antituberculous drugs.

Lupus vulgaris, the cutaneous type of tuberculosis, can involve the nose and can be nodular or ulcerative. Again, treatment is the same as systemic tuberculosis.

Leprosy

Leprosy is caused by the *Mycobacterium leprae* and is indigenous to developing countries. Nasal and sinus presentation is with symptoms of discharge, crusting, and nasal perforation. Diagnosis is made by culture of the organism. Treatment is as for systemic leprosy.

BONE DYSCRASIAS OF THE PARANASAL SINUSES

Fibrous Dysplasia

Fibrous dysplasia is a developmental abnormality of the facial skeleton with arrest of normal bone growth in the weaving phase and a concomitant appearance of disorganized, osteoid, and mesenchymal tissue. The disease manifests usually late in childhood, during the growth period, and tends to stabilize after puberty. In most cases only one bone is affected, the maxilla being the most common, although polyostotic forms may occur. The symptoms consist of a localized swelling that can be considerable, with typical radiographic findings. Usually the clinical and radiographic picture is all that is necessary for diagnosis, although this may be confirmed by biopsy. Of note, tearing may be due to bony closure of the lacrimal duct and dacryocystorhinostomy is usually curative.

There are differing opinions as to how aggressive a surgical approach is indicated. Generally, however, tumor-reducing surgery should be done to manage cosmetic abnormalities and functional impairments.

Ossifying Fibroma

Ossifying fibroma is a disease with many similarities to fibrous dysplasia. In contrast to that disease, it is encapsulated, and the onset of the disease is later in life. The treatment is surgical excision.

Paget's Disease (Osteitis Deformans)

Paget's disease is a replacement of normal compact cortical bone with hyperostotic vascular bone of the cancellous type. As with fibrous dysplasia, the diagnosis is made clinically and radiographically. Surgical treatment is directed at restoring a normal cosmetic and functional state. A rapid growth of pagetoid bone may be indicative of osteogenic sarcoma. As with other bony dyscrasias, if tearing is a problem due to closure of the nasolacrimal duct, dacryocystorhinostomy is usually curative.

SUGGESTED READINGS

1. Ballantyne J, Groves J. *Diseases of the ear, nose and throat,* vol 3, 4th ed. London: Butterworths; 1979.
2. Batsakis JG. *Tumors of the head and neck,* 2nd ed. Baltimore: Williams & Wilkins; 1974.
3. Dingman RO, Natvig P. *Surgery of facial fractures.* Philadelphia: WB Saunders; 1964.
4. English GM. Congenital anomalies of the nose, nasopharynx, and paranasal sinuses. In: English GM, ed. *Otolaryngology,* rev ed. Philadelphia: JB Lippincott; 1993.
5. English GM. Sinusitis. In: English GM, ed. *Otolaryngology,* rev ed. Philadelphia: JB Lippincott; 1988.
6. Kornblut AD, Wolf SM, deFries HO, Fauci AS. Wegener's granulomatosis. *Otolaryngol Clin North Am* 1982;15(3).
7. Lehman RH, Toohill RJ, Grossman TW, Belson TP. Rhinitis medicamentosa. In: English GM, ed. *Otolaryngology,* rev ed. Philadelphia: JB Lippincott; 1984.
8. Maniglia AJ, Goodwin WJ. Congenital choanal atresia. *Otolaryngol Clin North Am* 1981;14(1).
9. McDonald TJ. Granulomatous diseases of the nose. In: English GM, ed. *Otolaryngology,* rev ed. Philadelphia: JB Lippincott; 1990.
10. Mygind N, Malm L. Pathophysiology and management of allergic and nonallergic rhinitis. In: English GM, ed. *Otolaryngology,* rev ed. Philadelphia: JB Lippincott; 1992.
11. Rice DH. Chronic frontal sinus disease. *Otolaryngol Clin North Am* 1993;26(4).
12. Sofferman RA. Cysts and bone dyscrasias of the paranasal sinuses. In: English GM, ed. *Otolaryngology,* rev ed. Philadelphia: JB Lippincott; 1988.
13. Zinreich J. Imaging of inflammatory sinus disease. *Otolaryngol Clin North Am* 1993;26(4).

CHAPTER 30

Rhinoplasty Operation and the Lacrimal Drainage System

Kris Conrad and Jeffrey Jay Hurwitz

Rhinoplasty has become one of the most common cosmetic operations today. The results of the surgery are usually extremely gratifying, but nevertheless one may encounter at times less than optimal results and occasionally significant complications. There exists a concern among otolaryngologists, ophthalmologists, facial plastic surgeons, and plastic surgeons that some of these complications may be affecting the lacrimal system.

The lacrimal duct, sac, or even canaliculi are at risk by their proximity to the site of lateral osteotomies, which are never carried out under direct vision. Damage to the lacrimal drainage apparatus can occur during rhinoplasty operations, as evidenced by reports in the literature (1). The likelihood of such complications will depend on the particular technique used and it almost always affects the lacrimal sac rather than the canaliculi or the duct. The vulnerability of the lacrimal sac results from it not being completely protected by bone. Until recently, the lateral osteotomy was often performed with the use of a Joseph saw. This often led to extensive tissue disturbance. The straight line produced by such an osteotomy, disrespecting the natural curve on the face of the maxilla in the area of the nasomaxillary groove, could cut deeply through the thick bar of bone, which is the midline maxillary buttress protecting the lacrimal canal. With such a technique, greater likelihood of lacrimal drainage system injuries existed (2). Newer techniques utilize osteotomes rather than saws, and modification of the line of the osteotomy from straight to curved (Fig. 1). A number of factors relate to the risk of lacrimal damage:

1. Periosteal elevation, routinely performed by some surgeons to create a tunnel for the passage of an osteotome, may take place deep to the medial canthal tendon. The anterior wall of the sac is immediately posterior to the undersurface of the medial canthal tendon, thus being predisposed to shearing injury during periosteal elevation or when an instrument (a saw or an osteotome) is passed under the tendon.
2. The use of a curved osteotome without prior periosteal elevation is much less likely to create tissue disturbance deep to the medial canthal tendon. Such osteotomies have greater ability to follow a natural, safe course along the nasomaxillary groove in the pathway of least resistance (Fig. 2).
3. The maxillary bone is thicker close to the lacrimal fossa. This thickening is a part of the medial maxillary buttress, which should be lateral (posterior) to the properly performed curved, lateral osteotomy. Such an osteotomy is usually situated 4 to 7 mm medial to the lacrimal crest (3).

DISCUSSION

From the above considerations relating to the anatomy of lacrimal apparatus and the technical aspects of the modified curved, lateral osteotomy (4), it appears that serious injury to the lacrimal drainage system occurs infrequently as a result of modern rhinoplasty operations. In cases where epiphora has occurred postoperatively, it probably was related to postsurgical edema or

K. Conrad: Facial Plastic Surgery Unit, Department of Otolaryngology, Mount Sinai Hospital, and Department of Otolaryngology, University of Toronto Faculty of Medicine, Toronto, Ontario M5S 1A8, Canada.

J. J. Hurwitz: Oculoplastics Program, Mount Sinai Hospital; and Department of Ophthalmology, University of Toronto Faculty of Medicine, Toronto, Ontario M5S 1A8, Canada.

to a minor soft tissue injury that appears to have been exclusively in the area of the sac. Symptoms usually, but not always, subside completely within 3 months postoperatively without subsequent intervention. The previously used techniques of lateral osteotomy relying on the use of periosteal elevation and the application of saws have resulted, in some instances, in permanent lacrimal drainage obstruction requiring surgical correction. When lateral osteotomies are carried out in a curved manner with a curved osteotome, usually without periosteal elevation, the risk of lacrimal damage is further decreased.

It is advisable to observe the presence of bleeding into the conjunctival cul-de-sac immediately following a rhinoplasty. Such a clinical sign may represent bleeding from the packed nasal cavity through a patent nasolacrimal duct or indeed may be related to injury to the lacrimal sac. Should this occur, one may irrigate the system to prevent blood clot formation, which in turn may lead to organized scar and obstruction.

Lacrimal obstruction and the need for a dacryocyst-

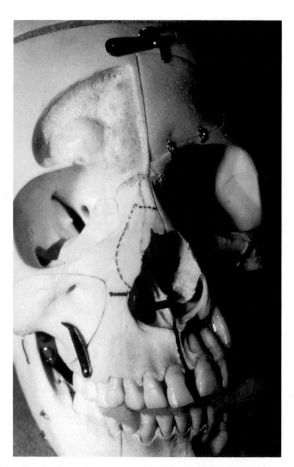

FIG. 2. Surface bony marking of modified curved lateral osteotomy.

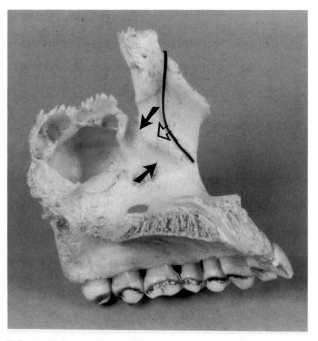

FIG. 1. Left maxilla showing lateral wall of nasal cavity and lacrimal canal (*black arrows*) protected anteriorly by medial maxillary buttress (*white arrow*). Note marked curved line of safe lateral osteotomy as seen on the inner aspect of the lateral wall.

orhinostomy following a cosmetic procedure such as a rhinoplasty is a devastating complication. Fortunately, modern modifications of the rhinoplasty procedure and attention to anatomic detail with awareness of the lacrimal system has even more significantly reduced this complication.

REFERENCES

1. Flanagan JC. Epiphora following rhinoplasty. *Ann Ophthalmol* 1978;10:1239–1242.
2. Flowers RS, Anderson R. Injury to the lacrimal apparatus during rhinoplasty. *Plast Reconstr Surg* 1968;42:577–581.
3. Thomas JR, Griner N. The relationship of lateral osteotomies in rhinoplasty to the lacrimal drainage system. *Otolaryngol Head Neck Surg* 1986;94(3):362–367.
4. Thomas JR, Griner NR, Remmler DJ. Steps for a safer method of osteotomies in rhinoplasty. *Laryngoscope* 1987;97:746–747.

CHAPTER 31

Lacrimal Trauma

Injuries and Management

Oleh Antonyshyn and Jeffrey Jay Hurwitz

A. Injuries to the Lacrimal System

The lacrimal drainage pathways may be involved through various types of injuries. The most common injury of the lacrimal system is through trauma. The trauma may involve sharp or blunt trauma to the soft tissues or the bony skeleton surrounding the nasolacrimal duct. The soft tissues may also be injured by lime burns, medications, etc. For the purpose of this chapter only those lacrimal injuries due to trauma will be discussed.

Traumatic injuries of the lacrimal system may be divided into two groups—those involving the punctum, canaliculi, and common canaliculus, and those involving the lacrimal sac and intraosseous lacrimal duct.

INJURIES TO THE PUNCTUM, CANALICULI AND COMMON CANALICULUS

Physiologic Principles in Consideration of Canalicular Injuries

The tears are pumped by the action of the orbicularis muscle pushing them along the upper and lower marginal tear strips to the lacrimal lake at the inner canthus.

The tears then pass by capillary action through the upper and lower puncta and then proceed along the canaliculi to the common canaliculus. Positive and negative pressure within the sac allows tears to be suctioned into the sac and, when the pressure changes within the sac, the tears are then propelled down through the nasolacrimal duct into the nose. A system of valves within the lacrimal drainage pathways usually prevents reflux of tears back into the palpebral aperture. It may well be that with forced orbicularis contraction, the tears pass all the way from the conjunctival sac into the nose and that the effect of changes of pressure within the tear sac do not have that much of a role to play. However, it is known that the orbicularis of the eyelids and the Horner's and Jones' muscles, which are in close proximity to the canaliculi, are important for draining of the tears through the system and ultimately into the nose.

Although it has, in the past, been suggested that the lower canaliculus "is for the patient to drain tears," and the upper canaliculus "is for the ophthalmologist," there is no question that the upper system is important for the drainage of tears through to the nose (1,2). The upper and lower puncta, when the eyes are closed, come to sit on the opposing eyelid and not in direct contact with each other. When the eye is open, the tears are suctioned into the puncta and then into the canaliculi. In studies where one canaliculus has been blocked and the tear flow measured through the other canaliculus, it has been shown that anywhere up to 50% of the tear flow goes through the unblocked canaliculus (3). There are also variations so that some patients might drain tears better

O. Antonyshyn: Plastic Surgery Unit, Sunnybrook Health Sciences Centre, and Department of Surgery, University of Toronto Faculty of Medicine, Toronto, Ontario M5S 1A8, Canada.

J. J. Hurwitz: Oculoplastics Program, Mount Sinai Hospital; and Department of Ophthalmology, University of Toronto Faculty of Medicine, Toronto, Ontario M5S 1A8, Canada.

through the upper canaliculus than the lower canaliculus, although it is felt that the lower canaliculus is probably more significant in the drainage of tears in most patients but maybe not by a significant amount. Linberg's studies suggested that plugging one punctum temporarily with a plug would not lead to significant tearing because enough tears would be drained through the other uninvolved punctum and canaliculus. These observations and publications (1,3) are extremely important in determining the indications for individual canalicular repair.

Etiology of Canalicular Lacerations

The common causes of canalicular obstructions are fights, falls, and traffic injuries. However, bites either by dogs or humans and scratches from other animals are quite common, especially in younger patients (4).

The lacerations may be due to sharp injuries or to avulsions. Avulsions may be due to trauma remote from the canaliculus. The avulsions look very much like direct lacerations to the canaliculus (5). In fact, the lacerations of the common canaliculus are probably most often due to avulsion injuries (6). The lateral portion of the canaliculus seems to be more resilient than is the medial portion and, therefore, most of the avulsions are found medially in the area of the common canaliculus or where the upper and lower canaliculi join the common canaliculus. In fact, the most common location of canalicular laceration seems to be beneath the anteromedial aspect of the caruncle, 2 mm in front of the junction with the lacrimal sac (7). The medial canthal tendon may often be avulsed, and this should be looked for clinically (8). The inferior canaliculus is lacerated almost four times as often as the upper canaliculus (9).

Clinical Assessment of the Eyelids and Canaliculi in Medial Canthal Trauma

Any laceration in the area of the medial canthus should have an assessment of the lacrimal system. The lower punctum should be dilated and a probe passed through the punctum. This should be done gently in the situation where there may be an unroofing of the canaliculus and part of the canalicular wall is indeed intact. One should observe at the slit lamp if there is any visibility of the probe within the depth of the laceration. One must also try to see if there is a visible medial cut end of the lower canaliculus within the lower lid (Fig. 1). In trying to identify this clinically, it is helpful to wipe the area with a cotton applicator and put some drops of Neosynephrine onto the defect to blanch some of the surrounding tissues. One may follow the eyelid margin medially from the punctum. The quadrangular aspect of the eyelid lateral to the punctum becomes triangular medial to the punctum, and this is often useful in trying to conceptualize the medial cut end of the lower canaliculus (Fig. 2). Similarly in an upper canalicular laceration, the same observations can be made on the upper lid (Fig. 3). If the lesion is due to a bite, the amount of necrotic material should be observed and one should determine whether there is any part of the eyelid missing.

Indications for Surgical Repair

If one canaliculus is obstructed and the eyelid is in good apposition to the uninvolved eyelid, tears may flow through the ipsilateral canaliculus if it is only the one canaliculus that is blocked (10). There is even the possibility that if one canaliculus is blocked, the other uninvolved canaliculus may increase the drainage of tears

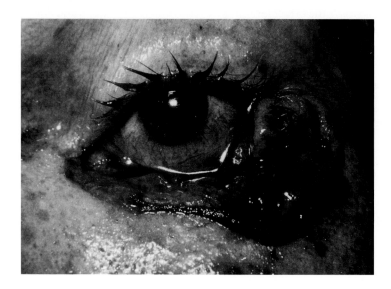

FIG. 1. Patient with lacerated eyelid and canaliculus. The lid has been torn laterally, but there are no missing pieces and both ends of the cut canaliculus can be seen on slit lamp.

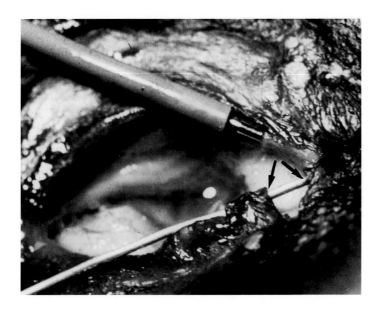

FIG. 2. Appearance of lower canalicular laceration in cadaver. The lateral end of the cut lower canaliculus can be seen and the probe can be passed through into the medial end of the cut canaliculus.

flowing through it (11). The decision as to whether repair is necessary or not should not be based on dacryocystography or lacrimal scanning, as this does little in the acute situation to help the surgeon. Because of the variability of tear flow from patient to patient, it is unpredictable as to whether any individual patient will have tearing if the lacerated canaliculus is left unrepaired (12). Therefore, it would seem prudent that if the canaliculus *can* be repaired, that one should at least attempt it at the same time as one would be attempting the repair of the lacerated eyelid. It has been reported that in 75% of the patients in whom an attempted inferior canalicular repair has failed, 75% of these patients did not have any tearing (13). To answer the corollary of this, we performed a study looking at patients who had been referred to us more than 5 days following the injury from a period of 5 days to 3 months, in whom the lid had been primarily

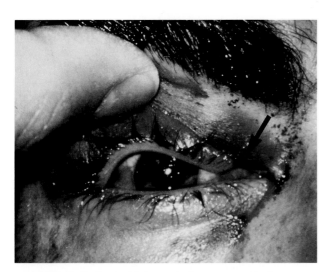

FIG. 3. Patient with lacerated upper canaliculus.

sutured and the canalicular laceration had not been addressed. In all these patients, there were no complaints of tearing even though a canalicular laceration had been documented. Because of the lack of symptoms and the delayed presentation of the patients to our department, after discussing the options with the patients, no repair was undertaken. All these patients were seen in follow-up approximately 1 to 3 months later and in none of these patients were there any symptoms of tearing. Of note is the fact that the eyelids had been repaired properly and were in good proximity to the globe and the upper lid. It would seem that if indeed the eyelids had been well repaired and the other canaliculus is functional, then the patient may indeed be tear-free on an ongoing basis without having to repair the canaliculus at a later date.

These observations suggest that if a canalicular laceration is a difficult one to repair, that is, if a piece of the canaliculus is missing or if there is severe infection and necrosis of the tissues, then one might argue to leave things to see how much tearing the patient has at a later date. As has been stated, if the patient does have tearing later on, the canaliculus can be attempted to be reconstructed. Alternatively, a simple dacryocystorhinostomy (DCR) might be performed to relieve the patient of epiphora (14) rather than inserting a permanent Jones bypass tube, but only if the ipsilateral canaliculus, eyelids, and the rest of the lacrimal system are normal. The DCR will augment the flow through the one remaining canaliculus.

When to Repair

If the injury is due to a bite, then tetanus toxoid must be used and the wound must be cleaned. The patient may have other injuries such as a lacerated globe or craniofacial or neurosurgical emergencies whereby the patient would be undergoing a general anesthetic. It is reasonable while the patient is under anesthesia to assess the lacrimal system and repair it if possible. However, it has been our experience that the easiest canaliculi to repair were those that had presented to us at least 2 or 3 days following the injury. The tissues tend to become somewhat avascular, and the medial cut end of the lower canaliculus or upper canaliculus becomes white and edematous, making it easy to view on the slit lamp. We feel that it is prudent, if possible, to schedule the repair electively and to perform the repair within 5 days following the injury. If the wound is necrotic, especially if it has been due to a bite, it is important to use prophylactic antibiotics and to clean the wound and revise the edges by removing the necrotic tissues.

If both the upper and lower canaliculi are lacerated, this usually occurs close to the common canaliculus. If this is the situation, or if the common canaliculus is lacerated, we prefer to let all the inflammation settle down and perform a canaliculodacryocystorhinostomy electively at a later date. We feel that it is extremely difficult, if both canaliculi or the common canaliculus have been lacerated, to be able to find the medial cut ends because there is usually a loss of supporting structure and there is the risk of doing further damage trying to pass a bicanalicular Silastic stent tube (6).

There is no urgency to repair the canaliculus or the eyelid. One may use cool compresses on the wound even if the lid is open, treat with prophylactic antibiotics, and bring the patient back electively to repair the eyelid and canaliculus.

Should an Upper Canalicular Laceration be Repaired?

Repairing an upper canalicular laceration is a debatable issue in the literature, but we feel that since an upper canaliculus is important in some patients for tear flow, and in fact may be even more important than the lower canaliculus in certain individuals, that if an upper canalicular laceration may be repaired easily, one should attempt this. Spoor suggests that with an upper canalicular laceration one should use a monocanalicular intubation so that there would be no possibility of damage to the lower canaliculus. However, he uses a bicanalicular intubation for repair of a lower canalicular laceration (15).

Punctal Injuries

Injuries to the puncta and canaliculi may be due to sharp or blunt trauma. If the punctum itself has a small laceration within it, it may end up functioning as a "three-snip" procedure and no repair might be necessary. If there is a large funnel across the punctum and proximal canaliculus, one may put in a stent suture in the proximal canaliculus while leaving the punctum open (16) (Fig. 4).

As with lower canalicular lacerations, late repair after 1 week has a much lower success rate.

Canalicular Injuries

Basic principles of canaliculus repair include:

1. The uninvolved canaliculus must not be damaged.
2. The common canaliculus must not be damaged.
3. The lacrimal sac and duct must not be damaged.
4. It must be remembered that if a canalicular repair is unsuccessful, that the patient may be rendered free of tears by simply performing a subsequent DCR without the insertion of a Jones bypass tube, so that tear drainage through the uninvolved ipsilateral canaliculus may be augmented (17). This has been shown by Jones to work in approximately two thirds of cases. Our success rate doing a DCR when one canaliculus is obstructed is approximately 70% to 75% (18).
5. The lids must be repaired so that there is good apposition between the lids and the globe and so that the lids will touch each other on eyelid closure, thus allowing tears to get through the uninvolved punctum.

For these reasons, if the canalicular repair is to be attempted, the plan should be to repair it without ultimately damaging tear flow through the other uninvolved canaliculus. It is obvious that in any given patient one cannot tell what the tear flow would be through each canaliculus and, therefore, if the canaliculus can be repaired without damaging the other uninvolved canaliculus, it should be attempted, no matter whether it is the upper or lower canaliculus that has been damaged.

Anesthesia

We prefer to perform this procedure with a general anesthetic if the patient is not cooperative, if we plan on putting in a bicanalicular stent, or if we feel that the patient will not be cooperative, especially if we are going to use a pigtail probe. However, most of the time we prefer to do this with local anesthesia.

Plan for Canalicular Repair

The key to the repair is to find the medial cut end of the canaliculus. This is best done by direct observation using magnification. Otherwise, it may be done by syringing material through the other uninvolved canaliculus to see where it exits from the medial cut end of the involved canaliculus (Fig. 5).

This can be done by using methylene blue, a whitish steroid sterile eye drop, or sodium hyaluronate tinted

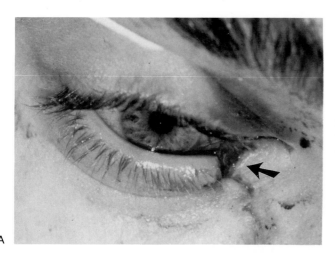

A

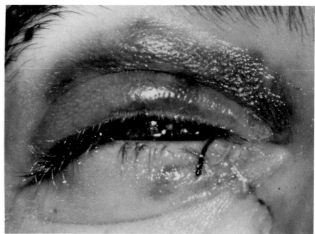

B

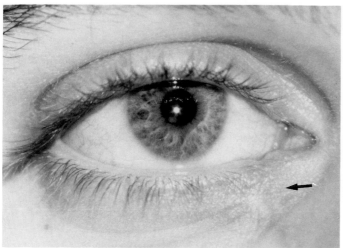

C

FIG. 4. A: Patient with laceration through punctum and vertical limb of canaliculus. **B:** Repair with direct suturing of canaliculi leaving a funnel at the punctum and a 0- silk suture sitting in the punctum as a stent. **C:** The stent has been left in for 2 months and then removed. This photograph is 3 months following the injury. The patient has no tearing and the canaliculus is open. (From Hurwitz et al., ref. 16, with permission.)

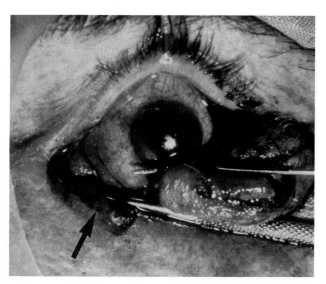

FIG. 5. Patient in Fig. 1 with torn lower lid and canaliculus. The probe can be seen to pass through the punctum and one can see the lateral cut end of the canaliculus. The punctal dilator is sticking into the medial cut end of the lower (*arrow*) canaliculus, which could be visualized 24 hours after the injury with slit lamp examination. This allowed for an easy repair.

with fluorescein (19,20). If the medial cut end can be found in this way, then it can be anastomosed to the lateral cut end. We strongly suggest that one should attempt to suture the canaliculi. If the medial cut end cannot be located with syringing, a pigtail probe (Fig. 6) may be used to pass through the upper canaliculus and exit through the medial cut end of the lower canaliculus (21,22). The type of pigtail probe that should be used is one that does not have a hook or knob on it, but should be the same diameter and caliber at its tip as at the shaft. This will minimize damage to the canaliculi on insertion and withdrawal. If a pigtail probe is used properly, it can help the surgeon find the medial cut end of the canaliculus (22,23). Then a Silastic tube can be put over the end of the pigtail probe, exiting through the medial cut end of the canaliculus, withdrawn through the system, and then passed through the lateral cut end of the canaliculus so that the loop of the tube will be within the common canaliculus and the free ends will be coming out of the puncta. This is the so-called ring intubation (annular) with the knot tied at the inner canthus. The knot is formed by tying the ends of the tube together, and then one can suture a nylon or silk suture around the tubes to

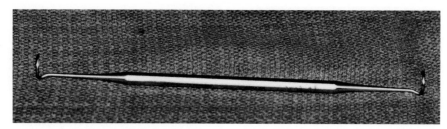

FIG. 6. A pig tail probe that can be passed through the uninvolved canaliculus, hopefully to exit through the medial cut end of the involved canaliculus.

hold the knot. The alternative is to use a modification of the technique of Crawford (24) to put a Vicryl suture through the cut ends at the inner canthus and glue them to the tubes so that there is no knot. If the surgeon does not have a good feel for the passage of the pigtail probe or if it is not successful the first time, it should not be used again. Similarly, the pigtail probe should not be forced through the system. If it does not go easily, its use should be abandoned.

A less traumatic technique of passing an instrument around from one canaliculus to the other has been described using cardiac catheterization technology. The cardiac catheter has a memory to it and is pliable enough that it follows the curvature of the canalicular system. This procedure entails the passage of a 20-gauge thin wall blunt entry needle (Cook Inc., Bloomington, IN) into the uninvolved canaliculus. A 0.53-mm gauge coral spring wire guide with a Teflon coating made of stainless steel with a 1.5-mm curve is then straightened and inserted in the hub of a 20-gauge needle. The wire guide is then advanced and manipulated until the curve of the wire goes around the turn at the common canaliculus and comes out the lateral cut end of the lacerated canaliculus (23). The catheterization technology is more expensive than the standard pigtail probe, but certainly would appear to have less potential for damage to unaffected tissues within the system.

With a single canalicular laceration, we would not advocate opening up the sac and trying a retrograde probing to find the medial cut end because this may indeed damage the common canaliculus. We would only open up the sac at a later date if we felt that a DCR or a canaliculodacryocystorhinostomy would be indicated (6).

It would seem that the single most important aspect in the canalicular repair would be the actual suturing of the edges of the torn canaliculus. This can be done with a 7-0 or 8-0 absorbable suture such as Dexon (Davis and Geck) or Vicryl (Johnson and Johnson). It is probably useful to pass a stent through the anastomosis to keep the passage open. We prefer to use three full thickness sutures through the canalicular edges. One suture is placed inferoposterior, one superoposterior, and one anterior. We prefer to place the two posterior sutures before passage of a stent, and the anterior after the stent has been passed. It is mandatory that if one wants to take the traction off the canalicular edges, that additional sutures be placed in the orbicularis muscle anterior to the canalicular sutures so that the anastomosis will not separate with orbicularis contracture. The traction suture may be placed through the orbital periosteum medially and tied to the tarsus just anterior to the vertical limb of the canaliculus (25). We have not tried to marsupialize the medial cut end of the canaliculus because we feel that this may interfere with apposition between the upper and lower lids on lid movement, and decrease the possibility of tears being suctioned through the remaining intact canaliculus.

Stents

Stents may be used in three ways:

1. bicanalicular Silastic intubation
2. annular Silastic intubation
3. monocanalicular intubation

1. The *bicanalicular Silastic stent* tube as described by Crawford (26). These tend to stabilize the lateral aspect of the laceration better than a monocanalicular intubation. However, on passing the tubes, it is mandatory that one not damage the other canaliculus, common canaliculus, sac, or duct. If damage occurs, and the canalicular laceration is unsuccessful, then one would be relegated to using a permanent bypass tube of the system because each canaliculus would not function, whereas otherwise with one functioning canaliculus, the patient may not tear, or may be repaired simply by a DCR without any permanent bypass. Certainly, the bicanalicular Silastic stent tube can be left in longer than any other stents because it is the best tolerated of the three types of intubation (Fig. 7).

2. *Annular intubation.* This is used when a pigtail probe has been used. The knot or the cut ends of the tube at the medial canthus may produce more irritation and possible granulation formation. This may be a problem and may preclude the length of time the tube may be left in place.

3. *Monocanalicular intubation* (Monaka-F.C.I., France) (Eagle Vision™ Memphis, TN). These tubes may be

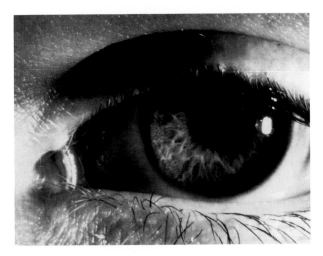

FIG. 7. A bicanalicular Silastic intubation (Crawford) following lower canalicular laceration.

passed along the canaliculus beyond the sutured anastomosis and into the sac. They fit in position at the punctum being held in the same fashion that a punctal plug would be held at the punctum when it is used to treat dry eyes. If the surgeon desires, a suture can be put through the plug at the punctum and sutured to the soft tissues around the punctum to be held in place. By using a monocanalicular stent, there is no possible damage to the other canaliculus, common canaliculus, sac, or duct. This seems to be a better stent than a suture stent or a metal rod (Figs. 8 and 9).

Whatever type of stent used, it seems that silicone is probably tolerated for the longest period of time within the system (27). One should try and leave the tubes in place if possible for approximately 3 months. We have found that a monocanalicular stent can be left in place for approximately 6 weeks, and it has been our experience that the stents tend to fall out at approximately this time. It is for this reason that we elect to suture the stent into place at the punctum to keep it in as long as possible. We do not use any metal rods in the system because it is more difficult to keep them in place for a longer period of time.

The passage of bicanalicular Silastic stents may sometimes be difficult and this becomes even more of a problem if there has been trauma to the nose. Ramocki et al. (15) state "there are times when it becomes in the best interest of everyone involved to abandon the attempt to repair (inability to locate the severed ends of the canaliculus or severe facial deformity precluding the possibility of passing the Crawford guide wires to the nose are absolute impasses to completing the repair) and plan for a secondary reparative procedure."

Our Plan for Repair of One Lacerated Canaliculus

1. Local anesthesia (perhaps general in an uncooperative patient)
2. At least 2 days after the injury
3. Locate the medial cut end on magnified examination and use tinted sodium hyaluronate to help
4. Suture the canalicular ends directly with 7-0 Dexon sutures (in our opinion this is the most important step)
5. Insert a stent tube, even though experimental studies by Conlon et al. (28) suggest that it is more important to insert stents than to suture the canaliculus. They feel that a stent will help to keep the cut edges of the canaliculus apart. We prefer to use a monocanalicular stent because we feel that this will be the one way that one can assure that the common canaliculus and sac and duct will be uninjured. There will also not be a problem with retrieving the tubes from the nose or with a knot of an annular fixation irritating the inner canthus. In the event that one cannot suture the canaliculus walls because there has been some tissue removed, a stent should be placed in the hope that there will be some epithelialization along the outer aspect of the stent if one can attempt to immobilize the lid.
6. Suturing of the adnexal structures. If the anterior limb of the medial canthal tendon has been disinserted, it is probably worthwhile to reinsert it. One may suture the medial edge of the tarsus to the posterior reflection of the medial canthal tendon (29).

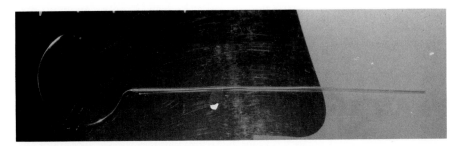

FIG. 8. The Eagle Vision monocanalicular stent. This stent has a metal rod inside the tube that acts as an introducer. This is passed through the laceration and the tube is pushed on the introducer into the canaliculus at the medial cut end.

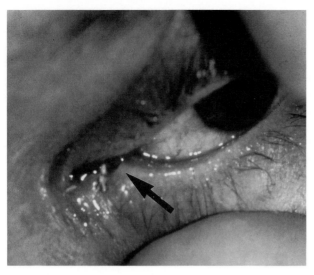

FIG. 9. A monocanalicular tube in place after a lower canaliculus repair.

Deep sutures must also be placed through the orbicularis to try and immobilize the lid.

7. Lid repair. The eyelid margin must be precisely approximated to avoid lid notching with subsequent cosmetic and functional defects. Because the lid contour is of utmost importance, the marginal sutures are placed first, regardless of how far the wound extends. A direct suture through the gray line on either side, equidistant from the cut end, is mandatory. We prefer to use a 5-0 Dexon (Davis and Geck) suture for this. Another suture may be placed through the lash line (full thickness) in the lower lid and full thickness except for the conjunctiva in the upper lid, to reapproximate the skeleton of the lids. Then 6-0 silk sutures may be used to close the skin after one suture of 5-0 Dexon through the distal aspect of the tarsus is inserted to keep the lid in good position (30). If there is tissue loss, or if one may have to debride the wound and treat the eyelid defect the same as one would a defect after tissue resection when a tumor has been excised. Direct suturing may sometimes be possible but often it is necessary to use a flap repair or grafts from distance sites.

8. Antibiotic ointment and shield. It is important to place a protective shield over the eye and have the patient wear this for a number of weeks. This prevents the patient from rolling over on the eye while sleeping and disturbing the anastomosis and/or the tube.

Postoperative Problems

1. *Loss of tube.* The tube may come out on its own, no matter what kind of tube has been used. This does not mean that the procedure is doomed to failure. One should wait and see if the patient has any tearing. The canaliculus can then be irrigated and one may be pleasantly surprised that the canaliculus may be patent, or if it is not patent, that the patient may not be tearing.

2. *Granuloma formation around tubes.* Any material in the lacrimal system, even silicone, may cause granuloma formation (31,32). A granuloma may not be a problem and when the tube is removed, the granuloma may be able to be snipped away. Even though there may be some bleeding when this is snipped away, and one is tempted to cauterize the base, we prefer not to cauterize the base because we do not want to put any cautery whatsoever in the area of the canaliculus.

3. *A slit canaliculus.* A slit canaliculus does not cause a functional problem in most patients (33). As well, the anastomosis site may open up and one may be able to see the medial cut end of the canaliculus, which functions as a separate punctal opening. One may be able to irrigate through to the nose. It would seem that this acts very much as a partially marsupialized canaliculus. This does not cause a problem as long as there is not a deep notch in the lid, which would interfere with tear flow through the upper punctum because of inability for the punctal surfaces to strike each other when the eyes close.

4. *Persistent tearing.* If the eye keeps watering afterward because the canalicular repair has not worked, if the other canaliculus and the rest of the system are normal, a DCR will relieve tearing symptoms in at least 70% of the patients. We would prefer to manage the patient this way rather than doing a resection of the eyelid to attempt to repair the canaliculi at a later date (34). We feel it would be more difficult doing a canalicular resection of the scar and a reanastomosis and having the anastomosis remain tight when a section of lid has to be removed. If the orbicularis is functioning well, we are concerned that with orbicularis contracture, the anastomosis of the revised ends might be disturbed.

Injuries of Both Distal Canaliculi or Common Canaliculus

These injuries are usually much more severe and often are due to avulsions. If both canaliculi are damaged, it is extremely difficult to pass monocanalicular stents through each canaliculus and have them function properly. As well, if both canaliculi are lacerated or if the common canaliculus is torn away from the lacrimal sac, the medial tissues of the nasolacrimal passages tend to retract medially so it is indeed very difficult to find the medial cut ends of the lacerated tissues. It has been our preference to perform a canaliculodacryocystorhinostomy wherein the sac may be opened and the lacerated ends of the canaliculi may be anastomosed to each other or more often directly into the lacrimal sac (6). After this is done, a bicanalicular Silastic stent tube is inserted and a DCR is performed. It is our philosophy that when we open the sac surgically, that we prefer to do a DCR to drain the sac into the nose, rather than merely to close the sac. We feel that if the sac is closed and not drained through a DCR, it has an increased risk of becoming scarred and obstructed. If one elects to do a caniculo-dacryocystorhinostomy, it does not have to be done immediately after the time of trauma, and often it is better to wait until the hemorrhage and edema subside so that the surgery can be done in relatively atraumatized tissues (6). A Jones bypass tube is hardly ever needed in this sort of situation. The same plan is operational when a common canaliculus is separated from the sac either by a direct laceration or by an avulsion.

INJURIES TO THE SAC AND DUCT

These will be covered in Sections B and C.

REFERENCES

1. Rabinovitch J, Hurwitz JJ, Chin-Sang H. Quantitative evaluation of canalicular flow using lacrimal scintillography. *Orbit* 1985;3:263.
2. Werb A. The lacrimal system. In: Smith B, Converse JM, Wood-Smith D, Obear MF, eds. *Plastic and reconstructive surgery of the eye and adenexa: proceedings of the second international symposium.* St. Louis: CV Mosby; 1987.
3. Linberg JV, Moore CA. Symptoms of canalicular obstruction. *Ophthalmology* 1988;95:1077.
4. Hawes MJ, Segrest DR. Effectiveness of bicanalicular silicone intubation in the repair of canalicular lacerations. *Ophthal Plast Reconstruct Surg* 1985;1:185.
5. Wulc AE, Arterberry JF. The pathogenesis of canalicular laceration. *Ophthalmology* 1991;98:1243.
6. Hurwitz JJ, Avram D, Kratky V. Avulsion of the canalicular system. *Ophthal Surg* 1989;20:726.
7. Zolli CL. Microsurgical repair of lacrimal canaliculus in medial canthal trauma. In: Hornblass A, ed. *Oculoplastic orbital and reconstructive surgery: eyelids,* vol 1. Baltimore: Williams & Wilkins; 1988.
8. Dortzbach RK, Angrist RA. Silicone intubation for lacerated lacrimal canaliculi. *Ophthal Surg* 1985;16:639.
9. Reifler D. The management of canalicular lacerations. *Surv Ophthalmol* 1991;36:113.
10. Meyer DR, Antonello A, Linberg JD. Assessment of tear drainage after canalicular obstruction using fluorescein dye disappearance. *Ophthalmology* 1990;97:1370.
11. Daubert J, Nik N, Chandeyssoun PA, El-Choufi L. Tear flow analysis through the upper and lower system. *Ophthal Plast Reconstruct Surg* 1990;6:193.
12. Hawes MJ, Dortzbach RK. Trauma of the lacrimal drainage system. In: Linberg JV, ed. *Lacrimal surgery.* New York: Churchill Livingstone; 1988.
13. Ortiz MA, Craushar MF. Lacrimal drainage following repair of inferior canaliculus. *Ann Ophthalmol* 1975;7:739.
14. Jones BR. A surgical cure of obstruction in the common lacrimal canaliculus. *Trans Ophthal Soc UK* 1960;80:345.
15. Ramocki JM, Nesi FH, Spoor TC. Management of injuries to ocular adnexa. In: Spoor TC, Nesi F, eds. *Management of ocular orbital and adnexal trauma.* New York: Raven Press; 1988.
16. Hurwitz JJ, Corin SM, Tucker SM. Punctal and vertical canaliculus lacerations. *Ophthal Surg* 1989;25:14.
17. Jones BR, Corrigan MJ. Obstruction of the lacrimal canaliculi. In: Rycroft PV, ed. *Corneo-plastic surgery.* London: Pergamon Press; 1969.
18. Rutherford S, Hurwitz JJ. A computerized programme for the assessment and management of lacrimal patients. *Ophthalmology* 1986;93:14.
19. Vila-Cora A. Hyaluronate facilitates passage of lacrimal probes for repair of lacerated canaliculi. *Arch Ophthalmol* 1988;106:579.
20. Seiff SR, Ahn JC. Locating cut medial canaliculi by direct injection of sodium hyaluronate into the lacrimal sac. *Ophthal Surg* 1989;20:176.
21. Kartch MC, French I. Pigtail probe for lacrimal canaliculus repair. *Am J Ophthalmol* 1971;72:1145.
22. Worst JGF. Method for reconstructing torn lacrimal canaliculus. *Am J Ophthalmol* 1962;53:520.
23. Corin SM, Hurwitz JJ, Corin WJ, Kazdan MS. Lacrimal catheterization. *Ophthal Surg* 1989;20:202.
24. Rutherford S, Crawford JS. A method of joining the ends of silicone tubes used in intubating the lacrimal system to ensure removal. *Ophthalmology* 1984;91:963.
25. Ahl NC. Traction suture for canalicular laceration. *Ophthal Plast Reconstruct Surg* 1994;10:189.
26. Crawford JS. Intubation of obstructions of the lacrimal system. *Can J Ophthalmol* 1977;12:189.
27. Kraft SP, Crawford JS. Silicone tube intubation in disorders of the lacrimal system in children. *Am J Ophthalmol* 1982;94:290.
28. Conlon MR, Smith KD, Cadera W, Shum D, Allen LH. An animal model studying reconstruction techniques and histopathological changes and repair of canalicular lacerations. *Can J Ophthalmol* 1994;29:3.
29. Jordan DR, Anderson SL, Thiese SM. The medial tarsal strip. *Arch Ophthalmol* 1990;108:120.
30. Kratky V, Hurwitz JJ, Avram DR. Management of eyelid and lacrimal trauma. *Ophthal Pract* 1989;7:5.
31. Dresner SC, Codere F, Brownstein S, Jouve P. Lacrimal drainage system inflammatory masses from retained silicone tubing. *Am J Ophthalmol* 1984;98:609.
32. Jordan DR, Nerad JA. An acute inflammatory reaction to silicone stents. *Ophthal Plast Reconstruct Surg* 1987;3:147.
33. Hurwitz JJ. The slit canaliculus. *Ophthal Surg* 1982;13:572.
34. Fox SA. *Ophthalmic plastic surgery,* 5th ed. New York: Grune & Stratton; 1976.

B. Nasoethmoid Complex Fractures: Current Principles of Diagnosis and Treatment

The nasoethmoid complex is a distinct anatomic region defined by the interorbital space and circumscribed by the anterior cranial fossa superiorly and the medial orbital walls laterally. Nasoethmoid fractures therefore potentially involve the cranial, orbital, and nasal cavities, as well as the lacrimal pathways. These injuries pose a significant challenge both diagnostically and therapeutically. Failure to recognize and adequately treat these injuries results in a significant aesthetic deformity and associated functional deficits.

PATHOLOGIC ANATOMY

The nasoethmoid region is situated in the central upper midface. The fragile and intricate skeletal framework

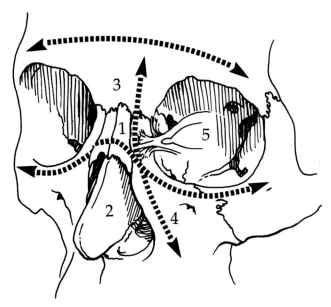

FIG. 10. Surface skeletal anatomy of the nasoethmoid complex. The nasal bones (*1*) and septum (*2*) have low impact resistance but provide dorsal nasal support. The nasal process of the frontal bone (*3*) and the frontal process of the maxilla (*4*) comprise the medial buttress. This is the main structural pillar of the central midface which, in concert with the supraorbital and infraorbital transverse buttresses (*dotted lines*), dissipates forces to protect the orbits and interorbital space. The lamina papyracea of the ethmoid (*5*) is extremely fragile and comprises most of the medial orbital wall.

that comprises the interorbital space is supported anteriorly by bilateral structural buttresses consisting of the frontal processes of the maxilla, nasal processes of the frontal bone, and paired nasal bones (Fig. 10). These central pillars serve as a supportive framework from which are suspended the relatively fragile nasal septum and medial orbital walls. Forces applied to the central midface are dissipated by these reinforced pillars, sparing the interorbital space and medial orbits. When forces are sufficiently high to disrupt the buttresses, the medial orbital walls and septum comminute readily, resulting in complete collapse of the central midface.

The roof of the nasoethmoid complex is made up of the floor of the anterior cranial fossa. Specifically, this consists of the fovea ethmoidalis, strengthened in the midline by the cribriform plate. These bones are thin and closely associated with the olfactory nerves and dura. Nasoethmoid complex fractures frequently extend into the anterior cranial fossa, potentially causing olfactory nerve injury, pneumocephalus, dural tears, or cerebral injury.

Within the interorbital space (Fig. 11) lie the paired upper nasal fossae separated by the septum and perpendicular plate of the ethmoid in the midline. The intervals between the nasal fossae and the medial orbital walls are occupied by the ethmoid labyrinths. These consist of multiple mucosa-lined air cells supported by a delicate

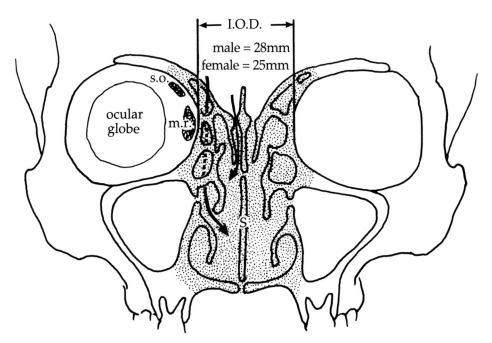

FIG. 11. Coronal section of the nasoethmoid complex. The interorbital space (*highlighted*) occupies the interval between the medial orbital walls laterally, the palate inferiorly, and the anterior cranial fossa superiorly. The interorbital distance (*I.O.D.*) must be re-established in any reconstruction. *Arrows* indicate potential sites of CSF leak through the disruptions in the posterior wall of the frontal sinus or cribriform plate. Relationship of medial rectus (*M.R.*) and superior oblique (*S.O.*) muscles to the medial orbital wall is demonstrated.

skeletal framework, which collectively drain their secretions into the middle meatus of the nasal cavity. Trauma to this area is frequently associated with septal displacement or disruption, causing nasal airway obstruction and loss of support to the nasal bones.

The medial walls of the orbit are composed of the lacrimal bone anteriorly and the lamina papyracea of the ethmoid bone posteriorly. These extremely thin and fragile bones form the lateral boundaries of the nasoethmoid complex. Fracture and posterior impaction of the nasomaxillary buttresses generally cause gross comminution and blowout of the medial orbital walls. Prolapse of orbital soft tissues into the medial wall defect predisposes to enophthalmos, muscle entrapment, and restricted ocular motility. Rarely, displacement of medial orbital fractures is lateral (blow-in), resulting in diminished orbital volume and proptosis.

The lacrimal drainage system is intimately related to the bone in this area. The lacrimal sac lies within the lacrimal fossa just inside the inferomedial rim of the orbit. The nasolacrimal duct itself runs an interosseous course within the maxilla before emptying into the inferior meatus of the nasal cavity. Disruption of the medial orbital rim in nasoethmoid fractures can therefore potentially cause obstruction of the nasolacrimal drainage apparatus.

The medial canthal tendon anchors the tarsal plate and the orbicularis oculi musculature to the medial wall of the orbit. At its point of insertion, the tendon splits into anterior, posterior, and superior limbs, attaching to anterior and posterior lacrimal crests. Functionally, it serves to pump secretions into the nasolacrimal duct and to keep the eyelids tangent to the globe. Morphologically, the medial canthal tendon maintains the configuration of the palpebral fissure and the intercanthal distance. Displacement of the medial canthus is a pathognomonic feature of nasoethmoid complex injury. Generally, fractures of the medial orbital rim and wall circumscribe a central bone fragment to which the medial canthal tendon is attached. Instability and displacement of this tendon-bearing bone produces the medial canthal dystopia. Avulsion of the medial canthal tendon from its bony insertion rarely occurs in the absence of direct laceration.

DIAGNOSIS

The presence of nasoethmoid complex injury can be detected on the basis of observed morphologic changes alone. However, the degree of instability and comminution can only be determined following bimanual physical examination and correlation with radiologic findings. Frequent involvement of the cranial, orbital, and nasal cavities further necessitates thorough neurologic, ophthalmologic, and intranasal examination.

Physical Examination

The physical examination begins with visual inspection of the central midface. The presence of stellate burst lacerations, edema, and periorbital ecchymoses should alert the examining physician to the possibility of underlying nasoethmoid fractures. Lacerations over the medial canthal region imply possible direct laceration to the medial canthal tendon or lacrimal system. Exaggerated depth of the nasofrontal angle and decreased projection of the nasal dorsum are indicative of posterior displacement of the nasal pyramid associated with nasoethmoid fracture.

Medial canthal position must be specifically assessed. The presence of canthal dystopia, i.e., a displacement of the medial canthus in any direction, identifies a displaced nasoethmoid fracture or avulsed tendon. Anthropometric evaluation of the medial canthus is done simply and effectively using a McCoy trisquare (Fig. 12). The position of the medial canthus is related to the facial midline and to the canthal line (a transverse plane through the lateral canthi) (1). This facilitates recognition of subtle asymmetries in both vertical and horizontal planes and permits quantitation of the degree of canthal displacement (Fig. 13 and Table 1).

When direct measurements are not possible, traumatic telecanthus is confirmed by identification of disproportions in periorbital morphology (2). Normally, the intercanthal distance is roughly equivalent to the palpebral fissure width and is approximately one half the interpupillary distance. Lateral displacement of the medial canthus following trauma increases the relative intercanthal distance while diminishing palpebral fissure width.

Palpation allows one to actively test the integrity of the medial canthal tendons and the degree of instability in the entire nasoethmoid complex. Gentle pressure on the nasal bones reveals the degree of support of the nasal dorsum. Collapse and prolapse of the distal nose into the pyriform aperture indicates gross disruption of the nasomaxillary buttresses and septum, and implies the need for bone graft reconstruction (Fig. 14). Palpation along the orbital rims reveals the site of orbital fractures. Intraoral examination consists of direct palpation along the pyriform aperture to determine the degree of medial buttress comminution and bimanual manipulation of the maxilla to rule out associated LeFort I, II, or III midface fractures. The occlusion is specifically evaluated.

The integrity of the medial canthal tendon attachment is tested by the eyelid traction test (Fig. 15). Lateral traction is applied to the eyelids and the tension and stability of the medial canthal tendon attachment are noted. If the eyelid margin does not become taut like a bow string, then a tendon avulsion is likely present. Subtle fractures of the nasoethmoid skeleton are further confirmed by a

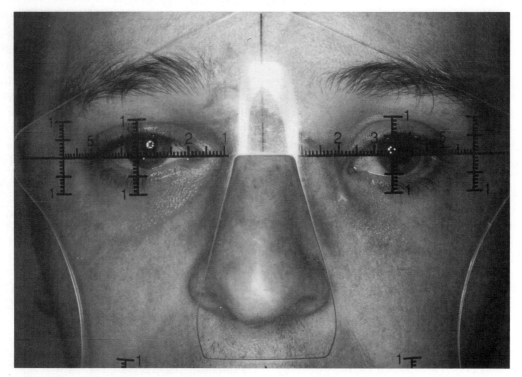

FIG. 12. The McCoy trisquare is a clear curved facial plane with a reference grid. The vertical axis is aligned with the facial midline. The transverse axis is aligned with the canthal line (between lateral canthi). In this patient, a left medial canthal dystopia, decreased palpebral fissure width, and hypoglobus are easily quantified.

bimanual examination. A Howarth elevator is placed intranasally against the lateral nasal wall directly opposite the medial canthal tendon attachment. An index finger is placed externally over the medial canthal tendon insertion. Stability is evaluated by assessing movement of

the canthus-bearing bone between the elevator and the index finger.

Nasal fractures are a consistent feature of nasoethmoid complex injury and the degree of both nasal bone stability and displacement are specifically evaluated. In-

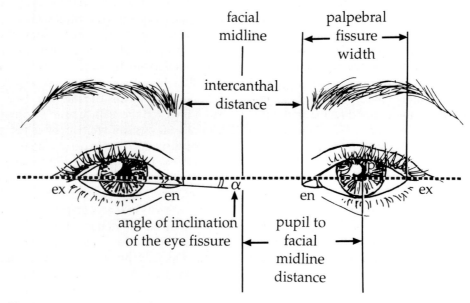

FIG. 13. Periorbital morphologic features. Landmarks commonly measured include *en* (endocanthion or medial canthus), *ex* (exocanthion or lateral canthus), and *P* (pupil).

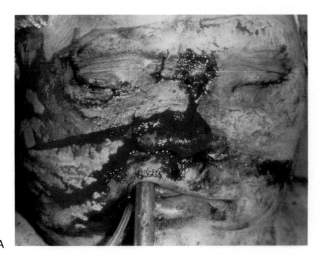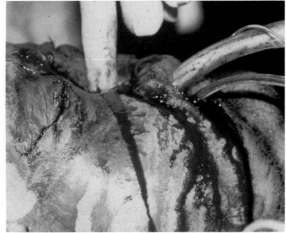

A   B

FIG. 14. Grossly unstable nasoethmoid fracture. **A:** Burst lacerations, flattening of the nasal dorsum, and obvious telecanthus are pathognomonic of nasoethmoid fracture. **B:** Collapse and prolapse of the nose with gentle pressure indicates total disruption of medial buttresses.

tranasal examination rules out septal hematoma and reveals septal dislocation and fracture.

Concomitant injury to the anterior cranial fossa may result in injury to the olfactory nerve fibers, tearing of the dura and cerebral spinal fluid (CSF) rhinorrhea, and potential intracranial injury. A complete neurologic examination is therefore mandatory. The sense of smell should be tested and documented. The presence of clear fluid nasal discharge should be assumed to be CSF rhinorrhea until proven otherwise. By leaning a patient forward, minimal amounts of discharge can be caught on a piece of filter paper. Pooling of blood and mucosal nasal secretions in the center of the collection site with formation of a clear circumferential rim produces a target appearance suggestive of CSF. If copious, the fluid can be collected and sent for glucose and protein analysis, or for beta II transferrin study, if available.

Ophthalmologic examination must include an assessment of visual acuity, pupillary reaction, visual fields, and intraocular pressure: observation of anterior and posterior chambers. Specific evaluation for enophthalmos or proptosis or other gross displacement of the ocular globe in a coronal plane is important. Full assess-

ment of ocular motility and documentation of diplopia are of paramount importance. Lacrimal irrigation is not performed clinically on the initial assessment.

Radiologic Assessment

Optimal radiographic visualization of the nasoethmoid region is provided by coronal computed tomography (CT) images. Coronal images clearly demonstrate fractures through the anterior cranial base, disruption of the medial orbital rim and medial orbital walls, and prolapse or entrapment of medial rectus muscle or orbital

TABLE 1. *Periorbital anthropometric norms[a]*

	Male		Female	
	Mean	SD	Mean	SD
Intercanthal distance (mm)	33.3	2.7	31.8	2.3
Palpebral fissure width (mm)	31.3	1.2	20.7	1.2
Pupil to midline distance (mm)	33.5	2.0	31.2	1.8
Palpebral fissure inclination (degrees)	2.1	1.9	4.1	2.2

[a] Based on normative data documented by Farkas et al., ref. 1.

SD, standard deviation.

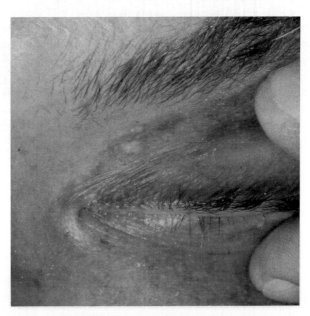

FIG. 15. Eyelid traction test. Lateral traction is exerted on the eyelids. Tensing of the eyelid margin and bow stringing at the medial canthal insertion rules out tendon avulsion.

soft tissues. Coronal images are particularly useful in comparative analysis of orbital dimensions.

Unfortunately, coronal images can be difficult to obtain in a patient with multiple injuries, potential cervical spine injury, or head injury. Coronal images require a cooperative patient who is able to maintain an extended head position for a prolonged period of time. With most acute trauma patients, it is therefore necessary to visualize the nasoethmoid region by axial CT scans. Axial CT scans do not provide sufficient information regarding the anterior cranial base, the orbital roof, or orbital floors. Under these circumstances, it is best to obtain 3-mm axial cuts, which can be subsequently reformatted into coronal images.

More recently, three-dimensional (3D) CT scans have been employed in the evaluation of nasoethmoid complex injuries. Three-dimensional images can be reformatted from standard axial CT scans. These images are particularly useful to demonstrate the degree of comminution, displacement, and rotation of the central fragment fracture. We find these 3D CT scans provide optimal information in terms of the degree of disruption of the central buttresses of the maxilla.

CLASSIFICATION AND GENERAL APPROACH TO TREATMENT

In formulating a treatment plan, the surgeon must be able to recognize the pattern of nasoethmoid injury, the status of the medial canthal tendon and central bone fragment, and the degree of disruption or loss of stability in the nasoethmoid complex. Two specific classification schemes are particularly useful in this regard.

Gruss (3), in a critical review of 104 patients with nasoethmoid injuries, classified fractures patterns into five types according to the extent of involvement of adjacent anatomical structures and the degree of inherent instability (Table 2). Type I injuries are isolated to the nasoethmoid region and retain adequate dorsal nasal support. Type II injuries involve the central maxilla and are characterized by gross disruption of the maxillary buttresses and cartilaginous nasal septum and loss of dorsal nasal stability. Type III injuries are extended nasoethmoid orbital fractures featuring direct extension of fracture lines to the frontal bone superiorly or to LeFort II and III fracture patterns in the maxilla. Type IV fractures consist of nasoethmoid fractures associated with grossly unstable and displaced fractures of the orbit, resulting in oculo-orbital displacement or orbital dystopia. Type V injuries are the most severe and represent central midface fractures with actual loss of bone substance.

Careful consideration of the clinical and radiologic findings allows the surgeon to accurately diagnose the pattern of nasoethmoid injury according to this classification scheme. This facilitates surgical planning by identifying the extent of injury and the degree of instability. Rational decisions can then be made regarding optimal incisions for exposure, the order of fracture segment reduction, and the necessity for immediate bone graft reconstruction.

Markowitz et al. (4) further classified nasoethmoid fractures according to the involvement of the central fragment, i.e., the fragment of bone on which the medial canthal tendon inserts. Three patterns of fracture are recognized (Fig. 16): Type I—single segment central fragment; Type II—comminuted central fragment with fractures remaining external to the medial canthal insertion; and Type III—comminuted central fragment with fractures extending into bone bearing the canthal insertion. Classification of the fracture pattern with respect to the central bone segment is clinically useful in that it provides guidelines for graded exposure and fixation appropriate to the degree of injury.

Immediate Reconstruction

Exposure

Reconstruction of the fractured nasoethmoid complex begins with an adequate exposure. Complete visualization of surrounding stable or uninjured segments of the craniofacial skeleton in addition to the nasoethmoid complex and medial orbital walls is required. Local lacerations generally do not provide adequate exposure and extension of these lacerations is therefore not appropriate. Such lacerations serve as an adjunct only, providing limited exposure of the immediately underlying fracture lines.

The coronal flap provides access to the superior aspect of the nasoethmoid complex, the entire upper and lateral craniofacial skeleton, and the roof and lateral and medial walls of the orbital cavity. In particular, use of the coronal flap provides a direct and safe access to the medial orbital wall. The anterior and posterior lacrimal crest can be clearly visualized and the insertion of the medial canthal tendon can be preserved.

TABLE 2. *Gruss classification of nasoethmoid injuries*

Type 1	Isolated bony nasoethmoid injury
Type 2	Bony nasoethmoid and central maxilla
	a. Central maxilla only
	b. Central and one lateral maxilla
	c. Central and bilateral lateral maxillae
Type 3	Extended nasoethmoid injury
	a. With craniofrontal injuries
	b. With LeFort II and III fractures
Type 4	Nasoethmoid injury with orbital displacement
	a. With oculo-orbital displacement
	b. With orbital dystopia
Type 5	Nasoethmoid injury with bone loss

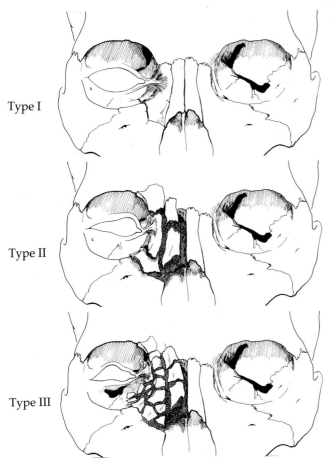

FIG. 16. Manson classification of nasoethmoid injuries. The classification is based on the involvement of the central segment, i.e., the region of the medial orbital rim and buttress, which bears the insertion of the medial canthal tendon. Type I, single fracture circumscribing the central segment; Type II, comminuted fractures of the central segment but external to medial canthal insertion; Type III, fractures extending into the medial canthal insertion.

Under certain circumstances, a neurosurgeon may be required to elevate a frontal bone flap to provide intracranial access to the nasoethmoid fracture (Fig. 17). This is generally done specifically for neurosurgical indications, i.e., a suspected major dural tear with a CSF leak, in the presence of compound or grossly displaced frontal bone fractures, or in the presence of intracranial injury requiring direct intervention. Concomitant intracranial exposure provides optimal access to the nasoethmoid complex and allows anatomic reduction of fractured segments of the supraorbital rims, glabella, and nasomaxillary processes.

Access to the inferior aspect of the nasoethmoid complex is obtained through lower eyelid incisions. We prefer to use subciliary incisions with elevation of skin muscle flaps. Periosteum is widely elevated to expose the inferior orbital rims, inferomedial aspect of the orbital cavity, and anterior surface of the maxilla. When frac-

ture lines extend into the lower midface, further access is provided by an upper buccal sulcus incision and wide subperiosteal elevation to expose the entire anterior and lateral surfaces of the maxilla.

Reduction Scheme

Once sufficient exposure of the craniofacial skeleton is obtained, displaced fracture segments are anatomically reduced. This is accomplished most effectively if a strategy for fracture reduction is consistently followed in all cases.

We prefer to identify stable, uninjured regions of the craniofacial skeleton first. This generally comprises the craniofrontal region superiorly and the orbitozygomatic or craniotemporal regions laterally, depending on the extent of the fracture. Facial bones in both these areas have a high impact tolerance and tend to fracture into large bone segments. Sequential anatomic reduction of fracture segments is therefore possible, allowing accurate 3D reconstruction of the facial skeleton.

In this fashion, upper and outer facial frames are constructed first (Fig. 18). Reconstruction of the supraorbital rims and glabella along the craniofrontal region provides a stable anatomic reference that defines the width of the orbital cavities, the location of the facial midline, and the location of the root of the nose. Anatomic reduction and rigid fixation of the zygoma bilaterally provides a stable reference dictating the vertical height of the orbital cavity, midfacial projection, and facial width.

Reconstruction of the nasoethmoid complex is undertaken after the upper outer facial frame is constructed. The nasoethmoid region is generally comminuted into multiple smaller bone fragments with or without actual bone loss and the availability of stable skeletal reference landmarks is extremely helpful in completing an anatomic 3D-accurate reconstruction of the nasoethmoid complex.

Rigid Skeleton Fixation

The principles of the rigid skeleton fixation applied to fracture management anywhere must be applied to the treatment of nasoethmoid fractures. These principles are as follows:

1. Rigid fixation is achieved only when the forces binding a fracture exceed the dynamic functional forces acting on the bone.
2. Reduction of fractures must be precise to maximize the contact surface area between opposing bone segments and thereby increase the frictional force between segments.

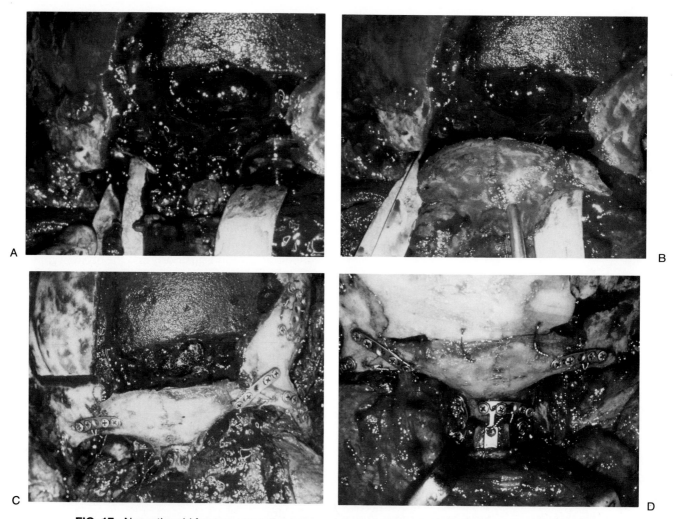

FIG. 17. Nasoethmoid fracture extending into craniofrontal region. **A:** Frontal craniotomy has been performed. Each malleable retractor protects the right and left orbital contents, respectively. The interorbital space (between retractors) is grossly disrupted and communicating with the cranial cavity. **B:** The fractured supraorbital bar is reduced. **C:** Supraorbital fractures are rigidly fixed. **D:** Nasoethmoid fractures are reconstructed.

3. In the upper nasoethmoid region, the only functional forces acting on fracture segments are those exerted by the orbicularis oculi muscle through the medial canthal tendon. Microplates (1.0- or 1.2-mm screw diameter systems) are therefore generally sufficient.
4. Lower nasoethmoid fractures, i.e., fractures of the medial buttresses of the maxilla, must resist transmitted forces of mastication and therefore larger plate systems (1.7-mm or 2.00-mm screw diameter) are most commonly used inferiorly.
5. With all the above systems, basic principles of rigid fixation are observed. At least two screws are required on either side of each fracture line for secure fixation. All micro- and miniplates must be accurately contoured to the 3D shape of the underlying bone such that these fixation systems are thoroughly and passively adapted to the underlying bone contour.

The specific approach to rigid fixation of nasoethmoid fractures is based on the pattern of nasoethmoid injury (5). Type 1 fractures are most effectively treated by anatomic reduction of the central segment, single microplate fixation at the glabella or frontal base, and single miniplate fixation at the medial buttress of the maxilla (Fig. 19).

Type II injuries are comminuted nasoethmoid fractures that circumscribe and spare a central canthal tendon–bearing bone segment. Such injuries are more difficult to treat because of the number of comminuted segments, the small size of these segments, and the inherent instability of the medial canthal tendon–bearing bone. Reconstruction requires sequential reduction of each bone segment to restore the nasomaxillary buttresses bilaterally. The method of fixation depends on the size of comminuted segments. Microplates can be em-

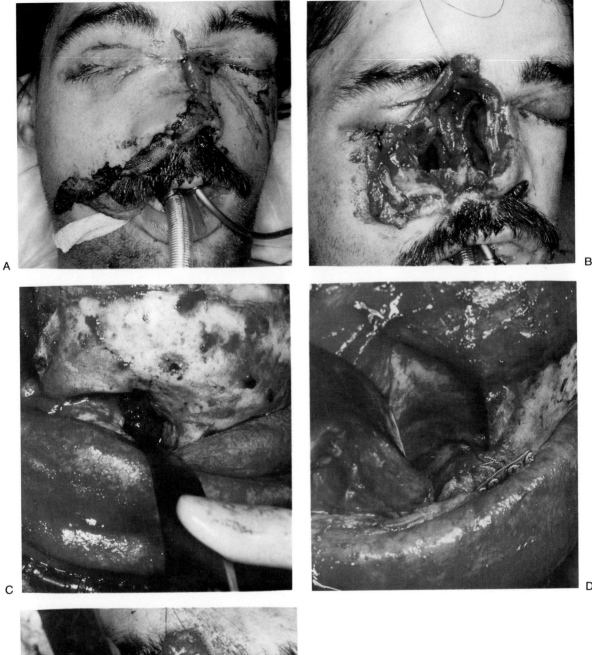

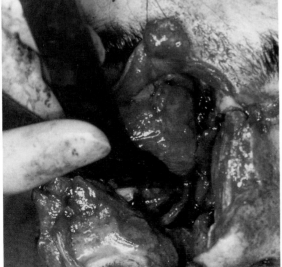

FIG. 18. A 30-year-old man with right nasoethmoid and orbitozygomatic fractures associated with a facial avulsion in a sawmill kickback accident. **A:** Gross right medial canthal dystopia. **B:** Opening of laceration reveals bone loss and absence of stable skeletal landmarks. **C:** Elevation of coronal flap and identification of stable supraorbital rim medially (malleable retractor protecting right orbital contents). **D:** Coronal flap extended laterally. The right temporalis muscle has been reflected to allow anatomic reduction of the fractured zygoma (note fracture line within temporal fossa and fixation plate at the lateral orbital rim). **E:** With the superior and outer facial frame reconstructed, reliable skeletal landmarks at the supraorbital and infraorbital margins are available to permit reconstruction of the inferomedial orbit.

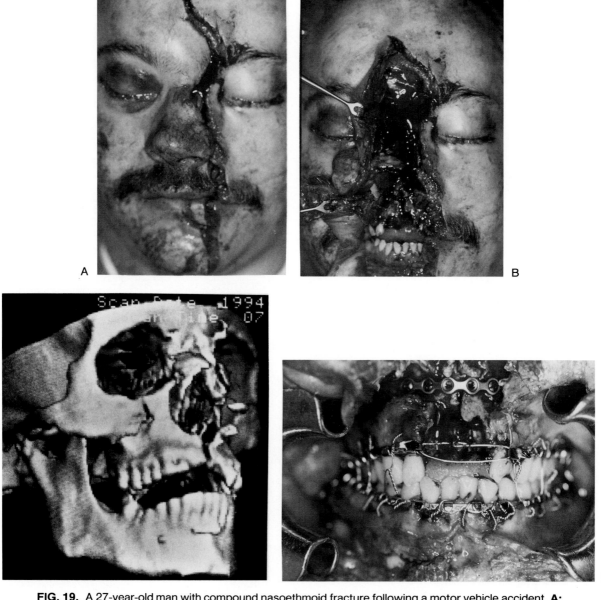

FIG. 19. A 27-year-old man with compound nasoethmoid fracture following a motor vehicle accident. **A:** Avulsive laceration left face. **B:** Retraction of the avulsion flap reveals a split of the palate, malocclusion, and nasoethmoid comminution. **C:** A 3D CT scan demonstrates bilateral Manson Type I nasoethmoid fractures associated with a right LeFort II maxillary fracture and split palate. **D:** Reconstruction begins with initial maxillomandibular fixation and rigid fixation of the maxillary fractures using 1.7-mm miniplates.

ployed to span the entire nasomaxillary buttress or, alternatively, multiple interosseous wires and a bridging plate across the junctional fractures can be used. The critical part of the procedure is to ensure anatomic 3D placement of the central canthal-bearing bone segment. The tendency to outward rotation or displacement of the central segment often requires placement of supplementary transnasal canthopexy wires posterior to the medial canthal tendon insertion. At all times the insertion of the medial canthal tendon is preserved and no attempt is made to dissect it.

Type III injuries are comminuted nasoethmoid fractures that transect or avulse the medial canthal tendon such that there is no sizable bone fragment to use in reconstruction. Under these circumstances, a formal medial canthoplasty must be performed. Fracture reduction is performed by sequential alignment of comminuted segments as described above. However, a formal transnasal medial canthopexy is absolutely necessary. Frequently such injuries are associated with marked comminution of the medial orbital walls and rims and bone graft reconstruction of the medial orbits is required

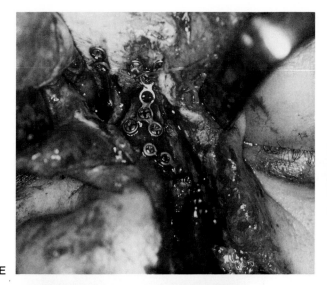

E

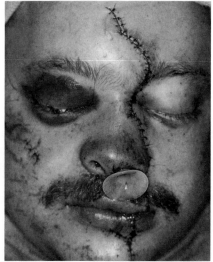

F

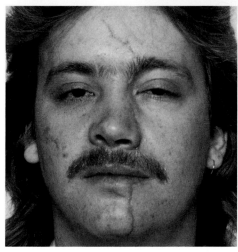

G

FIG. 19. (*Continued*). **E:** The central segments and nasal bones are anatomically reduced and fixed with 1.2-mm microplates. **F:** Immediately postoperatively, intercanthal distance and nasal projection appear adequately reconstructed. **G:** Three months postoperatively.

to provide an adequate skeletal fixation point for medial canthal tendon insertion.

Primary Bone Grafting

Primary bone grafting in the acute management of facial fractures was introduced and popularized by Gruss (3). The application of this technique is particularly indicated in comminuted unstable nasoethmoid injuries where actual loss of bone or the degree of bony comminution precludes anatomic fracture reduction and a stable 3D reconstruction.

Under these circumstances, the use of primary bone grafts serves to fill in bone gaps and thereby increases the stability of the reconstruction, to reconstruct deficiencies in the medial orbital walls thereby preventing prolapse of soft tissue contents, and to provide a skeletal base for

medial canthal tendon fixation. Primary bone grafts are also used in reconstructing dorsal nasal support in cases where this has been lost as a result of the injury. Such primary reconstruction provides a more stable result, maintains the 3D shape of the nasoethmoid region, and maintains soft tissue expansion during the healing phase.

Potential bone graft donor sites include the skull, iliac crest, and rib in order of preference. The skull provides an ample amount of bone graft material and is in the immediate operative site during coronal flap elevation. Split skull bone grafts can be harvested from the outer table of the skull. This is generally done over the nondominant hemisphere, posterior to the coronal suture line, and at least 2 cm lateral to the midline. Split skull bone graft is characterized by its inherent curvature, rigidity, and brittleness. It is primarily indicated for reconstruction of the medial orbital wall, localized deficiencies of the medial or inferior orbital rims, and constructing a dorsal cantilever strut for the nose.

When defects of the orbits span two or more adjacent walls of the orbital cavity, iliac crest or rib graft are preferable. In both techniques, the bone can be more effectively shaped and contoured to fit the requirements of the recipient site.

Primary bone grafts are employed for three specific purposes (Fig. 20):

1. Where isolated segments are missing along the nasomaxillary buttresses or along the adjacent inferior or superior orbital rims. Bony continuity is restored by the use of bone grafts. The bone graft is carved meticulously and precisely to fit into the skeletal defect as an inlay graft. Any contour irregularity will be clearly visible externally and must be avoided. The inlay graft is fixed rigidly using microplates. The use of bone grafts under these circumstances ensures normal external contour, maintains stability at the fracture site, and potentially speeds osteogenesis.

2. Where the medial orbital wall is comminuted, i.e, in Type III injuries, restoration of the medial orbital wall is required to prevent extraocular muscle entrapment or enophthalmos and to provide a skeletal base for medial canthal tendon attachment. It is imperative that the medial orbital walls be reconstructed in an anatomic position such that the normal interorbital

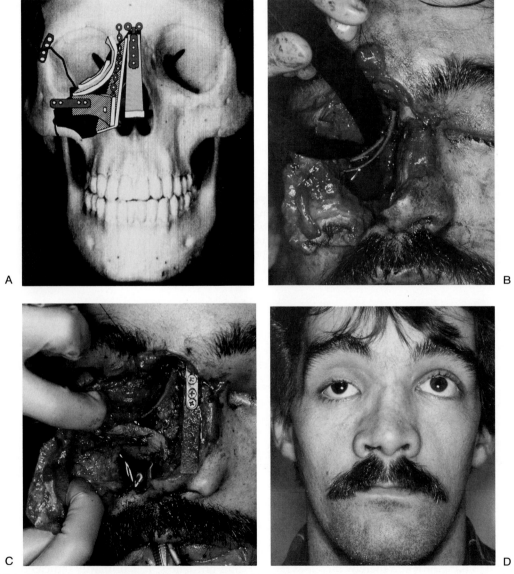

FIG. 20. Bone graft reconstruction of nasoethmoid orbital defect (same patient as shown previously in Fig. 18). **A:** Schematic diagram showing reconstruction. Stippled shapes are bone grafts. **B:** Split rib grafts are sequentially layered to reconstruct the medial wall and floor of the orbit. **C:** Split skull grafts are rigidly fixed to reconstruct the inferior and medial orbital rims as well as the nose in cantilever fashion. **D:** Postoperative result. Note residual ptosis of the upper lid and medial canthal dystopia.

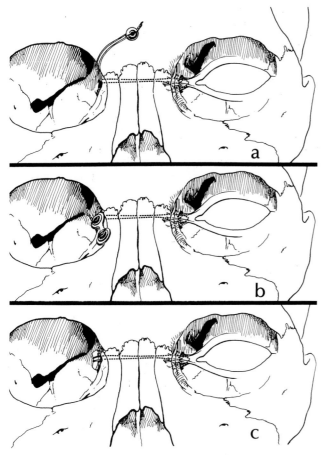

FIG. 21. Transnasal canthopexy techniques. The canthopexy wire approximates the medial canthal tendon to a fenestration in the medial orbital wall. The wires are passed transnasally into the contralateral orbit and fixed over a screw in the glabella (*a*), a fixation plate along the orbital rim (*b*), or a bone graft (*c*).

distance (distance between the medial orbital walls) is restored. Failure to do so will result in the medial canthi being fixed too far laterally and therefore will ensure telecanthus.

Bone grafts are shaped to the appropriate size for the medial orbital wall and are rigidly fixed in place by microplates both at the superior and at the inferior orbital rims. Calipers measure the distance between the two medial orbital walls; this should not exceed 25 mm.

3. In central maxillary fractures that destroy the perpendicular plate of the ethmoid, the septum, and the nasomaxillary buttresses, all dorsal nasal support is lost. This is an absolute indication for primary dorsal nasal bone grafting. Split skull bone graft is best employed for this purpose. The bone is fixed as a cantilever graft. Particular attention must be paid to details. The bone graft must be of adequate length, i.e., it must span the distance from the root to the tip of the nose to provide adequate support. Stabilization must be adequate and

is achieved by a single plate from the glabella to the dorsal nasal graft. Finally, it is imperative that the nasofrontal angle be maintained and not obliterated by the bone graft.

Medial Canthoplasty

Restoration of the premorbid medial canthal position is the single most important step in restoring premorbid nasoethmoid and orbital surface morphology. In Type I and Type II injuries, anatomic reduction of the tendon-bearing fracture segment generally ensures adequate placement of the medial canthus. However, in Type III injuries and in total avulsions or lacerations of the medial canthal tendon, restoration of medial canthal position is both technically challenging and susceptible to late failure.

The reconstructed medial orbital walls will provide the skeletal base for tendon reinsertion. Medial wall bone graft must be perfectly stable such that there is no ten-

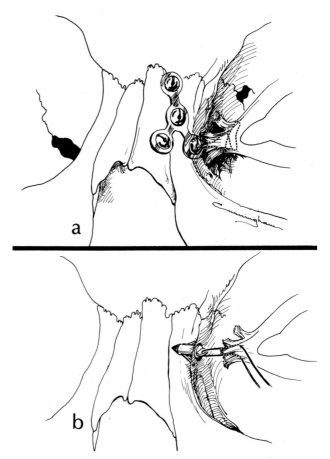

FIG. 22. Ipsilateral medial canthopexy techniques. The canthopexy wire approximates the medial canthal tendon to bone via a fixation device. This device can be a 1.2-mm screw in a microplate (**A**), rigidly fixed to the medial orbital rim, or a Mitek GII anchoring device (**B**).

dency for lateral displacement, and the distance between the medial walls must not exceed 25 mm.

Once an adequate skeletal foundation is provided, the 3D location of the medial canthal tendon insertion is precisely identified. Optimally, the tendon is inserted at the superior aspect of the posterior lacrimal crest. This ensures appropriate depth and vertical placement of the medial canthus. However, in grossly comminuted fractures where all adjacent anatomical landmarks are destroyed, placement is arbitrarily chosen at a point 5 mm posterior to the medial orbital rim, midway between the orbital roof and floor.

The techniques of canthal tendon fixation are varied (6) (Fig. 21). Classically, 3-0 stainless steel wire is used to secure the medial canthal tendon ends passed transnasally through a drill hole in the medial orbital bone graft to the contralateral medial orbit and secured distally over bone or bone graft in the contralateral orbit or over a central screw in the glabella. The transnasal wiring techniques offer the advantage of providing additional stability to the fractured medial orbital wall or medial wall bone graft by providing a posterior point of fixation. However, disadvantages include the need for dissection in the contralateral orbit and the mechanical disadvantage associated with a substantial length of wire. The wire can potentially stretch, leading to medial canthal drift.

An alternative means of medial canthoplasty consists of ipsilateral fixation of the medial canthal tendon to the medial orbital wall. These ipsilateral techniques isolate the dissection and fixation to the affected side only (Fig. 22). Multiple such techniques have been proposed previously but have not gained wide acceptance. We have in the recent past employed a Mitek GII anchoring device for this purpose, and have found it extremely effective.

CONCLUSION

Nasoethmoid complex injuries provide both a diagnostic and therapeutic challenge. Clinical and radiologic assessment must identify the degree of disruption and instability, and the extent of involvement of the cranial and orbital cavities. Optimal reconstruction then relies on adequate exposure, sequential reduction of unstable fragments, and immediate bone grafting of skeletal deficiencies to re-establish the 3D structure of the nasoethmoid complex.

REFERENCES

1. Farkas LG, Hreczko TA, Katic MJ. Craniofacial norms in North American Caucasians from birth (one year) to young adulthood. In: Farkas LG, ed. *Anthropometry of the head and face.* New York: Raven Press; 1994:241–333.
2. Holt GR, Holt JE. Nasoethmoid complex injuries. *Otolaryngol Clin North Am* 1985;18:877–998.
3. Gruss JS. Complex nasoethmoid-orbital and midfacial fractures: role of craniofacial surgical techniques and immediate bone grafting. *Ann Plast Surg* 1986;17:377–390.
4. Markowitz BL, Manson PN, Sargent L, et al. Management of the medial canthal tendon in nasoethmoid orbital fractures: the importance of the central fragment in classification and treatment. *Plast Reconstruct Surg* 1991;87:843–853.
5. Leidziger LS, Manson PN. Nasoethmoid orbital fractures. Current concepts and management principles. *Clin Plast Surg* 1992;19:167–193.
6. Crockett DM, Funk GF. Management of complicated fractures involving the orbits and nasoethmoid complex in young children. *Otolaryngol Clin North Am* 1991;24:119–137.

C. Management of the Lacrimal System Following Midfacial Trauma

IMMEDIATE MANAGEMENT OF THE LACRIMAL SYSTEM

At surgery for the open reduction and internal fixation of midfacial fractures, it is important that the lacrimal sac and duct be identified and any bone fragments be removed from their proximity. The membranous nasolacrimal sac and duct are usually quite resistant to external damage, but any resulting obstruction is probably due to external compression on the system by unreduced bone fragments (1). If, when the system is being inspected, one observes a laceration of the sac or duct, it is recommended that bicanalicular Silastic intubation of the nasolacrimal sac and duct be performed, without a dacryocystorhinostomy (DCR) (2).

Even though it has been suggested that a DCR could be performed at the time of the immediate repair (3), we feel that the success rate would be decreased because of the edema, hemorrhage, and anatomy distortion. If a subsequent DCR is to be performed, we prefer to wait approximately 4 to 5 months following the initial injury so that the edema and bone distortion is minimized, and any hardware may be removed without compromising the initial repair (4). If the patients present with telecanthus, there is an increased risk of a lacrimal obstruction and the subsequent need for a DCR. However, since this

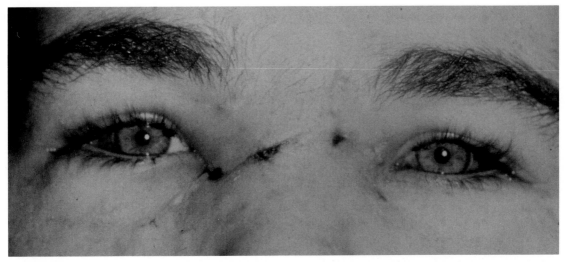

FIG. 23. Patient with telecanthus and tearing due to lacrimal obstruction. (From Nik et al., ref. 4, with permission.)

risk is not more than 50%, we prefer not to perform a DCR initially, but to inform the patient that a DCR may be necessary at a later date (4) (Fig. 23).

The patients may be observed for epiphora subsequently. Even in those patients with telecanthus who have early nasolacrimal block, approximately 20% of those will have the epiphora resolved spontaneously. The rest will probably require a DCR. Other causes of tearing may be due to punctal stenosis, ectropion, entropion, or wound infections (4).

We have been impressed that with severe midfacial trauma, if the lacrimal system can be identified and the bone fragments removed, that there is either no nasolacrimal obstruction postoperatively or, if there is, it often resolves spontaneously (5) (Fig. 24).

LATE MANAGEMENT OF LACRIMAL INJURY AFTER THE RECONSTRUCTION

If dacryocystitis presents postoperatively, it should be treated conservatively with systemic antibiotics and hot compresses. This usually leads to resolution, or fistulization. If tearing persists or dacryocystitis recurs, a DCR should be contemplated at a later date. With severe early dacryocystitis, a dacryocystotomy and external drainage of the sac is recommended if one does not wish to do an early DCR. We advocate waiting approximately 4 to 5 months after the trauma before performing a DCR. The patient, if tearing, is investigated with irrigation of the

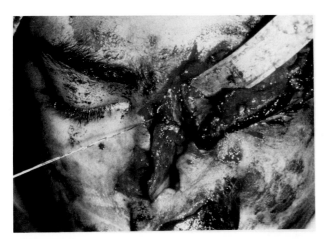

FIG. 24. Patient with severe midfacial trauma. Nasolacrimal sac and duct surprisingly intact (pointed out by probe). (From Nik et al., ref. 4, with permission.)

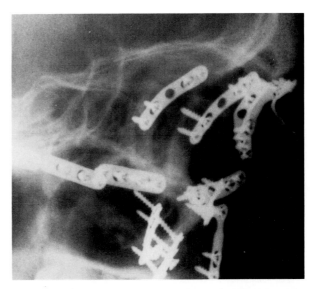

FIG. 25. Radiograph of patient following midfacial trauma and repair with miniplates and screws. (From Nik et al., ref. 4, with permission.)

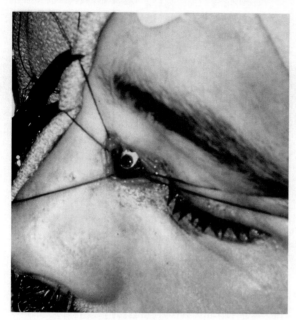

FIG. 26. At DCR surgery, a miniplate is encountered.

tween the sac and the nasal mucosa. If there is a large sac or a small sac, a DCR can usually be performed. The nasal mucosa may be opened and flaps of posterior sac and nasal mucosa can be anastomosed. We prefer in any trauma case to insert a bicanalicular Silastic stent tube and leave it in place for 3 months. We feel that in a post-traumatic case there is an increased risk of inflammation and potential for postoperative closure. The tubes help to hold the passage open. In certain circumstances, we will use in conjunction with the canalicular stent a rubber catheter, which is placed within the nose and sutured through the fundus of the sac onto the skin (see Chapter 36). This gives a larger opening between the anterior and posterior flaps (6). If there is a tiny scarred sac, or if there is no sac, a canaliculodacryocystorhinostomy may be performed (see Chapter 37). Often in these patients there is compromise of the space within the nose to perform a lacrimal procedure. If this is the situation, it makes it even more difficult to imagine that a Jones bypass tube could be placed and function properly. In this scenario, we prefer to enlarge the nasal opening by performing a turbinectomy, ethmoidectomy, or even septoplasty, and carry on with a canaliculodacryocystorhinostomy, rather than inserting a Jones bypass tube. We would only insert a Jones bypass tube at the primary procedure if indeed there was not enough canalicular tissue remaining to reanastomose with the sac and/or nasal mucosa.

If reconstructive lacrimal surgery fails, we would reassess the situation with another dacryocystogram. If there was enough residual sac, we would perform a repeat DCR. If there was no remaining sac, we would insert a Jones tube if there was a large enough nasal opening. If there is not enough of a nasal opening, we would probably do a canaliculodacryocystorhinostomy or insert a Jones tube in conjunction with a turbinectomy and/or septoplasty. However, we have found little need for second surgeries in these patients if the primary DCR is delayed for at least 4 months after the trauma and the immediate repair.

tear duct. If the tear duct is blocked, it is useful to get some imaging to determine the location of the sac, the site of obstruction, and the location of any hardware near the contemplated site of the DCR (Fig. 25). The proximity of these plates to the nasolacrimal system can be appreciated. Even if the patient is patent to syringing, a dacryocystogram may be useful to determine the size of the sac, and if the tearing is due to a distended (but patent) sac, a DCR is indicated.

The DCR begins in the traditional fashion. A skin incision is made and dissection is carried onto the bone of the frontal process of maxilla and the anterior lacrimal crest. If wires or plates and screws are encountered (Fig. 26), a window may be made in the appliance using an orthodontic cutter (Fig. 27). Bone is then removed be-

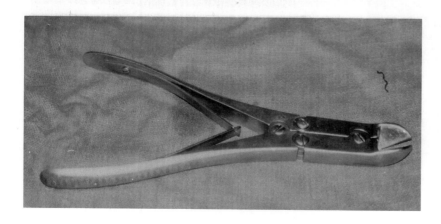

FIG. 27. An orthodontic plate and wire cutter are used to create a window in the hardware so that a DCR can be performed.

REFERENCES

1. Stranc MF. The pattern of lacrimal injuries and naso-ethmoid fractures. *Br J Plast Surg* 1970;23:339.
2. Crawford JS. Intubation of obstructions in the lacrimal system. *Can J Ophthalmol*. 1977;12:289.
3. Smith B, Nightingale JD. Fractures of the orbit: blow out and nasal orbit fractures. *Int Ophthalmol Clin* 1978;18:137.
4. Nik NA, Hurwitz JJ, Gruss JS. Management of lacrimal injury after naso-orbital ethmoid fractures. *Adv Ophthal Plast Reconstruct Surg* 1984;3:307.
5. Gruss JS, Hurwitz JJ, Nik NA, Kassel EE. The pattern and incidence of nasolacrimal injury in naso-orbital-ethmoid fractures: the role of delayed assessment and dacryocystorhinostomy. *Br J Plast Surg* 1985;38:116.
6. Hurwitz JJ, Archer KF, Gruss JS. Double stent intubation in difficult post-traumatic dacryocystorhinostomy. *Ophthal Surg* 1988;19:33.

CHAPTER 32

Pediatric Lacrimal Disease

Robert C. Pashby and Jeffrey Jay Hurwitz

The management of the epiphora in the infant necessitates the elimination of causes other than nasolacrimal apparatus difficulties (1–3). In the infant this sometimes is more difficult than it would seem, i.e., it is difficult sometimes without sedation to examine a child with a tearing, photophobic eye to determine if there is significant trichiasis or distichiasis or indeed foreign body or iritis.

DACRYOCYSTOCELE (AMNIOTOCELE)

Dacryocystocele presents at birth with redness and swelling of the lacrimal sac region (Fig. 1). It is important to rule out potential causes other than a dacryocystocele. It has been postulated that the fluid is amniotic rather than mucus, but nevertheless, it is irrelevant as far as treatment is concerned. Other causes would include hemangioma, encephalocele, orbital cellulitis, and even rhabdomyosarcoma. Imaging with ultrasound, computerized tomography (CT), or magnetic resonance imaging (MRI) can be done to aid one's clinical judgment before proceeding with appropriate treatment. If the child is ill or febrile, cultures of the conjunctiva and perhaps blood should be done. Once one has ruled out pathology other than nasolacrimal blockage, the usual treatment is conservative, with massage overlying the tear sac and topical antibiotic. One should show the parent how to massage over the tear sac and strongly suggest bilateral massage even in unilateral cases. The reason for this is that the

parent can gently grasp the base of the nose overlying the tear sac with his/her thumb and index finger and apply gentle rotary pressure over the tear sac; if the infant should move the parent's hand will move, thereby negating any chance of inadvertent corneal trauma with the parent's fingernail (2,4,5). If conservative management does not yield the anticipated result, a nasolacrimal probing may be required. It is unusual for conservative management to be unsuccessful in alleviating the situation if one waits long enough.

CONGENITAL NASOLACRIMAL OBSTRUCTION

Congenital nasolacrimal obstruction has been quoted in numerous sources (1,2,6,7) as being anywhere from 3% to 6% of newborn infants. The usual presentation is a wet discharging eye(s). Once other causes of the epiphora have been ruled out, massage as mentioned previously in the treatment of a dacryocystocele, along with appropriate antibiotic topical drops, is performed. If the baby has had an acute dacryocystitis, then as soon as the inflammation in the tear sac has subsided a probing is suggested if tearing persists and there is not resolution after a period of conservative management. However, the need to probe early, in our experience, is the exception rather than the rule (Fig. 2). If there is no acute dacryocystitis and the symptoms are not extreme, one should wait 12 to 18 months before probing. Numerous authors have quoted their statistics on these nasolacrimal probings and various successes and failures. It is generally felt that the membrane at the valve of Hasner will open by 1 year of age in 90% of children (7). Peterson and Rob reported spontaneous resolution in 89% of cases followed to 21 months of age. However, in those with symptoms that persisted beyond 9 months of age they found only a 43% resolution (8). Pollard (9) found a 41% resolution by 6 months and Katowitz and Welsh (10) found the success

R. C. Pashby: Department of Ophthalmology, Mount Sinai Hospital, and Oculoplastic Program, Hospital for Sick Children, and Department of Ophthalmology, University of Toronto Faculty of Medicine, Toronto, Ontario M5S 1A8, Canada.

J. J. Hurwitz: Oculoplastics Program, Mount Sinai Hospital; and Department of Ophthalmology, University of Toronto Faculty of Medicine, Toronto, Ontario M5S 1A8, Canada.

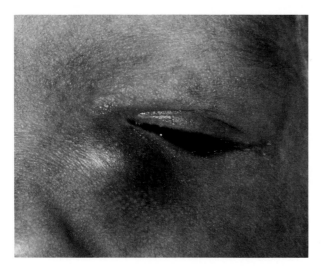

FIG. 1. Dacryocystocele (amniotocele) in a newborn. This resolved in 1 week with massage.

of their probings dropped from 98% success if performed before 6 months to 77% if performed after 13 months. Others (11) found 93.8% success with probings after 13 months. Interestingly, a Japanese study advocates probing as early as 2 weeks and states 100% success (12).

We generally feel that conservative management should be undertaken until 1 year of age. The only exception to this is the child with recurrent severe dacryocystitis, in whom a probing might be planned before 1 year of age during a "quiescent" phase. If the child presents even up to 5 years of age with a neglected congenital obstruction, we will still attempt a probing, and not intubation or a dacryocystorhinostomy (DCR). However, beyond the age of 2 years the success of probing decreases as the child gets older (13).

Nasolacrimal Probing Technique and Equipment

Numerous techniques of nasolacrimal probing are performed internationally by thousands of ophthalmologists with excellent results. Some are performed at a very young age, some at an older age, some are performed with simply bundling the child up without anesthesia, some are performed under sedation; our preferred method is under general anesthesia.

With the child under general anesthesia without endotracheal intubation and in the supine position, the ocular area is prepped with appropriate solution. The inferior punctum is dilated and in certain circumstances if there is a small punctum a simple straight pin can be used to dilate the punctum adequately so that the dilator may then be inserted. The dilator is passed vertically for 2 mm and then is turned medially while the lid is stretched in a lateral position to straighten the canaliculus. The dilator is then gently advanced along the inferior canaliculus and rotated gently. Following insertion of the dilator, a 00-size Bowman probe is passed in a similar fashion to the dilator but is passed along the entire horizontal length of the canalicular component to the common canaliculus, into the tear sac, until a bony hard stop is felt. The probe is then held gently against the bone and is turned in an inferior fashion, lying flat against the child's forehead. One does not want to pass this probe posteriorly. The probe is gently passed inferiorly until entry into the nasolacrimal canal is felt. The probe is then passed gently through the bony nasolacrimal canal until a firm stop is felt in the nose. At this point, to confirm that the system has been opened, a second probe, usually size 2 or 3 Bowman, is passed into the child's nose along the floor at the junction of the floor and the lateral wall of the nose to enter the inferior meatus. The probe is then moved superiorly to touch the tip of the first probe, which has been passed down into the inferior meatus. Metal to metal contact is felt and one can also see the probe inserted into the nasolacrimal system move back and forth as contact is made. The system is then dilated with a size 0 or 1 probe. The probe is then removed and an antibiotic drop is instilled into the conjunctival sac. To confirm patency, fluorescein-tinted saline may be syringed into the sac. If it can be retrieved via the mouth in the nasopharynx with a suction, the system has been rendered patent. The usual postoperative treatment entails insertion of an antibiotic drop two to three times daily for 2 to 3 days postoperatively. Decongestant nasal spray such as Naphazoline inserted into the inferior meatus may be used for 3 days to decongest the instrumented valve of Hasner. The parents are often cautioned that there may be a small amount of bleeding from the

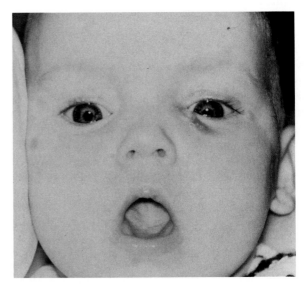

FIG. 2. Six-month-old baby with left congenital lacrimal obstruction and mild dacryocystitis. The infection resolved with penicillin, and epiphora ceased spontaneously at 10 months of age.

nose (which is not common) and sometimes there may even be a small amount of blood in the tear film. The child is usually reassessed in the office in 2 weeks' time.

There are many other techniques that have been described, including air insufflation of the system and the use of a nasal endoscopy to look into the nose and remove any membranes that are visible at the bottom end. Some authors have suggested that if one does indeed inject the fluorescein solution and it is not visible, that infracturing the inferior intubation will lead to success (14,15). To perform this maneuver, an artery forceps is passed through the nose along the lateral wall until it strikes the undersurface of the inferior turbinate. Then the turbinate is fractured toward the septum hopefully to pull any bone or soft tissues away from the valve of Hasner. We do not routinely do this on the first probing.

Failed Nasolacrimal Probing

If the nasolacrimal probing was felt to be successful by the surgeon, i.e., the system was felt to be patent, but yet the child continues to be symptomatic, one would likely then proceed to a repeat nasolacrimal probing. A dacryocystogram may be performed, but we do not do this routinely (13). A persistent block at the valve of Hasner can be cured in almost all cases, even at the time of a second probing, without intubation. However, only 40% of cases where the block is at the sac-duct junction can be cured with a probing alone. These cases might do well with intubations. One would wait a minimum of 3 months before considering another probing. The patient can be booked for a probing with a possible tube insertion. If the probing is easy and there is only a membrane to be "popped," silicone tubing is not necessary. If the probing was repeated and patency was obtained but the anatomy was felt to be abnormal or the probing itself was difficult, then insertion of silicone tubes is indicated. If the probing has been successful with an asymptomatic child but symptoms appear later, then silicone tube intubation is indicated (16–23). Balloon catheterization has been suggested by numerous authors as being an efficient and atraumatic way of dilating the nasolacrimal system in the area of obstruction (20). But since tubes are also inserted after dilatation, one cannot be sure whether the balloon, the tubes, or the probing cured the child. We feel that at this time balloon dilatation adds little to our treatment protocol. The length of time that the silicone tube is left in place is variable; many surgeons feel strongly that there is a definite time period that is necessary (23). We have found the usual 2- to 3-month length of time as being adequate. Sometimes when children pull these out after only 1 or 2 weeks, often success can be obtained. This would make one wonder whether the probing alone had cured the child when the tube had been in for only 2 to 3 weeks.

If one could not get through at all with a probe initially, or if on the second procedure one cannot pass the tubes, the surgeon should be prepared to perform a (DCR).

Congenital canalicular obstructions can be cured only infrequently by a probing. With congenital common canalicular or individual distal canalicular obstruction, silicone tube insertion is recommended. If this does not work, a canaliculodacryocystorhinostomy is recommended. Proximal canalicular obstruction usually requires a permanent bypass tube.

Technique of Nasolacrimal Silicone Intubation Using Crawford Lacrimal Intubation Set With Suture (Fig. 3A)

General anesthesia with endotracheal intubation is recommended. We have found the use of the Crawford Intubation set, which includes an indwelling suture, to be the optimum system for intubation in children. It is valuable in the following situations: failed probings, difficult probings with abnormal anatomy, at the time of craniofacial surgery to prevent nasolacrimal problems, and in cases of trauma. The technique that we have found successful over the years is the following: A standard probing is performed. The Crawford tube with an olive tip on the leading end and a swedged silicone tube with indwelling silk suture on the following end is passed as a standard probe through the system (Fig. 3B). A Crawford hook (Fig. 3C) is then inserted into the inferior meatus with the hook facing superiorly.

The Crawford hook has a flat spot on the handle indicating the direction that the hook is facing. The Crawford probe is then touched with the hook and one should identify whether the hook is medial or lateral to the probe. The hook is then turned 90° either medially or laterally to engage on the probe. The hook is held steady while the probe is pulled superiorly to engage the olive tip of the probe and lock it in the notch of the hook. The hook is then pulled out under the inferior meatus and externalized while the probe is held in a push/pull type of maneuver. At this point one may encounter a snagging of the tip of the hook on the inferior turbinate or the nasal mucosa and care must be taken not to use excessive force. If the angle of the inferior opening of the nasolacrimal duct is pointing exceedingly posteriorly, the difficulty can be encountered with pulling the probe out from this acute angle. Sometimes the exit is so acute and the system so tight that the swedged silicone may even be pulled off the probe. Once both Crawford probes have been passed and externalized through the nose, a snap with tips covered with silicone sleeves is used to clamp the silicone tube and indwelling suture such that it is fairly tight against the nose of the child (Fig. 3D). The silicone is then stripped from the indwelling suture im-

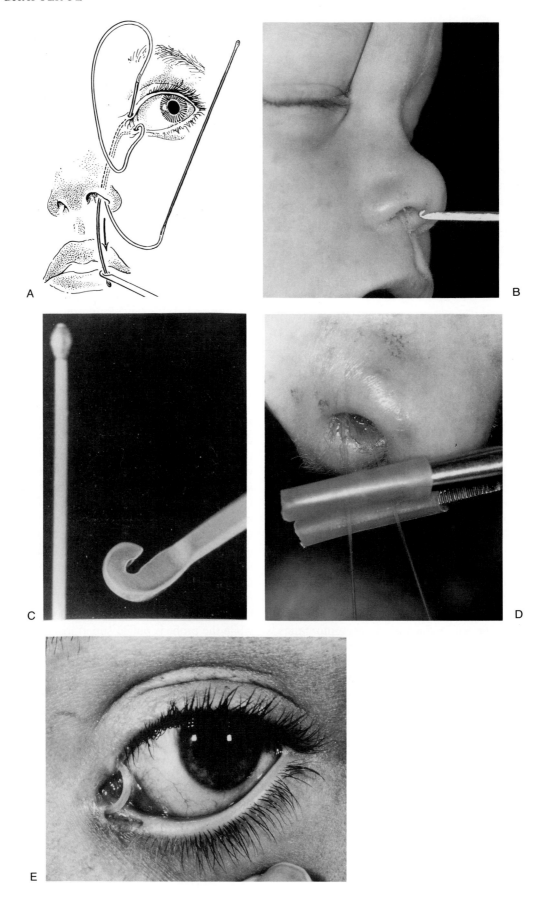

A

B

C

D

E

mediately adjacent to the clamp. The indwelling suture is then tied in numerous knots and the suture trimmed to an appropriate length. The clamp is released to allow the silicone and knot to retract under the inferior meatus. If it is too tight at the superior end between the punctum then a tying forceps is used simply to loosen the silicone slightly at the medial canthal region. A drop of topical antibiotic is instilled to the patient's eye. The patient is returned to the recovery room and is later discharged home on topical antibiotic drops two to three times daily for 3 to 4 days postoperatively. A postoperative reassessment is made in the office in about 2 weeks' time, at which point the position of the tube is assessed as well as whether the child is tolerating or having any irritation from the tubes. An office appointment is then made for 2 to 3 months later for removal of the tube in the office.

Removal of Silicone Tubing

The removal of the tube in the office is simple. One grasps the tube quickly at the inner canthus, pulls it laterally, clips the loop of the tube, and pulls out both ends of the silicone. Infrequently, the suture will stay in the system and this can be removed simply by grasping one end of the suture and pulling it out. Discomfort seems absolutely minimal for the children and we have not found anesthesia or sedation necessary. This inner suture modification of the Crawford tubing has negated the need to identify the tubing in the nose or pull knots of silicone through the puncta.

One may encounter complications with silicone tubes, namely, a tight tube "cheese wiring" the canalicular system (Fig. 3E), or a loose tube wherein the knot in silicone is externalized through the nose or where a loose tube may be pulled in front of the cornea. If the child has externalized the tubes, one may try to reposition the tube and secure it with a suture on the nasal skin. However, we have found it most efficient simply to cut the tube and remove it and hope that it has been in long enough to achieve patency. However, if one wishes to leave the tube in for a longer period, the simplest method is to tape the loop onto the side of the nose. We have been able to maintain tubes in place for as long as an extra 2 to 3 months in a few of these patients. If one has to repeat the procedure on these children, then either passing the inferior end of the tubes through a small retinal explant band or suturing the tubes into the nostril are methods of achieving more permanent fixation. If the tubes have been kept in the desired period of time, and the child has persistent epiphora after removal, a DCR is recommended after at least a 3-month waiting period.

Nasal Endoscopy

Nasal endoscopy can be performed by an otorhinolaryngologist or an ophthalmologist who has had some training in this area. This technique is useful if there is abnormal nasal anatomy or a mucosal flap overlying the distal end of the nasolacrimal duct. Under endoscopy this flap can be removed easily, usually leading to successful surgery and an asymptomatic child. Nasal endoscopy is a necessity with some of the tubes now on the market for retrieval of the tube at the distal end of the nasolacrimal duct. There have been reports of cystic intranasal masses that have been found to cause a blocked tear duct and even respiratory problems in some children (24), and these certainly would be best evaluated by endoscopic techniques.

DCR in Children

The ideal time to perform a DCR in a child is 4 years of age. At this age, the face is more adult size, and the scar, which grows with the face, will be cosmetically acceptable. However, we have performed DCR surgery in children as young as 1 year who had totally imperforate lower systems that could not be probed or tubed, and in whom recurrent dacryocystitis was troublesome.

Technique

A small incision is made on the side of the nose. Traction sutures are used to separate the soft tissues. Bone is removed between the sac and nasal mucosa as in the adult. In children there are usually few problems with ethmoids.

We prefer to suture posterior flaps of sac and nasal mucosa, and use a 7-0 polygalactin suture (2–3 sutures). The smaller needle facilitates suturing the flaps. The anterior flaps of sac and nasal mucosa may be sutured with this or

FIG. 3. A: Crawford intubation of lacrimal system. Both wires are passed through puncta and down into the nose. They are pulled out by the Crawford hook. (Courtesy of Dr. J. S. Crawford, Toronto.) **B:** Wires of Crawford tubes being pulled out of the nose with a Crawford hook. **C:** Close-up of olive-tipped end of Crawford rod on intubation set (*above*). Close-up of Crawford hook that engages the olive-tipped end of the rod. **D:** Artery forceps with rubber on ends grasps tubing once the rods have been removed. The tubing can be stripped from the indwelling suture. The suture is then tied, creating a closed loop with no knots in the tubing. This allows for easy removal. **E:** Crawford tube in place at inner canthus. Slight erosion of the punctum is noted.

a 5-0 polygalactin suture. Tubes are not necessary unless there is canalicular pathology, a reoperation, or trouble fashioning flaps. The skin is sutured with 6-0 absorbable catgut sutures. The eye or preferably the side of the nose is patched for 1 day. Garamycin ointment is used on the sutures and Cloxacillin is taken orally for 1 week if there is mucus or pus in the sac.

If there is bilateral obstruction, a bilateral DCR may be planned. Especially in a younger child, the question of blood loss becomes potentially significant. Even though we tell the parents we might have to abort the second side if there is too much bleeding on the first side, we have never had this happen.

Assuming that the child is healthy, with no anemia or cardiovascular problems, the blood volume should be 70 to 80 cc/Kg. Assuming a normal hemoglobin and blood volume, the child could conceivably lose up to 25% of the preoperative hemoglobin without needing to have a blood transfusion. This presupposes that during the operation the blood volume is being maintained by normal saline, albumen, or any other similar solutions.

The hemoglobin will change rapidly with bleeding if there is rapid hemodilution with the blood volume being maintained. As long as one maintains blood volume in the face of bleeding, the hemoglogin is as accurate as the hematocrit.

If bleeding is profuse, if the blood volume cannot be maintained, or if the hemoglobin drops below 25% of the original value, blood transfusion is recommended. One obviously tries to avoid giving blood with the recent fear of AIDS, hepatitis, etc. In practice, we have never had to transfuse a child intraoperatively (or postoperatively for that matter).

For a bilateral DCR, in a child 4 years of age or less (or in an older frail child), we will group and type, but not cross-match. Then, if blood is needed, it can be available in 10 minutes.

Absent Nasolacrimal Punctum

This abnormality may involve one or both puncta (6) (Fig. 4). Often, if one punctum is absent, the other normal punctum sometimes prevents symptoms of epiphora. Examination of infants with this problem is exceedingly difficult and often requires sedation or anesthetic to allow proper visualization of the eyelid and potential region of the punctum.

If the papilla is present then often, with the use of a straight pin or fine needle, the punctum can be opened. A routine nasolacrimal probing then should be performed to indicate patency of the remainder of the system.

If no papilla is visible it is possible to attempt to cut through the lid margin medial to where the punctum should be to identify any canalicular structure. If a canalicular structure can be visualized it could be marsupial-

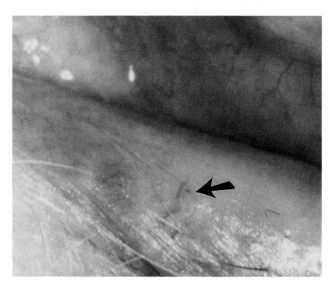

FIG. 4. Congenital absence of lower punctum. No papilla is present. A Jones tube was necessary to relieve epiphora.

ized to the conjunctival surface. A probing should be performed again to tell whether the remainder of the system is patent. However, if there is agenesis of the punctal region then likely there is agenesis of most of the proximal nasolacrimal apparatus. Therefore, we have usually found this maneuver to be unsuccessful and rarely attempt this. The child usually requires a DCR with insertion of a Jones tube as a bypass procedure.

Punctal Reduplication and Accessory Canaliculi

These congenital abnormalities may be asymptomatic. They usually occur along the mucocutaneous junction of the lid medial to the punctum. A true reduplicated punctum will have a papilla around it, with Hasner's muscle around the canalicular attachment to the system. This allows it to function normally (Fig. 5).

An accessory slit punctum is an accessory canaliculus, with no papilla and vestigial surrounding musculature. Therefore, even if there is a patent system to the nose through this slit, it rarely functions (Fig. 6). Dacryocystography is helpful in elucidating the connections of these accessory channels.

A congenitally slit punctum usually does not function. We have had little success marsupializing the canaliculus or suturing the slit, and have ultimately resorted to a Jones tube insertion in these patients (Fig. 7).

Bypass Tube Insertion in Children

The bypass tube that we prefer to use in children is the Pyrex glass Lester Jones tube. We insert the tube in patients with congenital punctal and canalicular agenesis, or slit puncta.

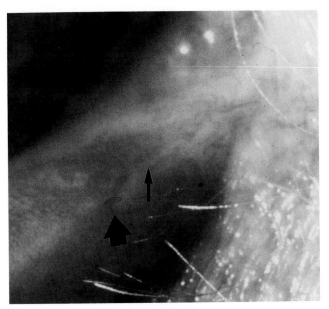

FIG. 5. An asymptomatic patient with a punctal reduplication as an incidental finding. (*small arrow*, accessory punctum, *big arrow*, normal punctum). (From Goldberg and Hurwitz, ref. 6, with permission.)

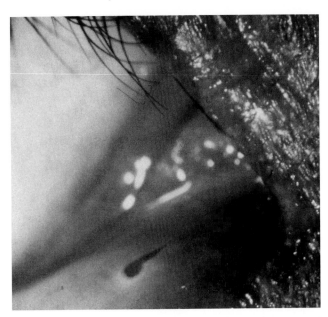

FIG. 7. Symptomatic congenital slit punctum. Attempts at suturing were unsuccessful. Epiphora was relieved with a Jones tube. (From Goldberg and Hurwitz, ref. 6, with permission.)

The Jones tube is a prosthesis, and there must be compliance of the patient and the parents if the procedure is to be a success. We prefer to wait until the child is approximately 10 to 12 years of age. However, we have inserted the tube in children as young as the age of 4 years in whom we felt compliance was possible. Because of sig-

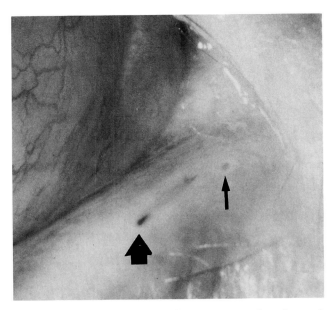

FIG. 6. Patient with accessory lower punctum (*small arrow*) medial to normal punctum (*big arrow*) on the edge of the eyelid, at the medial ends of a gutter connecting with the normal punctum. Epiphora was due to a lateral common canalicular obstruction and cured with a canaliculodacryocystorhinostomy (see Colorplate 8 following page 142). (From Goldberg and Hurwitz, ref. 6, with permission.)

nificant facial growth before the age of 4 years, even if a tube were to be inserted, it would have to be changed later for a longer tube.

In children, because the palpebral aperture is usually narrower, we prefer to use a 3.5-mm size ocular end. The 4.0 is too large and may erode the inner canthal tissues. The 3.0 mm tube is too small, and because the outer diameter of the shaft of the tube is 2.5 mm, the tube has a real possibility of slipping down into the nose. A suture placed through the suture hole in the neck of the tube and fixated at the inner canthus aids fixation.

The tube should be irrigated every 6 months to a year. The child, preoperatively, must be taught how to sniff water through the tube into the nose, so that postoperative cleansing of the tube can be performed on a regular basis.

Congenital Fistula (25–27)

A fistula communicating with the lacrimal sac or common canaliculus is not common (Fig. 8). One may notice a small fistula track below the medial canthal tendon and overlying the tear sac region. This is an epithelial connection between the sac or common canaliculus and the skin. If asymptomatic, no treatment is required. If symptomatic and the child has difficulty with excess tearing, then a surgical procedure can be performed. Our suggestion would be that under general anesthesia a nasolacrimal probing be performed. If patency of the system is found then a second probe is passed into the fistulous track and, using a #11 Bard Parker blade, a coring is done

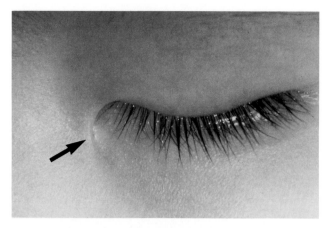

FIG. 8. Baby with symptomatic congenital fistula communicating with lacrimal sac. Probing of the nasolacrimal canal and excising the fistula relieved epiphora.

to remove the fistulous track around the inserted probe. An alternative method is to insert a hyfrecating needle into the fistula to obliterate the passage. Care must be taken not to damage the underlying lacrimal sac or common canaliculus with either method. We have had success with this simple technique. In 5 of our 14 cases, nasolacrimal intubation was also performed at the time of fistula excision if there seemed to be an abnormality in the remainder of the system. If, however, these measures are unsuccessful, these children would benefit from DCR and dissection of the fistulous tract. Preoperative dacryocystography is useful to demonstrate whether the fistula connects with the sac or the common canaliculus. Of interest is the fact that in our series of 14 we found that almost half these children suffered from Down syndrome (28).

Cranial Facial Abnormalities

Children with significant cranial facial abnormalities have an increased incidence of nasolacrimal problems. Children with Treacher-Collins syndrome frequently have problems, as do those with the Tessier midfacial cleft problems #3 or #4. Our suggestion for these children is a nasolacrimal probing at the time of their craniofacial surgery and intubation of the system if at all possible. This will hopefully reduce the problem of iatrogenic postoperative nasolacrimal problems.

REFERENCES

1. Isenberg J, ed. *The eye in infancy.* Chicago: Yearbook Medical Publishers; 1989:209–215.
2. Morin JD, Crawford JS, eds. *The eye in childhood.* New York: Grune & Stratton; 1983.
3. Welham RAN. In: Collin RJO, ed. *A manual of systematic eye lid surgery.* New York: Churchill Livingstone; 1982.
4. Stager D, Baker JD, Frey T. Office probing of congenital nasolacrimal duct obstruction. *Ophthal Surg* 1979;23:482–484.
5. Pashby RC, Sullivan TJ, Clarke M, Morin JD. Management of congenital dacryocystocoele. *Aust N Z Ophthalmol* 1992;20(2): 105–109.
6. Goldberg A, Hurwitz JJ. Congenital abnormalities of lacrimal drainage; management of difficult cases. *Can J Ophthalmol* 1979;14:106.
7. Hurwitz JJ. Paediatric nasolacrimal obstruction. *Ophthal Practi* 1987;5:64.
8. Peterson RA, Robb RM. The natural course of congenital obstruction of the nasolacrimal duct. *J Paediatr Ophthalmol* 1978;15: 246–250.
9. Pollard J. Tear duct obstruction in children. *Clin Paediatr* 1979;18:487–490.
10. Katowitz JA, Welsh MG. Timing of initial probing and irrigation in congenital nasolacrimal duct obstruction. *Ophthalmology* 1987;94:698–705.
11. El-Mansour JH, Calhoun JH, Nelson LB, Harley RD. Results of late probing for congenital nasolacrimal duct obstruction. *Ophthalmology* 1986;93:1052–1054.
12. Ishikawa C, Tamaka H, Toibanam. *Folia Ophthalmol Jap* 1990;41:940–944.
13. Hurwitz JJ, Welham RAN. The role of dacryocystography in the management of congenital nasolacrimal duct obstruction. *Can J Ophthalmol.* 1975;10:346.
14. Harris WE, Wilkins RB. A useful alternative to silicone tube intubation in congenital nasolacrimal duct obstructions. *Ophthal Surg* 1988;14:666–670.
15. Wesley RE. Inferior turbinate fracture in the treatment of nasolacrimal duct obstruction and congenital nasolacrimal duct anomaly. *Ophthal Surg* 1985;16:368–371.
16. Lyon D, Dorzbach RK, Lemke BN, Gonnering RS. Canalicular stenosis following probing for congenital nasolacrimal duct obstruction. *Ophthal Surg* 1991;22:228–232.
17. Pashby RC, Rathbun JE. Silicone intubation of the lacrimal drainage system. *Arch Opthalmol* 1979;97:1318–1322.
18. Kraft SP, Crawford JS. Silicone tube intubation in disorders of the lacrimal system in children. *Am J Ophthalmol* 1982;94:290–299.
19. Crawford JS. Intubation of obstructions of the lacrimal system. *Can J Ophthalmol* 1977;12:289–292.
20. Becker BB, Berry FD. Balloon catheter dilatation in paediatric patients. *Ophthal Surg* 1991;22(7):750–752.
21. Kushner BJ. Congenital nasolacrimal system obstruction. *Arch Ophthalmol* 1982;10:597–600.
22. Quickert MH, Dryden RM. Probes for intubation in lacrimal drainage. *Trans Am Acad Ophthalmol Otolaryngol* 1970;74:431–433.
23. Migliori ME, Putterman AM. Silicone intubation for the treatment of congenital lacrimal duct obstruction: successful results removing tubes after six weeks. *Ophthalmology* 1989;95:792–795.
24. Given TR, Mertz JS, Stuss-Isern M. Congenital nasolacrimal ducts cysts in dacryocystocoele. *Ophthalmology* 1991;98:1238–1242.
25. Birchansky LD, Nerad JA, Kersten RC, Kulwin DR. Management of congenital lacrimal sac fistula. *Arch Ophthalmol* 1990;108:388–390.
26. Welham RAN, Bergin DJ. Congenital lacrimal fistulas. *Arch Ophthalmol* 1985;103:545–548.
27. Pashby RC, Sullivan TJ, Clarke M, Morin JD. The surgical management of congenital lacrimal fistulae. *Aust N Z J Ophthalmol* 1992;20(2): 190–194.
28. Pashby RC, Sullivan TJ, Clarke M, Brazel S, Morin JD. Congenital lacrimal fistula associated with Down syndrome. *Am J Ophthalmol* 1992;112:215–216.

CHAPTER 33

Introduction and Philosophy

Jeffrey Jay Hurwitz

For centuries, surgeons have treated patients with tearing due to lacrimal drainage pathway obstructions. If one examines the literature over the past hundred years, there have been described a host of various procedures used in the treatment of patients with epiphora. As Jones and Wobig stated in their textbook on surgery of the eyelids and lacrimal system (1), many of the procedures that have been described in the literature have not withstood the test of time. In fact, it would seem that many of the authors describing certain procedures no longer use these procedures but have returned to the standard operations used by most surgeons.

The external dacryocystorhinostomy (DCR) described in the early 1900s by Toti (2) has withstood the test of time and is indeed the "gold standard" today. It is against this procedure that all operations *can* and *must* be compared.

The area of lacrimal surgery lies somewhere between that practiced by the ophthalmologist on one hand and by the otolaryngologist and plastic surgeon on the other. The otolaryngologists (and to a certain extent the plastic surgeons) feel extremely comfortable operating in the nose. However, they are certainly much less comfortable working around the palpebral aperture and the globe, and certainly the investigation both clinically and radiologically of patients with epiphora and lacrimation does not fall within their scope. On the other hand, the ophthalmologist is fully comfortable examining and diagnosing the nature of the tearing problem but does not have the experience in most cases to work in the nose. Therefore, lacrimal surgery through the years has not been a major concern for any of these three disciplines. As well, in most health care jurisdictions, the importance of afflictions of the lacrimal system has not been given

much significance. Therefore, reimbursement for these procedures has not, by and large, been substantial, and the surgeons from these specialties have preferred to perform surgery that is more mainstream for their own individual skills.

This issue has been even more apparent by the division of the speciality of "eyes, ears, nose and throat" (E.E.N.T.) into ophthalmology and otolaryngology. Fortunately, there have been a small group of ophthalmologists who are interested in lacrimal problems who have taken these patients on as a major area of interest.

To patients with tearing problems and diseases of the lacrimal drainage pathways, these problems are real and they are as interested in having them investigated properly and managed appropriately as patients with any other condition elsewhere in the body. Unfortunately, just as ophthalmologists and otolaryngologists have not been interested in surgery for these patients, they also have not been terribly interested in the investigation of these patients. Indeed, it is as important that these patients are investigated properly as it is for the cataract patient presenting to the ophthalmologist, and the patient with a hearing problem presenting to the otolaryngologist. It is no longer appropriate to tell the patient with a tearing problem "let's open up your canaliculus and see if that helps—if it doesn't then may be we can tighten up your lid—if this doesn't then maybe we can do a DCR." The diagnosis must be properly made and the appropriate treatment must be instituted. Conway (3) discusses, from results of a survey of a group of ophthalmologists, how to handle patients with "functional obstructions," that is to say, patients who have tearing and who are patent to syringing. The vast array of responses such as operating on the lid, the punctum, the lacrimal system, the lacrimal system with a DCR, the lacrimal system with tubes, etc. show that these patients have probably not been properly investigated most of the time, and that the rationale for surgery has not taken into

J. J. Hurwitz: Oculoplastics Program, Mount Sinai Hospital; and Department of Ophthalmology, University of Toronto Faculty of Medicine, Toronto, Ontario M5S 1A8, Canada.

account the results of any investigation. The lacrimal patients have definite problems and should be managed in a definite way.

Many health care jurisdictions have forced ophthalmic surgery to move to the outpatient setting. Certainly, cataracts are most often done in the outpatient setting in many areas nowadays. Lacrimal surgery has been lumped with other ophthalmic procedures and in many areas the surgeon is forced to do lacrimal surgery in an outpatient setting. Many surgeons have therefore, worrying that they will have to send their patients home the same day, been forced to change their techniques that had been working quite well and in many cases to compromise their surgical plan. Certainly, with the move to outpatient surgery, many surgeons now perform their drainage pathway procedures under local anesthesia rather than with general anesthesia. This in many cases has also forced the surgeon to compromise the surgery done under local anesthesia where it is perceived that one does not have as much control to do the operation that otherwise would have been planned. Many surgeons in the outpatient setting, especially with the patient under local anesthesia, do not feel comfortable performing the standard DCR and instead would prefer merely to intubate the system and hope that this works.

However, the move to outpatient surgery has not been all bad. Techniques have indeed been formulated to perform surgery on many patients under local anesthesia. Changes in technique, *without compromising* the surgical plan, have been elucidated for performing full DCRs under general anesthesia in those patients who would have to go home the same day.

Newer techniques with media appeal have been designed in an attempt to attract patient interest. Some of these procedures such as using the laser for DCR surgery, eyelid surgery, and even blepharoplasty surgery increase the cost of instrumentation for the procedure, and may not withstand the test of time or measure up to the "gold standard" of the commonly performed procedures. Indeed, the recent enthusiasm for using laser technology for DCR surgery has waned, as only a small number of patients presenting with lacrimal sac obstruction could indeed be treated by a laser DCR (those with potential stones, tumors, ethmoid problems, small sacs, common canaliculus or canalicular problems being ruled out),

and also as longer term success rates decreased and were not acceptable.

The resurgence of interest in performing DCRs intranasally (not necessary with the laser) has been compared to the change of technique in performing cataract surgery with a phaco-emulsification technique as opposed to the manual extracapsular technique. The intranasal approach has been around for many years and an elegant description was published by Jones in 1951 (4). It is basically this technique that is being resurrected, probably because of the development of the nasal endoscope. The lacrimal surgeon must be comfortable in the nose and must have some facility to do intranasal surgery as well as external surgery. Intranasal surgery will probably withstand the test of time as an adjunct to external DCR and will be a part of the armamentarium of the procedures performed by the lacrimal surgeon. The ratio of internal to external surgery that any individual lacrimal surgeon will perform will vary from surgeon to surgeon, and how well intranasal surgery withstands the test of time and measures up to the "gold standard" of the external DCR.

In the chapters on lacrimal drainage surgery, the external DCR is described extensively. Indications for surgery, preoperative assessment, anesthesia (both general and local), informed consent, and preoperative and postoperative management are extensively described. In later chapters, modifications of this procedure such as endonasal surgery, endonasal laser surgery, canaliculodacryocystorhinostomy for some canalicular obstructions, and conjunctivodacryocystorhinostomy with Jones tubes for other forms of canalicular obstructions are also described. There also are descriptions of modifications for the treatment of patients with lacrimal sac tumors, following lacrimal trauma, and surgery for reoperation.

REFERENCES

1. Jones LT, Wobig JL. *Surgery of the eyelids and lacrimal system.* Birmingham, AL: Aesculapius Publishing; 1976.
2. Toti A. Dacryocistorhinostomia. *Clin Mod* 1904;X:33–34.
3. Conway ST. Evaluation and management of "functional" blockage. *Ophthal Plast Reconstruct Surg* 1994;10:185.
4. Jones LT, Boyden G. The rhinologist's role in tear sac surgery. *Trans Am Acad Ophthalmol Otolaryngol* 1951;34:654.

CHAPTER **34**

Anesthesia for Lacrimal Surgery

Chidambaram R. Ananthanarayan, Ernest M. Hew, and Jeffrey Jay Hurwitz

Anesthesia for lacrimal surgery presents unique challenges. The anesthesiologist must provide safety, akinesia, profound analgesia, minimal bleeding, avoidance or obtundation of the oculo-cardiac reflex, proper control of intraocular pressure, and smooth emergence while watching for drug interactions. In addition to having technical expertise, the anesthesiologist must have a thorough knowledge of relevant anatomy, physiology, and pharmacology (1,2).

Most patients undergoing lacrimal surgery are either younger than 10 years or older than 55 years of age. In children, operations on the ocular adnexa especially related to the lacrimal apparatus are common. They are usually done under general anesthesia.

The airway must be protected from obstruction as the anesthesiologist is usually remote from the operative field.

In adults, general or local anesthesia may be used, but many factors are involved in this decision. Additional preparations include identification and control of underlying disease states such as asthma, diabetes, nephropathy, hypertension, coronary artery disease, thyroid and parathyroid dysfunction, and bleeding diathesis. The patients should be prepared emotionally for the recovery period as they will awaken and may have one eye patched, and one or both nasal passages packed.

Patients presenting for lacrimal surgery may be at the extremes of ages with coexistent medical diseases and congenital syndromes in children (1).

Extraocular procedures such as dacryocystorhinos-

tomy (DCR) surgery require greater control of the oculo-cardiac reflex. This may occur in sinus surgery as well as lacrimal surgery, even though the rectus muscles are not being manipulated.

Surgery on the lacrimal system may be classified under extraocular adnexal surgery; the special considerations for these operations include the following: safety, adequate analgesia, potential for major blood loss, control of oculo-cardiac reflex, drug interactions, hypotensive anesthesia, and smooth emergence.

PREOPERATIVE PREPARATION

Patients must be prepared carefully. Most patients accept that surgery and anesthesia have inherent risks, and often they appreciate a candid explanation of potential complications. A thorough history and physical examination are the sine qua non of current patient care. It is also common to classify the physical status according to the American Society of Anesthesiologists (ASA) Classification scheme (3) (Table 1).

The advantages of this classification are twofold:

1. It allows the anesthesiologist and others to compare the outcomes (complications or death) within and between institutions based on one standard criterion.
2. It provides the anesthesiologist with a quick summary of the physical status of the patient. In many centers, ASA I, II, III, and well controlled IV are accepted for outpatient procedures with local anesthesia, sedative techniques, or even general anesthesia.

A complete list of the drugs (both systemic and topical) currently being used by the patient should be recorded so that potential drug interactions and side effects can be anticipated. The following is a brief summary of some drug interactions and side effects that can be expected and the measures that may be taken to combat them.

C. R. Ananthanarayan and E. M. Hew: Department of Anesthesia, Mount Sinai Hospital, and Department of Anesthesia, University of Toronto Faculty of Medicine, Toronto, Ontario M5S 1A8, Canada.

J. J. Hurwitz: Oculoplastics Program, Mount Sinai Hospital; and Department of Ophthalmology, University of Toronto Faculty of Medicine, Toronto, Ontario M5S 1A8, Canada.

TABLE 1. *ASA status*

I. Healthy patient
II. Mild systemic disease
III. Severe systemic disease, but not incapacitating
IV. Severe systemic disease that is a constant threat to life
V. Moribund. Not expected to live 24 hours irrespective of the operation

ASA, American Society of Anesthesiologists.

Drug Therapy in Relation to Anesthesia (4)

Analgesics

Aspirin

May cause a bleeding tendency because of functional impairment of platelets. Try to stop aspirin 14 days before surgery. Occasionally platelet transfusions are required in emergency surgery. If in doubt, do a bleeding time (normal <8 min) before surgery, but recognize that this test is *not* infallible.

Antibiotics

Aminoglycosides

Clindamycin, gentamicin, kanamycin, neomycin, and streptomycin can cause nondepolarizing neuromuscular block on their own. They may potentiate curare-type muscle relaxants and may worsen muscle diseases such as myasthenia gravis and muscular dystrophies. Muscle block may be reversed with calcium and/or neostigmine. Monitor neuromuscular function in the perioperative period.

Cephalosporins

Cefazolin, cefotaxime, and cefotetan can cause allergic reactions. Vancomycin can cause hypotension; therefore, administer by slow infusion at a rate of 10 mg/min.

Anticholinesterases

Echothiophate eye drops or organophosphate insect spray may prolong the action of depolarizing muscle relaxants and choline esters and local anesthetics of ester type.

Anticoagulants

Coumarin derivatives—extreme bleeding, occult bleeding (GI tract) causing anemia and hypovolemia. Obtain coagulation screens. Avoid regional anesthesia if coagulation is abnormal. Reverse coumadin with vitamin K and heparin with protamine sulfate in emergency surgery.

Antidepressants

Lithium Preparations (Lithane, Eskalith)

Can cause nausea, vomiting, sodium diuresis, and muscle weakness; use relaxants carefully. Serum therapeutic level of lithium <1.8 mmol/L.

Monoamine Oxidase Inhibitors (MAOs)

Isocarboxazid (Marplan), pargyline, phenylzine (Nardil), and tranylcypromine (Parnate) cause increased synaptic catecholamine levels. Alarming hypertensive crises as a result of interactions with direct or indirectly acting sympathomimetic amines. Prolonged effect of other drugs because of decreased metabolism resulting from enzyme inhibition. Watch for hypertension, hypotension, bradycardia, diaphoresis, convulsion, coma, respiratory depression, or hyperpyrexia. Fatal interaction with opioids, particularly Demerol, may occur but this is very rare. It was recommended that MAO inhibitors be discontinued at least 2 weeks before surgery. Recently, new evidence suggests that it is safe to proceed with anesthesia and surgery in the usual way.

Tricyclic Antidepressants

Amitriptyline (Elavil), doxepin (Sinequan, Triadapin), imipramine (Tofranil), and nortriptyline (Aventyl) at therapeutic doses cause prolonged sleeping time and minor electrocardiogram changes. Cardiac and elderly patients may show myocardial depression. Response to vasopressor agents may be exaggerated. Anesthetic risk is probably less than MAO inhibitors.

Antidiabetic Agents

Insulin

The risk of hypoglycemia is increased if long-acting insulin is used and the patient is maintained NPO. Administer half the regular dose of long-acting insulin on the morning of surgery. Change from long-acting to short-acting injectable insulin if necessary. Start intravenous (i.v.) infusion with D5W in the morning and obtain fasting blood sugar.

Oral Agents

For clorpropamide (Diabinese), metformin (Glucophage), and tolbutamide omit oral agents before surgery and obtain fasting blood sugar.

Antihypertensive Agents

Clonidine (Catapres), guanethidine, hydralazine (Apresoline), methyldopa (Aldomet), minoxidil, prazosin (Minipress), reserpine, propranolol (Inderal), labetalol (Trandate), prazosin, acebutolol, atenolol, metoprolol, pindolol, nadolol, sotalol, and timolol all cause hypotension and potentiate anesthetic agents. All these agents should be taken up to and including the day of surgery with sips of water.

Currently there is the trend of same-day admission and surgery, and therefore patients are seen by the family physician or the anesthesiologist in a clinic, assessed, and the appropriate laboratory work-up ordered. The patients are given written instructions regarding what medications should be continued in the perioperative period. The patients are advised to take their cardiac and antihypertensive medications with sips of water on the morning of surgery. Aspirin and other antiplatelet drugs should be stopped 2 weeks before surgery so that platelet adhesiveness may return to normal.

Lacrimal procedures are generally associated with little pain. Therefore, premedication should be directed toward allaying anxiety and promoting adequate sedation, amnesia, and antiemesis. With the current practice of same-day admission, premedication is no longer given except to an occasional patient.

Anesthesia

Probing and syringing in an adult is often an office procedure and can be done with topical anesthesia using tetracaine eyedrops. Sometimes if the patient is extremely anxious, or mentally handicapped, or is a child, general anesthesia becomes necessary.

LACRIMAL ANESTHESIA IN CHILDREN

Operations to relieve blockage of nasolacrimal duct (probing) are usually required in children after the age of 12 months, although sometimes the children are younger or mentally deficient. Saline is syringed through the duct after probing. This fluid enters the nasal cavity and the pharynx, and unless suctioned rapidly away, it may be aspirated by the unconscious anesthetized patient. Occasionally, the mucus in the lacrimal sac is so copious that this too may be aspirated.

Induction of general anesthesia may be inhalational (using nitrous oxide, oxygen, and a potent inhalation agent such as isoflurane, halothane, or ethrane) or by i.v. thiopental or propofol. Maintenance of anesthesia may also be either by inhalational or i.v. agents, or a combination.

Although face masks and laryngeal masks may be used to provide inhalational anesthesia, it is preferable to use endotracheal intubation to protect the airway and limit aspiration risks as well as allowing surgical access.

Probing in children is usually a short procedure, about 5 minutes, and, thus, succinylcholine, unless specifically contraindicated (e.g., by a family history of pseudocholinesterase deficiency, or malignant hyperpyrexia), is the muscle relaxant of choice.

One may decrease the risks of aspiration:

1. By having a suction catheter positioned in the mouth and suctioning continuously during probing and irrigation
2. By placing the child head-down and on the side to promote drainage out of the mouth. This maneuver is especially important when face-mask anesthesia alone is used
3. By not extubating or removing the laryngeal mask until reflexes have returned and the child is able to protect the airway

LACRIMAL SURGERY IN ADULTS

Dacryocystorhinostomy (DCR) often requires general anesthesia, but it may be performed with local anesthesia, with or without sedation.

General Anesthesia

General anesthesia has the advantage of airway control as well as blood pressure control. The major problem in lacrimal surgery is bleeding. General anesthesia is indicated when there is a language barrier and in very young, uncooperative, extremely nervous and anxious patients. The usual monitoring includes electrocardiogram, automatic blood pressure measurement, pulse oximeter, and end-tidal carbon dioxide monitor and temperature. An i.v. infusion is started with a balanced salt solution. The common induction agents used today include thiopental 4 to 5 mg/Kg body weight, or propofol 2 to 2.5 mg/Kg body weight. Endotracheal intubation is accomplished with a muscle relaxant and anesthesia is maintained with a mixture of nitrous oxide and oxygen, inhalational agents, muscle relaxants, and small doses of opioids with controlled ventilation in order to maintain slight hypocarbia end-tidal carbon dioxide tension at 30 to 35 mmHg. An oral right atrial enlargement (RAE) tube is used because it is preformed and gives the surgeon better access. One can also use a reinforced tube in place of the RAE tube but caution should be exercised with any tube because of the possibility of kinking. Alternatively, one can also use a total i.v. technique with propofol and opioids. A throat pack is often inserted after endotracheal intubation to minimize spillage of blood and secretion into the trachea. Occasionally to facilitate surgery, blood pressure is lowered with i.v. labetalol using increments of 10 to 15 mg to achieve a satisfactory arterial pressure, usually 80 mmHg in a previously normotensive patient. If the patient is initially hypertensive, say 170/90 mmHg, it is prudent to limit the induced hypotension to 70% of the patient's accepted normal systolic and diastolic blood pressure. The choice of inhalational agents is based on the underlying disease as well as the presence or absence of arrhythmias. Generally, most anesthesiologists avoid using halothane in adults whenever the surgeon uses local anesthesia with adrenaline because halothane sensitizes the myocardium to catecholamines and the risk of dangerous arrhythmias is then too great. Halothane has been used safely in children (with cleft palates and lips) who have had adrenaline infiltrated for vasoconstriction perioperatively. The relative safety of halothane and adrenaline in children is probably related to the absence of coronary artery disease in this age group.

To control oozing (and blood loss) at surgery, it is usual to position the patient head-up so that venous flow from the operative site is facilitated. Caution should be exercised in old patients as well as patients with critical valvular stenoses who cannot compensate for any lowering of blood pressure.

Deliberate reduction of blood pressure is common in some types of surgery, but it is only occasionally indicated in ophthalmic operations, for example, vascular tumors of the orbit and less commonly in surgery on the lacrimal apparatus. Many pharmacologic agents given singly or in combination may be used to lower the blood pressure. A list of the common agents and their relevant pharmacology is given below (5). Direct arterial blood pressure monitoring by an indwelling arterial line is helpful if the more potent agents such as nitroprusside and nitroglycerine are used. It is impossible to say one technique is always best to effect lowering of the blood pressure because much depends on the sensitivity of the patient to the different agents. This, in turn, may be influenced by other medications that the patient may be taking, for example, beta-blockers, calcium channel blockers and angiotensin-converting enzyme (ACE) inhibitors.

Antihypertensive Agents (6)

Sodium Nitroprusside

Sodium nitroprusside (SNP) continues to be the most widely used drug to produce hypotension because of its rapid onset, consistent effect, and short half-life (2–3 min). It dilates primarily the resistance vessels (arterioles) either by interfering with sulf-hydryl groups or by blocking intracellular calcium activation.

Some adverse effects from SNP infusion include cyanide and thiocyanate toxicity, rebound hypertension, in-

tracranial hypertension, coagulation abnormalities, pulmonary shunting, hypothyroidism, and decrease in myocardial, liver, and skeletal muscle oxygen reserves.

Thiocyanate toxicity occurs in those with compromised renal function. Recent evidence suggests that either captopril (Capoten, an ACE inhibitor) or trimethaphan (Arfonad, a ganglion-blocking agent) can be used concurrently with SNP to reduce the dosage of SNP and thus the risk of cyanide toxicity. Systemic and pulmonary hypertension may occur after abrupt withdrawal of SNP secondary to increased pulmonary vascular resistance.

Cyanide toxicity occurs when the SNP dose exceeds 0.5 mg/Kg per hour in 24 hours or exceeds 1 mg/Kg within 2.5 hours. It is more likely in patients who are nutritionally deficient in cobalamin (vitamin B12). Fifty milligrams of nitroprusside in 250 mL of D5W gives a concentration of 200 g/mL. The bag and tubings are shielded with silver foil to prevent deactivation of nitroprusside. The usual dose is 0.25 to 4 g/Kg per minute and does not exceed 10 g/Kg per minute.

Nitroglycerine

Nitroglycerine (NTG) dilates predominantly the capacitance vessels. It also has a short half-life, 2 to 3 minutes, and has no clinically toxic metabolites. Resistance to NTG has been reported in some patients receiving nonvolatile anesthetics, and therefore this agent is not always effective. The usual dose is 0.25 to 5 g/Kg per minute. Fifty milligrams in 250 mL D5W gives a concentration of 200 g/mL. Some of the drug gets absorbed into the plastic tubings. In high doses it dilates the arteriolar bed as well.

Trimethaphan Camsylate (Arfonad)

Trimethaphan camsylate is a ganglionic blocking agent that produces sympathetic ganglion block, resulting in both relaxation of resistance and capacitance blood vessels. It has a short half-life (2–3 min) so it is easy to control, but onset of action is slightly slower. However, its histamine-releasing property and its ganglion-blocking effect may induce bronchospasm. The intracranial pressure may also increase. Myoneural blockade has also been reported with an Arfonad infusion. Overall this drug is not the agent of choice. As it produces ganglionic blockade, pupils are dilated and this should be taken into account in evaluating the patient following surgery. The other side effects include paralytic ileus and urinary retention. Simultaneous administration of Arfonad and nitroprusside is synergistic and avoids the problem of tachyphylaxis. The usual dose is 2.5 to 3 g/Kg per minute. Five hundred milligrams of Arfonad in 250 c.c. of D5W gives a concentration of 2 mg/mL.

Inhalational Agents (Halothane/Enflurane/Isoflurane/Desflurane)

All these agents can be used to lower blood pressure, and all are capable of doing so in a dose-related fashion, but the mechanism of lowering the blood pressure is different with each agent. Halothane lowers the blood pressure by depression of myocardial contractility as well as sensitizing the heart to catecholamines. Enflurane lowers the blood pressure both by myocardial depression as well as vasodilation. Isoflurane depresses the myocardium least among inhalational agents, but its predominant effect is the relaxation of the resistance vessels. Desflurane is a relatively new inhalational agent that lowers blood pressure primarily by inducing vascular relaxation similar to isoflurane. Currently, isoflurane is the inhalational agent most commonly used to produce deliberate hypotension.

Hydralazine (Apresoline)

Hydralazine is an arterial dilator that can also be used in combination with a beta-blocker. Fifty milligrams in 250 mL D5W gives a concentration of 200 g/mL; the dose range is 0.5 to 2 g/Kg per minute.

Adenosine Triphosphate

Adenosine triphosphate (ATP) has recently been used to induce hypotension. The advantages are prompt onset of action and short duration. ATP is metabolized to adenosine and phosphate. Adenosine is the active agent that causes vasodilatation. It is metabolized to uric acid. There is a recent report that adenosine may adversely affect cerebral autoregulation. ATP is a relatively new agent. Its place, therefore, is not yet established.

Esmolol and Labetalol

Esmolol and labetalol are commonly used. Esmolol is a short-acting (half-life of 9 min) cardioselective beta-adrenergic blocker. It is used in combination with inhalational agents or by itself as i.v. boluses (50–100 mg in adults) with or without a continuous infusion.

Labetalol (Trandate) is a combined alpha- and beta-adrenergic blocker and is considered the drug of choice in treating cocaine-induced hypertension and pre-eclampsia. The action of beta receptors is four times stronger than that on alpha receptors. It is widely used to treat hypertension in the perioperative period. It is given in increments of 10 to 20 mg (0.25 mg/Kg) (in adults) intravenously and it is always effective provided an adequate dose is given. One may give more than 100 mg over 20 minutes with little fear of toxic effects. Labetalol

is a useful drug to lower the blood pressure. As an infusion it can be given at 2 mg/min 40 mL of Trandate added to 250 mL of balanced salt solution or D5W giving a concentration of 200 mg in 250 mL or 2 mg/3 mL; administration is at a rate of 3 mL/min or 2 mg/min. The side effects can be due to excess blockade, postural hypotension, syncope, hepatocellular damage, skin rash, conjunctival drying, and severe bradycardia.

One can also use Demerol in increments of 20 to 40 mg or a combination of Inderal or hydralazine as well as nitroglycerin and nitroprusside infusion. An arterial line is helpful if the last two mentioned agents are used. Like any ophthalmic procedure, the extubation must be smooth to minimize coughing. Coughing is controlled at extubation primarily by timing the anesthetic. Ideally, the patient's oropharynx should be suctioned thoroughly, preferably under vision, and the throat pack removed. All this is performed while the patient is anesthetized and still paralyzed by muscle relaxants. When one is sure that bleeding from the nose and DCR site has been controlled, the reversal agents for the muscle relaxants are given and the patient is allowed to awaken from the general anesthetic. An i.v. bolus of Xylocaine 1.5 mg/Kg, given at least 3 minutes before extubation, may be helpful to suppress coughing (6). It is also preferable to give an antiemetic in these patients as there is a high incidence of postoperative nausea and vomiting. One can give small doses of droperidol (Inapsine) 0.75 to 1.25 mg intravenously. The management of these patients is the same as any other cases in the Post-Anesthesia Care Unit (PACU)—oxygen therapy, pain control, and antiemetics, combined with careful monitoring.

Propranolol (Inderal)

Propranolol was the first widely used beta-adrenergic blocker introduced. Ramoska et al. describe a lethal hypertensive case as a result of unopposed alpha-stimulation after administration of propranolol to treat cocaine-induced hypertension (7–9). More specific beta-adrenergic blockers are now available. They are more cardioselective, for example acebutolol, metoprolol, atenolol, and esmolol, and are theoretically safer. Their actions are more rapid and more predictable than propranolol, and thus the latter is now less commonly used in anesthesia, although it is still widely used as an oral antihypertensive agent.

Local Anesthesia

If local anesthesia is employed, the choice of patient and the patient's understanding of the procedure is crucial for success. i.v. sedation and added inspired oxygen via face mask are used as supplements when necessary.

Xylometazoline nasal spray is administered before

surgery for decongestion of the nasal mucosa. When the patient arrives in the operating room and after the i.v. line and all the monitors are in place, we spray the nostril with 10% Xylocaine spray, limiting the dose to 4 to 6 mg/Kg body weight. The patient is then given a light neurolept with midazolam (Versed) in increments of 0.25 mg to a maximum of 2 mg and alfentanil 250 to 500 μg or fentanyl 25 to 50 μg, depending on the patient's cardiorespiratory response. If the patient still appears anxious, restless, tachycardic, and hypertensive, one may add i.v. propofol in 10-mg increments until satisfactory sedation is achieved. One must be sure the patient is not hypoxic. One can also use other combinations of sedatives, hypnotics, and opioids. The surgeon administers the local nerve block with Xylocaine and epinephrine 1:100,000. We have used this technique for the past 3 years in elderly patients who have significant cardiac and respiratory disease and who are poor candidates for general anesthesia. We have found the patients to be quite comfortable with this treatment and have not had any complications.

Local Anesthesia Plus Sedation

Local anesthesia is often supplemented with titrated doses of a sedative, hypnotic, tranquilizer, narcotic, or neuroleptic agent. An ideal sedative hypnotic should provide a calming effect, analgesia, sedation, and anterograde amnesia. It should depress coughing, gagging, and laryngospasm in procedures irritating the oropharynx yet keep the patient cooperative. There are several agents in our armamentarium that can achieve some or all these conditions. In ophthalmic procedures, we have to be careful not to obtund protective airway reflexes, especially when the face is completely covered with drapes. As well, the patients should remain cooperative and pain free. Unfortunately, we do not yet have the absolutely ideal agent to predictably induce a safe neurolept analgesic state.

Many patients prefer to be sedated and have no recollection of a procedure performed under local/regional block. Many agents are used to induce this state: sedatives/hypnotics, such as benzodiazepines (diazemuls, diazepam), thiobarbiturates (thiopental, methohexital), phenols (propofol), phencyclidines (ketamine), opioids (fentanyl, alfentanyl, sufentanyl, morphine, Demerol) and inhalation agents (nitrous oxide, N_2O, enflurane, isoflurane) (6).

The hypnotics in common use are the barbiturates and phenols. Barbiturates of intermediate-lasting class are often used for overnight sedation. These include pentobarbital (Nembutal), and secobarbital (Seconal). Sometimes they are given with sips of water in the morning, 1 to 2 hours before surgery, to allay anxiety and apprehension. The usual dose is 1 to 1.5 mg/Kg. Barbiturates are seldom used for i.v. sedation because of lack of control of sedation as well as the depressant effects on the respiratory and cardiovascular systems. The most popular hypnotic currently is propofol (Diisopropylphenol). It has revolutionized anesthetic practice in the last 5 years. Propofol, being a short-acting phenol, has a very short half-life, and is rapidly and completely broken down with no active metabolites. The patients awaken after propofol sedation or anesthesia with a clear mind and minimal nausea and vomiting.

Hypnotics

Propofol (Diprivan)

Propofol produces a dose-dependent central nervous system (CNS) and cardiovascular system (CVS) suppression as well as ventilatory depression similar to thiobarbiturates. The onset of action is almost identical to thiopental although slower, but the major difference is the recovery profiles. Recovery is much faster with fewer side effects such as nausea, vomiting, headaches, and hangover. Often, there is pain on i.v. injection of propofol. The severity depends on individual pain threshold and the site and speed of injection. The intensity of pain can be decreased by using a large vein, injecting slowly, and adding Xylocaine 20 to 40 mg to a mixture of 200 mg propofol. The terminal elimination half-life of propofol is 1 to 3 hours, which is significantly shorter than that of thiopental (10–12 hours). The usual sedative dose of propofol for an average adult is 10 to 20 mg initially and 25 to 50 g/Kg per minute as an infusion (10–12).

Barbiturates

Thiopental (Pentothal) and Methohexital (Brietal)

Pentothal was introduced in 1934 and is the gold standard for i.v. induction agents. The elimination half-life, 10 to 12 hours, can contribute to a prolonged recovery time. Although the distribution phase kinetics of thiopental and methohexital are similar, redistribution is a major factor determining the duration of sedation after a single bolus. The more rapid recovery of complex psychomotor function seen after methohexital probably is a result of more rapid metabolism. Methohexital is to be preferred when more rapid recovery is desired, particularly if larger or repeated doses are necessary, as in i.v. sedation. Methohexital is associated with a faster return to consciousness, greater stability in solution, less tissue irritation, and shorter periods of hypotension. However, Dundee (13) found that there is a higher incidence of excitable phenomena such as coughing and hiccoughing with Methohexital.

Sodium Pentobarbital (Nembutal) and Secobarbital (Seconal)

Sodium pentobarbital and secobarbital are relatively short-acting barbiturates used as sedative hypnotic preanesthetic medications as well as amnesic agents in obstetric patients. Rectal administration provides mild sedation and sleep when oral administration is not feasible or contraindicated.

They are contraindicated when there is idiosyncrasy, respiratory depression, and latent or manifest porphyria. They are not recommended in the presence of pain as it might lower the pain threshold and in elderly patients who are prone to confusion and restlessness after hypnotic agents. The concomitant use of alcohol and other sedatives potentiate the effect of barbiturates.

As a preanesthetic medication or night-before sedative, 100 to 200 mg are given. Barbiturates induce liver enzymes and may decrease the blood concentrations and clinical efficacy of other concomitant drugs administered, so one should monitor the dose of anticoagulants, theophylline, steroids, digoxin, oral contraceptives, griseofulvin, dilantin, propranolol, quinidine, testosterone, and tricyclic antidepressant drugs.

Phencyclidines

Ketamine (Ketalar)

Ketamine is of questionable benefit for outpatient sedation anesthesia. Thompson et al. (14) found that ketamine-treated patients were less alert, had more headaches, dizziness, and suffered from "weird dreams" when discharged. Often the dreams were frightening and unpleasant. Concomitant administration of diazepam or droperidol can reduce the incidence of dreams, but these may delay discharge from the postanesthetic care unit. There is also a significant increase in nausea and vomiting following ketamine use (15).

In a recent study (16) in children, it was found that recovery times were not prolonged after ketamine 2 to 3 mg/Kg intramuscularly. This dose in the 1- to 5-year age group promotes a smooth mask induction within 3 to 7 minutes. Hallucinations and nightmares did not seem to occur with low-dose ketamine in children.

Benzodiazepines

Benzodiazepines are currently the most popular sedative hypnotic and tranquilizers: chlordiazepoxide (Librium), diazepam (Valium), nitrazepam (Mogadon), and oxazepam (Serax). Valium raises the seizure threshold and is ideal for patients with seizure disorders. They can depress CNS, medullary respiratory, and vasomotor centers in a dose-related fashion.

Midazolam (Versed)

Midazolam is a water-soluble benzodiazepine that induces sedation, hypnosis, and amnesia (Table 2). This drug produces less pain at the i.v. injection site in comparison to diazepam. This is because of water-solubility available in HCl form with a pH of 3.5. After injection it becomes lipophilic and assumes a pH >6 and this property enables the drug to cross the blood–brain barrier and exert its effect on the CNS. After intramuscular (i.m.) injection, its bioavailability is 90%. Midazolam is 95% protein-bound and distributed mainly to muscle and fat. It is metabolized in the kidney and its estimated half-life is 2 to 3 hours following i.m./i.v. injection.

The dose varies between individuals and should be reduced in the elderly by 30%. The initial i.v. dose is 15 to 30 g/Kg over 5 seconds; 2 to 3 minutes later, if necessary, give 25% of the initial dose, with a maximum total of 100 g/Kg.

The dose should be titrated in the elderly, debilitated patients, those receiving adjuvant drugs such as narcotics and other CNS depressants, patients with chronic obstructive pulmonary disease, hypotension, heart disease, and renal disease, and patients who are obese, alcoholic, or benzodiazepine users, who all may require higher doses.

Diazepam (Valium)

Diazepam is an anxiolytic, sedative hypnotic, muscle relaxant, and anticonvulsant (Table 2). It is mediated through facilitation of action of gamma aminobutyric acid (GABA) in the CNS. Diazepam acts selectively on postsynaptic neuronal pathways and may inhibit or augment transmission, depending on the endogenous function of GABA. Diazepam is well absorbed after oral administration and peak blood levels are achieved in 1 hour. About 99% is bound to plasma proteins. The reported half-life is 24 to 96 hours depending on the age and clinical status of the patient. The older and the sicker the patient, the longer the half-life of the drug. Diazepam is metabolized in one hour by N-demethylation and converted to N-dimethyloxazepam and N-methyloxazepam,

TABLE 2. *Comparative pharmacology of benzodiazepines*

	Diazepam	Lorazepam	Midazolam
Dose (mg)	5–20 iv or im	1–4 po or sl	2–7 iv or im
Onset of action (min)	2–5	5–15	1–2
Duration of action (min)	45–60	60–120	40–50
Amnesic action	++	+++	+++
Venous sequelae	++	+	−

iv, intravenously; im, intramuscularly; po, by mouth; sl, sublingually.

which are then metabolized to oxazepam, conjugated with glucuronic acid, and excreted in the urine.

It is usually given intravenously in increments and titrated to response. The dose is 50 to 150 g/Kg. Large veins are used in the forearm or elbow as it is an irritant to veins. An alternative formulation, diazemuls, is now used to reduce this side effect.

Diazemuls

Diazemuls is an emulsified preparation of diazepam that has been introduced for quite some time. The main advantage is that the incidence of pain and venous sequelae is far lower than for diazepam. Diazepam has to be released from the oil phase of diazemuls' emulsion before it can exert a therapeutic affect. The peak blood levels are reached 15 minutes after i.v. administration, but diazepam and diazemuls have a long half-life, depending on the age of the patient, from 20 hours at age 20 years to 80 hours at age 80 years. The active metabolite, N-dimethyloxazepam, has an even longer half-life of 50 to 120 hours. This has implications when it is used in elderly, debilitated patients and in patients with significant hepatic and renal dysfunction. It is not recommended for status epilepticus because of its delayed onset of action.

Lorazepam (Ativan)

Lorazepam has similar actions to midazolam, diazepam, and diazemuls, but differs in that it is available as a sublingual tablet (Table 2). When given by this route, it is readily acceptable to patients as a premedication and its onset of action is fairly rapid. Its duration of action is clinically longer than that of diazepam or midazolam. It has a marked amnesic effect and in some cases the amnesia is unpredictable in its duration. It does prolong the time to awaken after general anesthesia.

Conscious Sedation

The term "conscious sedation" was first used by Bennett (17) and refers to the supplementation of local/regional anesthesia with i.v. agents that depresses consciousness minimally while maintaining protective reflexes. The aim of conscious sedation is to maintain adequate sedation with minimal risk, relieve anxiety, and provide amnesia and relief of pain from noxious stimuli.

Conscious sedation is an art that is learned by experience (18,19). Originally developed for dentists and oral surgeons for office use, it is becoming popular in outpatient as well as inpatient anesthesia together with local/regional block. As defined by the Dental Association, conscious sedation emphasizes that the patient must be able to respond rationally to commands, and maintain his/her own airway patent. Shane (20) has described an iv anesthetic technique called "IV amnesia" using a combination of opioid, anticholinergic, ataractic, and barbiturates given in small increments.

Opioids are often used in combination with tranquilizers as part of the so-called neurolept-analgesia technique. It is common to use i.v. fentanyl ($0.5–1.0$ μg/Kg) in increments with i.v. midazolam (Versed, $2–7$ μg/Kg).

Droperidol (Inapsine) may be given as an antiemetic; a dose of 0.125 mg is all that is required in an adult for this action.

Combinations of other narcotics—morphine, Demerol, sufentanyl, alfentanyl—and other tranquilizers—Valium, low-dose thiopental (10–25 mg), low-dose propofol (10–20 mg)—may be used effectively and safely in selected patients. Some factors that might influence the drug combination chosen are the individual cost of the agents, the experience of the anesthetist, and the patient's general condition.

The technique must be tailored to each patient. During conscious sedation, the anesthesiologist, or other qualified personnel, should monitor the level of consciousness by speaking to the patient frequently, reassuring the patient, and warning them of stimulating events about to take place, such as injection of local anesthetic agents, tourniquet inflation, etc. The patient should be encouraged to take occasional deep breaths. One should use drugs that have a shorter elimination half-life and high clearance rate. The ASA standards of basic monitoring apply for conscious sedation techniques. These include monitoring of blood pressure, electrocardiogram, pulse oximetry, and end-tidal carbon dioxide (capnometry).

When does conscious sedation become general anesthesia? This is often difficult to answer. The potential for central nervous, cardiovascular, and respiratory depression is an ever-present danger of sedation techniques. Individual tailoring of doses according to the patient's clinical status is mandatory.

Whenever conscious sedation is employed, facilities for oxygen administration, airway management, and cardiopulmonary support must be available. As well, drugs to antagonize the central effects of sedatives and opioids should be on hand. These include naloxone (Narcan), flumazenil (Anexate), and physostigmine (Antilirium). Naloxone (adults: 0.4 mg/amp) is usually diluted in 10 mL of saline and injected in increments of 1 to 2 mL (40–80 μg). Caution should be exercised in using Narcan because it suddenly arouses and is a sympathomimetic and can cause hypertension, tachycardia, angina, myocardial ischemia, infarction, and acute pulmonary edema.

Flumazenil is a benzodiazepine antidote specific for Valium, Librium, and Versed, and is given in increments of 0.1 to 0.2 mg to the desired end point.

Physostigmine, a nonspecific arousal agent, is an anticholinesterase agent used to reverse general anesthesia, tricyclic antidepressant, barbiturate, diphenhydramine (Benadryl), and scopolamine (Hyoscine) overdose.

Anesthetic Concerns with Cocaine

Cocaine, introduced in ophthalmology in 1884 by Karl Koller, has limited topical ocular use because it can cause corneal pits and erosion. However, as the only local anesthetic that produces vasoconstriction and shrinkage of the mucous membranes, cocaine is commonly used in a nasal pack during DCR. The drug is so well absorbed from mucosal surfaces that plasma concentrations comparable to IV administration are achieved and, because cocaine interferes with catecholamine uptake, it potentiates sympathetic activity (21–23). Historically, epinephrine had often been mixed with cocaine in the hope of augmenting vasoconstriction. This practice is potentially dangerous and may be lethal, as cocaine is a potent vasoconstrictor and its combination with epinephrine may trigger life-threatening dysrhythmias and hypertension. It has been shown in some studies that cocaine, without added topical epinephrine, does not sensitize the heart to endogenous catecholamines during halothane or enflurane anesthesia (24). However, animal studies have shown that following some treatments with exogenous epinephrine, cocaine facilitates the development of epinephrine-induced cardiac arrhythmias during halothane anesthesia, so it is advisable not to use halothane in situations when epinephrine is used by the surgeon and, if halothane is used, caution should be exercised in the amount of epinephrine injected.

The normal maximal dose of cocaine used in clinical practice is 200 mg for a 70-Kg adult or 3 mg/Kg. However, 1.5 mg/Kg is the preferred dose because this dose has been shown not to exert any clinically significant sympathomimetic effect in combination with halothane. Although 1 g is considered as the lethal dose, considerable variation occurs. Furthermore, systemic reactions have been reported with as little as 20 mg.

Myers described two cases of cocaine toxicity during DCR (23), emphasizing that cocaine is contraindicated in hypertensive patients or in patients receiving drugs such as guanethidine, reserpine, tricyclic antidepressants, or MAO inhibitors. If serious side effects occur, labetalol should be used to counteract the symptoms.

SUMMARY

Today, the introduction of better induction agents (propofol), more potent ultra-short acting opioids (alfentanil, sufentanil), newer muscle relaxants (mivacurium, vecuronium, tracrium, rocuronium), and a better understanding of their pharmacology and their interactions allows safe conduct of anesthesia and surgery in patients for lacrimal surgery. The use of newer antiemetics such as ondansetron (Zofran), which is devoid of central effects, permits a smoother and more pleasant awakening. Minimal postoperative nausea and vomiting is certainly welcomed by all patients. Surgical and anesthetic practice, however, continues to evolve with the increasing influence of changing economics and patients' expectations.

REFERENCES

1. Donlon JV. Anesthesia for eye, ear, nose and throat surgery. In: Miller, R, ed. *Textbook of anesthesia*. New York: Churchill Livingstone, 1990;2001–2023.
2. McGoldrick KE. Anesthesia and the eye. In: Barash PG, Cullen BF, Stoelting RK, eds. *Clinical anesthesia*, 2nd ed. Philadelphia: JB Lippincott, 1992.
3. Dripps RD, Lamont A, Eckenhoff JE. The role of anesthesia in surgical mortality. *JAMA* 1961;178:261.
4. Philip C, Larson JY. Evaulation of the patient and preoperative preparation. In: Barash PG, Cullen BF, Stoelting RK, eds. *Clinical anesthesia*, 2nd ed. Philadelphia: JB Lippincott.
5. Benda AA, Hartung J, Kass LS, Cottrell JE. Neurophysiology and neuroanesthesia deliberate hypotension. In: Barash PG, Cullen BF, Stoelting RK, eds. *Clinical anesthesia*, 2nd ed. Philadelphia: JB Lippincott, 1992.
6. Warner LO, et al. Intravenous lidocaine reduces vomiting. *Anesthesiology* 1988;68;618.
7. Gay GR, Loper KA. Control of cocaine induced hypertension with labetalol. [Letter] *Anesth Analg* 1988;67;92.
8. Rappolt RT, Gay GR, Inaba DS. Propranolol: a specific antagonist to cocaine. *Clin Toxicol* 1977;10:265.
9. Ramoska F, Sacchett AD. Propranolol-induced hypertension in treatment of cocaine intoxication. *Ann Emerg Med* 1985;14:1112.
10. MacKenzie N, et al. Propofol for IV sedation. *Anaesthesia* 1987;42;3.
11. Scamin FL, Klein SL, Choi NW. Conscious sedation for procedures under local anaesthesia. *Ann Otol Rhinol Laryngol* 1985;92;21.
12. McCarthy FH, Solomon AL. Conscious sedation: benefits and risks. *JADA* 1984;109;46.
13. Dundee JW. Clinical studies of induction agents: a comparison of eight intravenous anaesthetics as main agents for a standard operation. *Br J Anaesth* 1963;35;784.
14. Thompson GE, Remington JM, Millman BS, et al. Experiences with outpatient anesthesia. *Anesth Analg* 1973;52;881.
15. Wetchler BV. For ambulatory surgery patients, use ketamine with caution. *Same Day Surgery* 1984;8(1):11.
16. Hannallah RS, Patel RI. Low dose intramuscular ketamine for anesthesia pre-induction in young children undergoing brief procedures in outpatients. *Anesthesiology* 1989;70:598.
17. Bennett CR. *Conscious sedation in dental practice*, 2nd ed. CV Mosby: St. Louis; 1978.
18. Wetchler BV. Outpatient anesthesia: conscious sedation. In: Barash PG, Gullen BF, Stoelting RK, eds. *Clinical anesthesia*, 2nd ed. Philadelphia: JB Lippincott, 1992.
19. Shane SM. *Conscious sedation for ambulatory surgery*. Baltimore: University Park Press; 1983.
20. Shane SM. Intravenous amnesia for total dentistry in one sitting. *J Oral Surg* 1966;24:27.
21. Ritchie JM, Greene NM. Local anesthetics. In: Gilman AG, Goodman LS, Rall TW et al., eds. *The pharmacological basis of therapeutics*, 7th ed. New York: Macmillan; 1985.
22. Barash PG, Kopriva CJ, Langou R, et al. Is cocaine a sympathetic stimulant during general anaesthesia? *JAMA* 1980;243:1437.
23. Meyers EF. Cocaine toxicity during dacryocystorhinostomy. *Arch Ophthalmol* 1980;98;842.
24. Chung B, Naraghi M, Adriani J. Sympathetic effects of cocaine and their influence on halothane and enflurane anesthesia. *Anesthesiol Rev* 1978;5:16.

CHAPTER 35

Regional Anesthesia for Lacrimal Surgery

Jeffrey Jay Hurwitz

Regional anesthesia is desirable in patients who do not want or cannot have general anesthesia, and in elderly patients. There is generally less bleeding, and the rehabilitation after the procedure is much smoother than with general anesthesia. To obtain satisfactory analgesia, the patient must be comfortable and feel a minimum amount of pain.

The nerve supply to the area of dacryocystorhinostomy (DCR) surgery is threefold. The area superior to the lacrimal sac region is supplied by the infratrochlear nerve. The lower part of the sac and duct on the anterior surface is supplied by the nasociliary nerve, and the more inferior and lateral aspects supplied by the infraorbital nerve. The infratrochlear and nasociliary nerves are branches of the first division of the trigeminal nerve, and the infraorbital nerve is a branch of the second division of the trigeminal nerve (Fig. 1). The distribution on the lateral wall of the nose is essentially the infratrochlear nerve superonasally, and the infraorbital nerve inferolaterally (Fig. 2).

PREOPERATIVE MEASURES

The patient should be told preoperatively that he will able to communicate with the surgeon, but he will be mildly sedated. He should be told that there might be "fluids" going down the back of his throat, and that he will either swallow these or spit them out through his mouth if he wishes. He will feel little pain but will feel the surgeon moving instruments in the surgical site.

J. J. Hurwitz: Oculoplastics Program, Mount Sinai Hospital; and Department of Ophthalmology, University of Toronto Faculty of Medicine, Toronto, Ontario M5S 1A8, Canada.

INJECTION TECHNIQUE

Following sedation, four areas of regional anesthesia are addressed (Fig. 3):

1. *Subcutaneous injection in surgical site.* Two percent Xylocaine with epinephrine is given on the side of the nose under where the skin incision will be. Before injecting the local anesthesia it is important to advance the needle into the desired site and withdraw the plunger to make sure that one is not in the angular vein. Pressure over the area will diffuse the anesthesia.

2. *Peri-infraorbital nerve injection.* Rather than injecting the anesthetic under the inferior orbital rim directly into the infraorbital nerve, we prefer to inject subcutaneously over the orbital rim and then advance the needle toward the side of the nose. Once it hits the side of the nose, we withdraw the plunger to make sure we are not in the angular vein, and then inject a bolus of local anesthesia. We keep injecting as we draw the needle laterally and out through the skin. We then press over the area to diffuse the local anesthesia around the inferior orbital rim to the area of the infraorbital nerve.

3. *Infratrochlear nerve injection.* One can reach the infratrochlear nerve by injecting through the skin in a posterior direction just superior to the anterior limb of the medial canthal tendon. A #25 needle is used for this purpose. One moves the needle posteriorly, directly backward, for approximately 2 cm. One then withdraws the plunger to make sure one is not in a vessel, and then injects approximately 1 to 1.5 cc of Xylocaine with epinephrine on withdrawal. The pupil may occasionally be seen to dilate. This is due to the epinephrine effect. The patient's vision should be checked periodically during the procedure because it is possible for the infratrochlear injection to involve a vessel and cause some bleeding. We have also tried

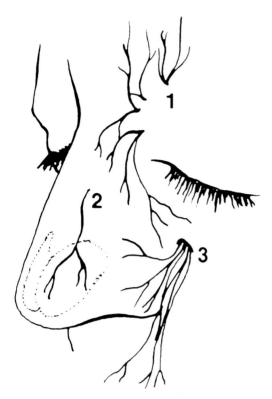

FIG. 1. Nerve supply to the region of a DCR. External surface. **1:** Infratrochlear nerve. **2:** Nasociliary nerve. **3:** Infraorbital nerve. (From Kratky et al., ref. 1, with permission.)

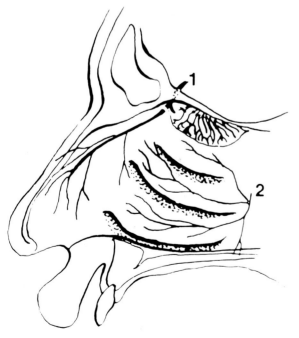

FIG. 2. Nerve supply to lateral wall of the nose in region of DCR. **1:** Infratrochlear nerve. **2:** Infraorbital nerve. (From Kratky et al., ref. 1, with permission.)

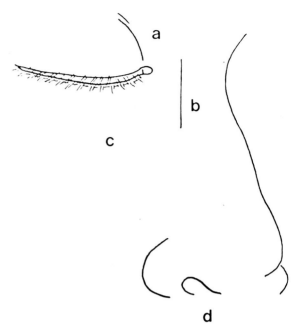

FIG. 3. Sites of regional anesthesia. **A:** Infratrochlear block. **B:** Local anesthesia from subcutaneous injection around site of skin incision. **C:** Para-infraorbital nerve block. **D:** Nasal mucosal anesthesia (possible sphenopalatine ganglion block). (From Kratky et al., ref. 1, with permission.)

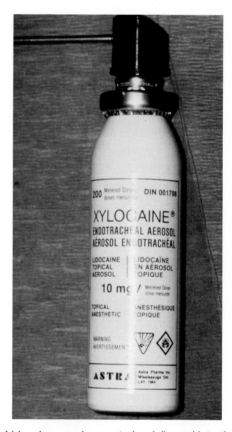

FIG. 4. Lidocaine nasal spray to be delivered into the middle meatus at the beginning at the DCR. With the patient moving the head, at the time of delivery, some of the Lidocaine probably gets back to the sphenopalatine ganglion to increase the anesthesia. (From Kratky et al., ref. 1, with permission.)

to perform DCRs under local anesthesia without the infratrochlear injection because of the fear of a hemorrhage posteriorly (especially in one-eyed patients), but have found the anesthesia to be not quite as good.

4. *Topical application of anesthesia:*
   a. *Ocular anesthesia.* Drops of Tetracaine are given on the cornea to anesthetize the cornea, conjunctiva, and punctum.
   b. *Nasal anesthesia.* Using a nasal spray to deliver Xylocaine (Fig. 4), two puffs are given three times—one as soon as the patient enters the room, one before the patient is draped, and one immediately before the surgery is about to start. More spray may be given into the wound itself just before one is about to incise the nasal mucosa. The maximum of dose of Xylocaine (Lidocaine) should not exceed 5 to 7 mg/Kg in a healthy adult. This represents 25 ml of a 2% solution. Each spray delivers approximately 10 mg of Lidocaine to the mucosa.

We do not use any cocaine because we are concerned about the additive effect of cocaine and epinephrine, especially in the older patient. In fact, we find we get adequate decongestion of the nasal mucosa due to our preoperative xylometazoline spray. Two applications of this 0.1% solution are given 2 hours, 1 hour, and one-half hour preoperatively to the nasal mucosa. The xylometazoline does not have the same additive effect with epinephrine as does cocaine.

SURGICAL MODIFICATIONS IN REGIONAL BLOCK DCR

During the procedure the face is left open so the patient does not feel claustrophobic and can communicate with the surgeon. The nose is not packed preoperatively. The patient under local anesthesia may be troubled by intranasal manipulation (but not always), and this should be kept to a minimum. The technique of removing bone must be modified slightly and can be done comfortably if the head is not mobilized as the bone is being removed. Constant communication with the patient is useful and tends to prevent restlessness, gagging, and anxiety (1). One need not compromise the surgery because the patient is awake.

CONCLUSION

Regional anesthesia in lacrimal surgery can be performed with intravenous sedation, regional anesthesia, and patient preparation to give satisfactory results in most situations to the patient and the surgeon.

REFERENCE

1. Kratky V, Hurwitz JJ, Ananthanarayan C, Avram DR. Dacryocystorhinostomy in elderly patients. Regional anaesthesia without cocaine. *Can J Ophthalmol* 1994;29:13.

CHAPTER 36

Dacryocystorhinostomy

Jeffrey Jay Hurwitz

Dacryocystorhinostomy (DCR) is an operation performed for obstructions within the nasolacrimal sac and duct. The external DCR is the "gold standard" against which all other operations must be compared. The success rate of this surgery when performed for the appropriate condition, with appropriate investigation, should be well over 90% (1).

INDICATIONS

1. Epiphora due to obstruction within the nasolacrimal sac and duct in an acquired obstruction
2. To relieve lacrimal sac infection before intraocular surgery (2)
3. Discharge and conjunctivitis in an older patient due to lacrimal sac obstruction
4. A mucocele of the tear sac
5. A "diagnostic" procedure to determine if a swelling is due to a tumor or a mucocele (if it is not certain with radiologic investigation). If it turns out to be a mucocele, a DCR can be performed
6. Incomplete obstructions with significant impairment of tear flow to cause annoying epiphora. Balloon catheter dilatation may help dilate a stenosis in the short term, but long-term results are not yet available (3). However, even though balloon dilatation may gain more of a role in the future, we still prefer to do a DCR in these patients
7. Chronic dacryocystitis (one should try to avoid a DCR in a patient with acute dacryocystitis). One should attempt to wait until the infection has been eliminated (4)

J. J. Hurwitz: Oculoplastics Program, Mount Sinai Hospital; and Department of Ophthalmology, University of Toronto Faculty of Medicine, Toronto, Ontario M5S 1A8, Canada.

8. Congenital nasolacrimal sac-duct obstruction that cannot be cured by probing (or probing with tubes).

CONTRAINDICATIONS

1. *Lacrimal sac tumor.* One should not open into the nose if a tumor of the lacrimal sac exists; instead, a dacryocystectomy should be performed. When frozen section is obtained, if one cannot be certain as to whether the lesion is benign or malignant, it is best to err on the side of not doing a DCR but only a dacryocystectomy. A common canaliculorhinostomy can always be performed at a later date if tearing is a problem.

2. *Adnexal lesions growing into the lacrimal sac.* When a basal cell carcinoma involves the canaliculi and the lacrimal sac, it is probably best to not perform a DCR and drain the tears into the nose, for fear of spreading malignancy into the nose.

3. *Acute dacryocystitis.* If acute dacryocystitis has been localized to the sac and cannot be controlled with antibiotics, one should perform a dacryocystotomy to settle down the infection. We have had some cases in which we have treated the patient with intravenous antibiotics and performed a DCR successfully. However, we would prefer in cases of pericystitis or dacryocystitis, with orbital cellulitis, not to perform a DCR and wait until the infection localizes in the sac or is eradicated. If there is any question of infection preoperatively, we prefer to treat the patient with antibiotics before the DCR (5). The exception to this would be a dacryocystitis with posterior cellulitis and orbital abscess, where immediate surgery is necessary.

4. Age of the patient. A DCR is probably contraindicated in children less than 1 year of age. This congenital obstruction should be treated by probing. There does not seem to be an age that is too old to have a DCR, especially since this can be done under local anesthesia. We

have operated on a number of patients in their 90s and two patients who were in their 100s.

PREOPERATIVE ASSESSMENT

The full investigation of the patient including the history of symptoms, the physical examination of the ophthalmic and lacrimal and adnexal regions, and the motivation for surgery should be determined.

Through a complete history and physical examination and the use of ancillary radiologic tests, it must be determined whether complete or incomplete obstruction exists, and where it is located. As well, it must be ascertained whether the obstruction within the drainage pathways is indeed what is causing the patient's symptoms. The duration of symptoms is extremely important. Before one undertakes a lacrimal drainage procedure, which is a significant procedure, the patient must be bothered enough by the tearing and/or discharge to be motivated to have the procedure. We certainly prefer that a patient have symptoms at least for a minimum of 2 to 3 months before performing surgery.

Almost all lacrimal obstructions are operable, and the success rate is usually quite high. However, the more lateral the obstruction exists within the pathways, the less the success rate of the surgery (1).

A complete general history regarding the health of the patient and the medications the patient is currently taking is important. One must decide whether the surgery, if it is to be performed, is to be under local or general anesthesia. We irrigate, in the office, all our patients from a diagnostic point of view. If the patients cannot tolerate the simple procedure of irrigation, then it is extremely unlikely that they will be able to have a DCR performed under local anesthesia being fully awake or somewhat sedated (there are exceptions, however, to this rule). We try to persuade our older patients to have the procedure done under a local anesthesia, and with our younger patients, we get them involved in making the decision as to local or general anesthesia. We also try to determine whether the patient can be done in the outpatient facility or should have a bed available to stay overnight. Much of the determination as to whether the patient stays overnight is based on the time of day that the patient is having the surgery, the amount of time necessary (with nursing care) to recover from a general anesthesia or sedation, the social situation and home support of the patient, and the potential for immediate postoperative bleeding. The latter is seldom an issue because most postoperative hemorrhages, in our experience, occur between the fourth to seventh days postoperatively with clot retraction, as opposed to a persistent bleed as the patient leaves the operating room.

Patients with heart problems, asthma, etc. should be seen by an anesthetist preoperatively, and the anesthetist should help in the planning as to the type of anesthesia used, and whether the patient should stay overnight. A history of medications is important. If the patient is on acetylsalicylic acid (ASA) or nonsteroidal anti-inflammatories, it is useful to have the patient off these for at least 2 weeks before and after the operation. It is well known that even one ASA within a 2-week period before surgery can decrease the platelet adhesiveness and cause increased bleeding. If a patient is on warfarin (Coumadin), one would have to reverse the anticoagulation effect and prepare the patient for surgery as an inpatient.

Even though some cataract surgeons do not stop warfarin, there is an increased risk of bleeding. Certainly, periocular bleeding with the warfarin is less serious than the major life-threatening potential complications in these patients without the warfarin (6).

Since a DCR nose bleed can be life-threatening on its own, we feel the warfarin should be stopped preoperatively. Warfarin loses its effect in 5 days, and does not need to be stopped longer preoperatively or postoperatively. Its effect can be reversed by vitamin K. Warfarin has a half-life of 37 hours. Warfarin can be stopped 5 days before surgery, and the patient anticoagulated with heparin (half-life of 5 hours). The heparin can be discontinued immediately (5 hours plus) before surgery, and recommenced (5 hours plus) after surgery. It can be reversed with protamine sulfate.

The "prothrombin time" test measures prothrombin (Factor II) as well as Factor VII. When warfarin is stopped, there is a different rate of synthesis of vitamin K–dependent factors. Factor VII returns to normal faster than factor II. The prothrombin time is more sensitive to factor VII. Therefore, a "normal" prothrombin time does not necessarily mean the Factors have all returned to normal. However, it is the best test available (6).

Specific questions must be asked as to whether the patient is a smoker, drinks alcohol to excess, and has had nasal or sinus problems. Certainly, these situations may cause increased friability of the nasal mucosa and lead to more bleeding. Of course, the history of previous surgery on the nose, sinuses, or tear ducts is important, and we also like to ask if the patients have had previous ocular surgery because certainly one would not want to put any pressure on the eye if recent intraocular surgery has been performed. A question of trauma to the face is extremely important because the nasal bones may be altered in their anatomy, or there may be hardware that had been inserted at the time of facial repair. These patients require good preoperative imaging.

It is important to determine whether the patient is having unilateral or bilateral symptoms. If the symptoms are bilateral and asymmetrical, it must be determined whether the patient would like to have a DCR performed on both sides at the same sitting. Appropriate investigation is important to make this decision. Certainly, a bilateral DCR can be performed at one sitting if indicated

(7). Not only can both sides be done at the same sitting, but it is possible for two surgeons to work simultaneously and perform a bilateral DCR without significantly increasing the operating time.

The question of blood loss is important. The patient does not need to be crossed and typed for blood transfusion. The exception to this would be a patient under 4 years of age having a bilateral DCR, or in a patient who is a suspected bleeder. It is mandatory that the surgeon ask about problems with respect to bleeding and bruising. If necessary, the patient should be sent to a hematologist for prothrombin time (PT) and a full blood work-up. The question of hypertension is extremely important when one considers postoperative bleeding. The blood pressure should not only be normal, but it should be stable and the medication for hypertension control should be noted. The patients often come into the hospital with nothing to eat or drink from midnight the night before and do not take their antihypertensive medication in the morning. It must be stressed that the patient take the antihypertensive pill with a sip of water in the morning when coming in for the operation.

Preoperative blood work: A hemoglobin assessment is routine. A chest x-ray is probably not necessary, and a cardiogram is performed routinely in patients over the age of 50 years and in smokers. In smokers, it is probably useful to get a chest x-ray as well.

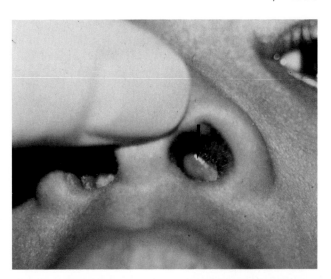

FIG. 2. When one looks up the nose before a DCR, one might find abnormalities such as a nasal polyp (*arrow*), which is seen here. As well, the size of the nasal opening and the position of turbinates and the septum are important to the surgeon.

Referral to an otolaryngologist is not part of our preoperative work-up. We examine the nose ourselves, and if a DCR is planned, there are specific things that we look for. We look for the size of the nasal opening, that is, the distance between the nasal septum and the lateral nasal wall and turbinate (Figs. 1 and 2). We determine the size of the inferior turbinate and, if we do not see beyond it, we often decongest the inferior turbinate to have a look into the middle meatus. One should look for chronic granulation within the nose and, obviously, if there are any signs of inflammation or tumors present. In the latter instance, a referral to an otolaryngologist preoperatively is important. If there is a nasal septal deviation toward the side of the surgery, one could theoretically have a submucous resection of the septum performed by an otolaryngologist. However, we find that the problem is not so much at the lower end of the nose where the septum is mainly cartilaginous, but up higher adjacent to the middle meatus, an area not usually addressed with a routine submucous resection by an otolaryngologist (8). If there is a lot of crusting we usually instruct the patient to lavage the nose. This is done by sniffing in forcibly a solution made up of 1 L of warm water and a tablespoon of baking soda, which is deposited on the hand and snorted into the nose while the other nostril is held closed. With forcibly blowing the nose, the crusts can usually be expelled onto a tissue. We instruct patients to get a vaporizer or humidifier to have postoperatively for 2 weeks to give more moisture to the air. This is especially important in a patient who has signs of atrophic rhinitis or other drying conditions of the nose (9).

It must be determined whether other procedures can or should be done in conjunction with the DCR. If the punctum is everted, a punctal eversion procedure can be

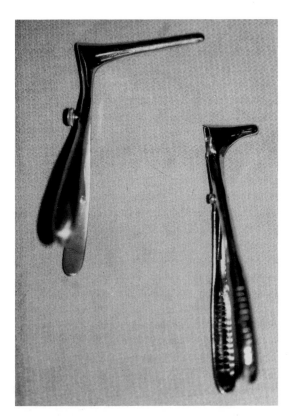

FIG. 1. A nasal speculum is important in the preoperative work-up of every lacrimal drainage surgery patient.

performed. If the lid is lax and there is a lacrimal pump dysfunction secondary to tearing, then a lid tightening procedure can be performed in conjunction with a DCR.

INFORMED CONSENT

The patient should be counseled as to the etiology of the problem that has caused tearing, discharge, or mucocele. The nature of the surgical procedures should be outlined. The question of local versus general anesthesia and inpatient versus outpatient setting should be discussed with the patient. The patient should be told that in almost every situation the procedure is elective and optional. The exception to this rule would be when there is an orbital abscess with posterior cellulitis secondary to a fulminant dacryocystitis. Certainly, a person may live with a lacrimal sac mucocele or a watery eye, or even discharge for that matter. Some patients would rather have repeated attacks of dacryocystitis and treat them with antibiotics than have a definitive operation to cure the problem. The patient should be counseled and then the ultimate decision is up to the patient. If the patient is to have a cataract operation, the precataract surgery DCR is an optional situation, but we must recommend that if the patient does not have the DCR, the cataract should not be performed.

The patient must be told that this is an operation mainly on the nose and that there may be a nose bleed during the first 2 weeks following the procedure. We have never had postoperative hemorrhage following this period of time. It is most unusual that nose bleeds occur immediately after the surgery, and when they do occur, they seem to come on at about 4 to 7 days following the surgery because of clot retraction, much as one finds with a secondary bleed from a hyphema. The patient must be told that if there is bleeding, the measures that can be taken at home are pinching the nose, ice packs, and rest. However, it must be emphasized that should a severe nose bleed occur, the patient would have to come to the hospital and have the nose packed. The patient may also have the need, if nasal packing does not work, to have embolization or ligation of the anterior ethmoidal artery. It is a question how much one wants to get into the discussion preoperatively, especially the potential for a blood transfusion. We routinely tell the patient that they may have a bad hemorrhage afterward, but it is most unusual for this to happen, and that we can get the bleeding stopped if it occurs. We tell the patients that this is an operation mainly on the nose, and even though orbital hemorrhages have been reported during DCR (10), we do tell the patients there is a risk that bleeding may occur behind the eye. However, we reassure the patient that we have not had any patient lose any vision because of this. This would be analogous to mentioning to patients who are to undergo cosmetic blepharoplasty that there is a risk of losing vision (or blindness), and that we have never seen this happen (even though it has been reported), and that there is probably more of the risk of them being injured driving to the hospital than there is losing vision from this procedure. This allows us to inform the patients of the remote possibility of this rare occurrence, without turning them off to the operation.

We tell the patients as well that because it is an operation on the nose, that they must not blow the nose for approximately 2 weeks postoperatively (for fear of a nose bleed being precipitated). We also mention that after the operation when they do blow their nose it is normal that they may be able to blow some air back from the nose through the puncta in front of the palpebral aperture. We tell them that this indeed is a good thing and it means that the DCR is open (11). It may seem that this is a trivial side effect of which to warn the patients, but it is such frequent occurrence, and since the patients may complain about this afterward, it is best that the surgeon warn them about it preoperatively. It is important to realize as well that if tubes are placed within the system, that the patient most of the time will not be able to blow back air, and that this effect might occur after the tubes are removed.

The patients should be told that with the external DCR that there will indeed be a scar on the side of the nose. The scar does tend to fade over a period of 3 months, and we tell the patients that they will be using some ointment and emollients to place on the sutures, and then after the sutures come out, to massage actively onto the side of the nose. It would seem that the pressure of massage tends to break up any scar tissue contracture and decrease the scar. We have been gradually decreasing the size of our incisions to now be approximately 8 mm, and the resulting scar is usually quite small, blends into the side of the nose, and becomes imperceptible. We tell the patients that if there is a persistent scar, and this is unusual, that one could theoretically inject the scar with some steroids or do a small plastic procedure in the office to revise it (V-Y plasty), but this is exceptionally rare.

The patients always ask how long it will take to heal. We tell the patients they may have some bruising for a week or two (depending on their age, smoking, etc.), but we tell them that the healing process is approximately 3 months until the scars contract and the wounds heal (12).

We tell the patients that there may be a temporary tube inserted at the time of the surgery. The purpose of this tube is to hold the passage open and not to drain any tears. We tell the patients that although tears may percolate around the tube and tearing will be decreased, that they can expect that there may be some tearing until the tube is taken out. We tell them that the tube usually lies quietly and causes no irritation, but they may sense the tube in the inner canthus and use a lubricating drop to help with any irritation. We also tell them that if they stick a finger in the nose, they may feel the tube and we mention that this is not a foreign body and not to try and pull it out.

We tell patients that with a DCR the success rate is "90% to 95%" or even more. We mention, however, that there is no 100% guarantee that this procedure will eliminate the tearing, even though the odds are very high. We tell the patients that they will have the sutures removed 1 week postoperatively, and that we will have to irrigate the system at least once, and possibly twice, postoperatively if all is well, and perhaps more frequently if there is any stenosis developing within the system postoperatively. We tell them that in the small percentage of patients in whom the system does not stay open, that usually we are able to eliminate the tearing with an office procedure or, failing that, with an intranasal procedure with or without tubes in the operating room. It is unusual that we have to perform any secondary surgery, but this does occasionally occur.

Last of all, we write on our charts who else was present in the room while the informed consent was being given. This is extremely important if a patient has a different native language than the surgeon. We then ask the patient if he wants to have the surgery. If he is unsure, we write on the chart that the patient will think it over and call if he wants to have the procedure done. Even though it is usually more convenient to book the patient for surgery while he is present in the office, it is much more prudent to have the patient think about it and come back at a later date to have the surgery scheduled. We feel that it is important that if surgery is to be done, that patient must want to have the surgery.

PSYCHOLOGICAL ASSESSMENT

The patients must have a good idea as to why they are having the surgery and whether they are psychologically prepared to undergo the operation. The surgeon does not usually have an extended period of time to get to know the patient well. However, it is sometimes possible for the surgeon to determine if the patient has a severe form of neurosis, personality disorder, or psychosis (13). The surgeon might tend to turn off toward a patient whom he considers to have any of these psychiatric problems, but most patients who have a subsequent "surgical-psychiatric team" approach to treatment will have a positive response to the surgery.

The question of a scar may pose a problem to a patient who is exceptionally concerned about esthetics. Male patients seem to have as much concern as female patients (14). The surgeon can reassure the patient that even though the nose may be sore, and that in some cases placing eyeglasses on top of the scar may cause a little bit of discomfort, that this will be alleviated with time. Similarly, the scar should settle down with time, and blend into the side of the nose. The patient's concern of a scar is one reason that some surgeons have been looking toward performing intranasal surgery.

If a patient feels more comfortable with the surgeon and the surroundings, the patient's attitude and perceptions of the surgery will improve greatly (15). However, there are some patients who may become extremely aggressive toward the surgeon or there may be a poor rapport between the surgeon and the patient. There is certainly no obligation to operate on patients in whom the concerns are solely cosmetic. However, patients with lacrimal obstructions will have functional problems as well and it is certainly more difficult for the surgeon to refuse to operate. Some patients, however, are best not operated on if there is poor rapport, and should be referred either to another surgeon or possibly may be helped by psychological assessment (16).

The surgeon must try to predict how dissatisfied the patient will be if the surgery does not work or even if it does work, if it does not match up with the patient's expectations. In these days of law suits, the surgeon is also fearful that the dissatisfied patient, if not handled properly, will institute a law suit. To minimize the dissatisfaction of the patient, maintain the rapport with the patient, plan for further treatment if necessary, and to minimize the risk of law suits:

1. the surgeon should attempt to understand the patient and his concerns
2. the surgeon should not try and promote his trade
3. the surgeon should immediately disclose any "mistakes"
4. if in doubt surgery should not be done
5. there should be no guarantees
6. if there are any questions a consultation should be sought
7. the surgeon should never speak poorly of his colleagues or give the patient the impression that the surgeon is arrogant
8. extreme caution should be used when attempting new or unproven procedures
9. the surgeon should be aware of what of is printed in the chart (17).

PREOPERATIVE MANAGEMENT

Preoperative Medications

If the patient has had a pre-existing dacryocystitis, then the patient is put on oral cloxacillin 250 mg every six hours. If the patient has pericystitis or orbital cellulitis, then the cloxacillin is given intravenously. If the patient is allergic to penicillin, either cephalosporins or erythromycin 250 mg every six hours is given. We commence the oral antibiotics approximately 3 days preoperatively.

Preoperative Decongestants

We premedicate the patients with naphazoline nasal spray, a very effective decongestant. It is given 2 hours, 1 hour, and one-half hour preoperatively. Two puffs are given in the nostril on the side of the contemplated surgery. This is usually sufficient to decongest the mucosa. Overdosage of these drugs may occasionally cause central nervous system stimulation and the patients may experience excitation, headache, insomnia, and irritability. Tachycardia, although unusual, may occur (18). If cocaine is to be used as well preoperatively, it has been shown that the administration of naphazoline or other decongestants such as oxymetazoline before application of nasal cocaine decreases the blood level and cardiovascular side effects of the latter by reducing the nasal mucosal blood flow. We use the decongestant nasal spray regardless of whether the patient is being operated under local or general anesthesia.

When surgery is being performed under general anesthesia, one or two small neurosurgical patties measuring 1×1 cm are soaked in 5% cocaine and placed directly into the middle meatus on the lateral wall above the inferior turbinate. This is the site of the surgery, and there is no need to decongest the rest of the nose. Certainly there are potential problems from cocaine toxicity. Cocaine inhibits the reuptake of norepinephrine and increases the effect of endogenous and exogenous epinephrine. We do not use any local anesthesia with epinephrine if we are using cocaine. Toxic reactions have been reported with as little as 20 mg of intranasal cocaine even though reactions are unusual in dosages under 3 mg/Kg (19). The cocaine is absorbed by the nasal mucosa and can be recovered in the urine of patients for up to 72 hours after surgery (20). We feel that the preoperative decongestant nasal spray seems to play more of a role in decongestion than the administration of the cocaine. In fact, we have not noticed any difference in the appearance of the nasal mucosa when we have used cocaine and when we have not used cocaine. For these reasons, we are using cocaine less frequently even with patients under general anesthesia. We have totally eliminated the use of cocaine in conjunction with epinephrine when a patient is being operated on under local anesthesia. The bayonet forceps used when placing the neurosurgical patties should only place the patties above the inferior turbinate. This will eliminate the chance of pushing the patties too far superiorly in the roof of the nose with the potential risk of violating the cribriform plate and causing cerebrospinal fluid (CSF) leak.

Draping

During the procedure, traction sutures, rather than a retractor, are used to open the wound because this gives better exposure. For this reason, the drapes must be put on very securely, leaving the nose and the eye of the operated side open. Thus, when the traction sutures are clamped down to the drapes, they will be held snugly and the wound will stay open.

Positioning of the Patient

The patient is placed in reverse Trendelenburg position. This is a head-up, feet-down position. This facilitates venous outflow from the head and neck region and decreases bleeding in the area.

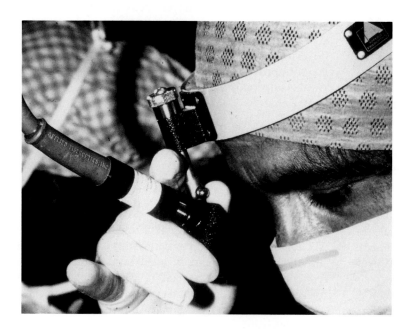

FIG. 3. Illumination for the surgeon in DCR surgery using fiberoptic head light.

Preparing of the Operating Tray

A bipolar cautery is mandatory for this procedure. We also prefer to use two separate suctions draining to separate bottles. This is helpful so that suctioning can be used directly into the wound, and also up the nose. It is also helpful to have a second suction in case one suction plugs and the other suction can be used while the nurse is cleaning the plugged suction.

Illumination

Fiberoptic illumination gives the surgeon the best visualization of the operative field (Fig. 3). Operating loops are a useful adjunct in surgery performed on the canaliculi or in helping the surgeon dilate an extremely stenotic punctum. A chip camera may be mounted on the headlight (Madison Medical, Canada) to give the same video display on a screen that the surgeon is able to see in the

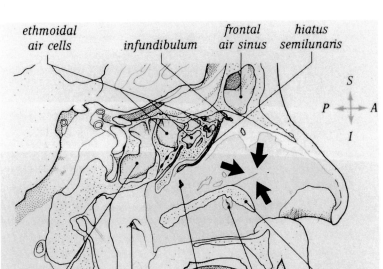

A

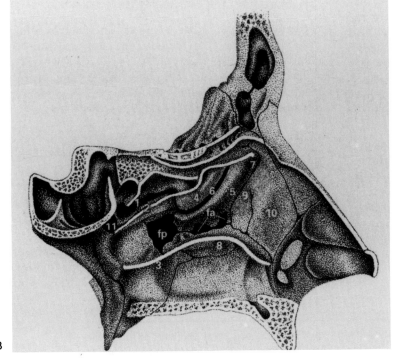

B

FIG. 4. A: Regional anatomy of the DCR. Site of DCR opening (*arrows*) on lateral wall of nose. B: Bony structures of the lateral nasal wall. *1,* edge of resected superior turbinate; *2,* edge of resected middle turbinate; *3,* edge of resected inferior turbinate; *4,* ethmoidal bulla; *5,* uncinate process; *6,* hiatus semilunaris between the ethmoidal bulla and the uncinate process; *7,* agger nasi; *8,* inferior turbinate bone; *9,* lacrimal bone; *10,* processus frontalis of the maxilla; *11,* sphenopalatine foramen; *fa,* anterior (inferior) nasal fontanelle; *fp,* posterior nasal fontanelle.

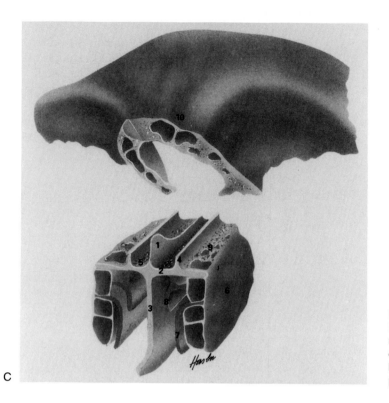

C

FIG. 4. (*Continued.*) C: Diagram of the ethmoidal bone. Important structures: *1,* crista galli; *2,* anterior face cribriform plate; *3,* perpendicular plate of ethmoid; *4,* lateral extent cribriform plate; *5,* cribriform plate; *6,* ethmoidal labyrinth. (From Stammberger and Hawke, ref. 82, with permission.)

field. This greatly facilitates teaching and interest of the nurses who otherwise would not be able to see what is going on.

Surgical Goals

The goal is to make an epithelial lined tract so that the sac will cease to exist as a structure, and the common canaliculus drain tears directly into the nose. To do this, one needs an epithelium-lined tract that is best performed, in our opinion, by suturing posterior flaps of sac and nasal mucosa, and suturing anterior flaps of sac and nasal mucosa. If flaps are excised or not sutured, it is our opinion that this leaves the epithelialization to establish a new tract to chance, and we prefer to create the new tract. However, it must be emphasized that in suturing flaps, one must not compromise the size of the opening. In a similar fashion, one must determine whether an adequate opening has been achieved, or whether a stent (with its potential complications) should be used to keep the passage open during the healing process.

The DCR works by three factors:

1. the orbicularis pump involving the canaliculi and common canaliculus (lacrimal pump)
2. respiration
3. gravity

There is a slight increase in tear flow through a DCR when one compares this to a normal patient never having had a lacrimal problem (21). Therefore, it is extremely important that the orbicularis, which is the chief part of the lacrimal pump, be respected.

Anatomy of the DCR: A knowledge of the location of the DCR opening to the adjacent nasal structures is mandatory (Fig. 4).

Specific instruments: We prefer that certain instruments be available for the procedure, that is, punches, elevators, probes, and tubes (Fig. 5).

DCR TECHNIQUE

Skin Incision

We prefer to make a skin incision on the side of the nose medial to the angular vein (Fig. 6A). The angular vein sweeps around laterally, and if one makes the incision medial to the angular vein there is less chance of violating it and causing a hemorrhage. The skin incision should be made through skin only. The skin incision

FIG. 5. Important instruments for DCR. **A:** Kerrison punch for removing bone. **B:** Rollet's Rougine (*arrow*) and Traquir's periosteal elevators. **C:** Punctal dilators. Tiny tapered dilator (*arrow*) is excellent if tiny puncta. **D:** Beyer punch for removing bone from nasolacrimal canal.

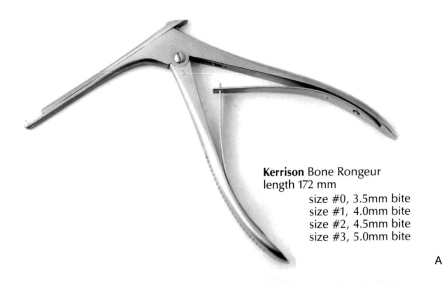

Kerrison Bone Rongeur
length 172 mm

    size #0, 3.5mm bite
    size #1, 4.0mm bite
    size #2, 4.5mm bite
    size #3, 5.0mm bite

A

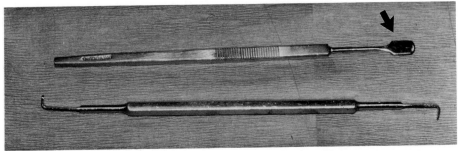

B

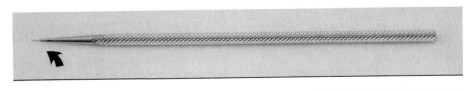

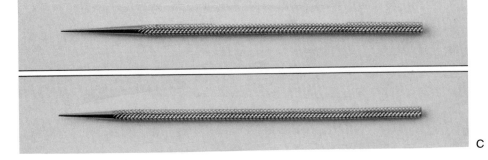

C

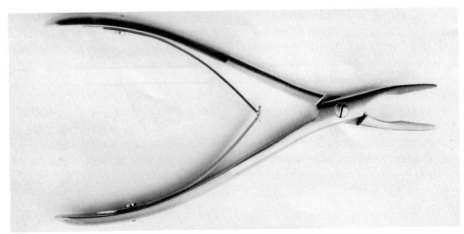

D

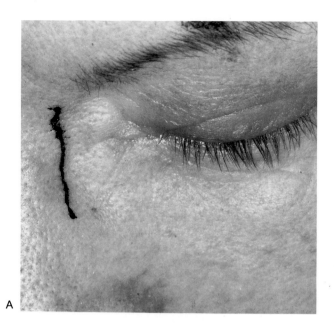

FIG. 6. A: Skin incision on the side of the nose for DCR surgery. The incision should be straight and well away from the inner canthus. B: The lines of Langer (*arrows*). Standard DCR incision (*thick line*) and eyelid DCR incision (*thin line*). C: Relaxed skin tension lines. Standard DCR incision (*thick line*) and eyelid DCR incision (*thin line*). (Figs. B, C from Freeman, ref. 83, with permission.)

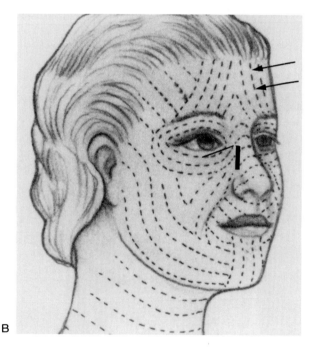

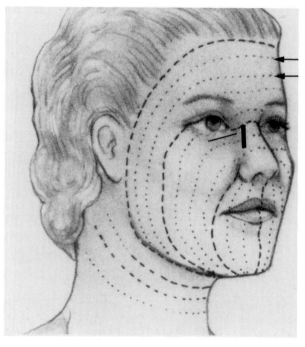

should start at the level of the medial canthus and proceed inferiorly. We have been able to decrease the size of our skin incision placed in the proper position on the side of the nose to approximately 8 to 9 mm if we wish to make as small a scar as possible, for example in a young woman with a small nose. This incision, therefore, usually is placed approximately 10 to 12 mm medial to the medial canthus. If one makes the incision over the angular vessels, which may be more medial than usual, this is not a problem because the incision goes through skin only, and one is able to identify the vessels without a problem. If one desires a larger incision, a multiple Z-plasty incision may decrease the resulting scar.

In a patient in whom there is an epicanthal fold, the incision must be made medial to the epicanthus and then it is usually hidden nicely. If previous surgery has been performed and there is a scar on the side of the nose, we usually go through the original incision to perform our DCR.

We have also performed some DCRs using the infralash incision starting just medial to the medial canthal tendon and then proceeding along the lower lid crease (22). This incision has a theoretical advantage of being in the relaxed skin tension lines (Fig. 6B,C). However, we have not been impressed that the scar is any better than our modified incision that we make on the side of the

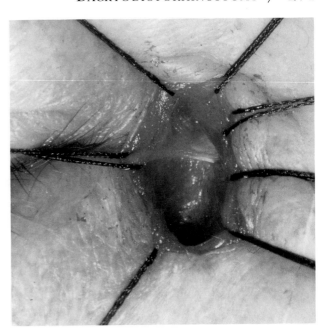

nose. Also the exposure, especially getting to the common internal punctum, is not as good. The incision needs to be a lot longer than our standard incision on the side of the nose, and we worry about the fact that the incision comes over the common canaliculus, which may potentially lead to pericanalicular scarring and subsequent closure of the lower canaliculus or common canaliculus. For this reason, we have gone back to using our standard approach on the side of the nose but have modified it to decrease the size and have been happy with the cosmetic results.

Handling the Angular Vessels

If the angular vessels are in the way under the skin incision, the bipolar diathermy at the superior aspect of the incision and the inferior aspect of the incision is used to close off the vessels. If needed, the vessel can be transected half way between the superior and inferior aspects of the cauterized vessel.

Exposure

We prefer not to use any sort of retractor that might compromise some of the space and the exposure. We prefer to use traction sutures (Fig. 7), which are 4-0 silk sutures that are placed initially on the medial and lateral aspects of the subcutaneous tissues, and the wound separated horizontally. After this, the orbicularis is separated vertically so that there is a plane between the orbital and palpebral heads of the orbicularis. To do this, the muscle does not have to be cut. This gets one directly down to the periosteal plane without having cut anything but the skin, and not having done any harm to the orbic-

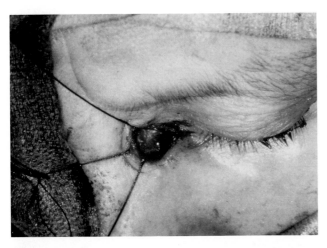

FIG. 7. Traction sutures are used to open up the wound. Dissection is carried out after the skin incision and after the angular vein has been moved out of the way laterally, to separate the muscle fibers so that the medial canthal tendon can be exposed.

FIG. 8. The medial canthal tendon can be seen after the muscle bellies have been separated.

ularis. Then two more 4-0 silk traction sutures are placed at the superior and inferior aspects of the wound subcutaneously just on the medial aspect of the apices of the incision. This pulls the wound medially. The sutures are snapped down to the drapes, which have been previously firmly attached, and the wound is held open with nothing inside it.

Incising the Periosteum

A sharp periosteal elevator such as a Rollet's Rougine (see Fig. 5) (Dixey Instruments, London) can be used to incise the periosteum and then separate the periosteum medially and push it in a medial direction so there will be no periosteum overhanging the rhinostomy. If there is, some of the periosteum can be excised. Using the Rollet's, the periosteum can then be deflected laterally. The plane of cleavage must be between the bone of the lacrimal fossa and the periosteum overlying the lacrimal sac. We prefer to do a "hand over hand" technique using the Rollet's in one hand and a suction (a #9 French), in the other hand to mobilize the sac laterally. The initial incision with the Rollet's into the periosteum to cut the periosteum and the anterior limb of the medial canthal tendon should be made just anterior to the anterior lacrimal crest (Fig. 8). If it is made inferiorly as well, there is more room to get the instruments between the bone and the periosteum to mobilize the sac laterally (Fig. 9). It must be remembered that the lacrimal sac has a layer of periosteum overlying it when one performs this maneuver.

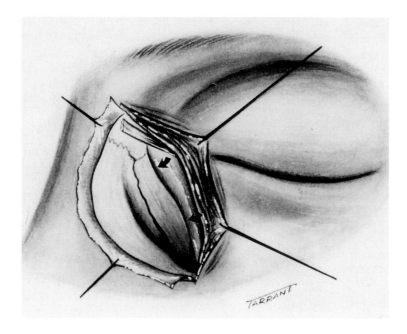

FIG. 9. Artist's diagram of mobilizing the sac laterally after incising through periosteum so that the frontal process of maxilla and the lacrimal bone can be identified. The sac (*arrows*) is retracted laterally. (Courtesy of Mr. Terry Tarrant, London, UK.)

Medial Canthal Tendon

Initial descriptions of DCR suggested that the medial canthal tendon should be left unviolated. Pico (23) stated that anterior limb of the medial canthal tendon should be cut to give access to the fundus of the lacrimal sac and allow for an easier DCR. We certainly would agree with this statement. It would seem that this would be necessary to fulfill Lester Jones' dictum that there must be 5 mm free of bone in all directions from the common canaliculus opening (24). However, the anterior limb of the medial canthal tendon is a landmark to the most inferior

projection of the cribriform plate of the ethmoid bone. We know that a multiplicity of fine olfactory nerves, with dural sheaths around them, run through the cribriform plate, and violation of the cribriform plate could cause a CSF leak (Figs. 10 and 11). Some surgeons feel that one should leave the medial canthal tendon to act as a landmark to the cribriform plate in order to prevent a CSF leak (25). We feel that leaving the tendon intact would decrease the ease of performing a DCR. As well, CSF leak has been a complication that we have not yet had to deal with. The medial canthal tendon has a free lower end and a reflected (or attached) upper end. The tendon

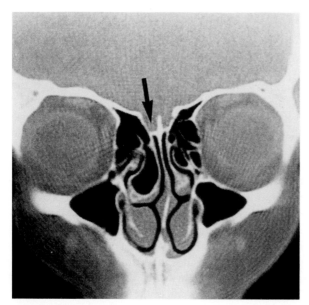

FIG. 10. Demonstration of a low position of the cribriform plate. (From Stammberger and Hawke, ref. 82, with permission.)

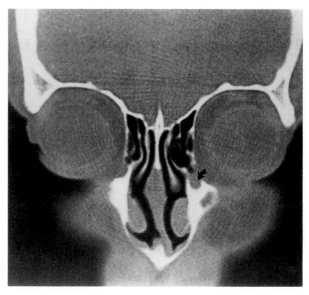

FIG. 11. CT scan showing relationship of cribriform plate to DCR opening (*arrow*).

tends to fan out anterior to the anterior lacrimal crest and has a vertical limb that goes quite superiorly (26). We therefore feel that it would be difficult to disinsert all the anterior limb of the medial canthal tendon. We snip, with a blunt scissors, the 4 mm or so of medial canthal tendon that would overly the sac, up to the fundus of the sac. Certainly, there is no need to cut any higher. This has been recently emphasized by Bartley (27). This would also give the surgeon the indication as to where the most superior recess of the lacrimal fossa would lie, as it is certainly unnecessary to remove bone higher than that (28).

Bone Removal

Even though many different methods for removing the bone of the lacrimal fossa and anterior process of maxilla have been described, such as the use of a drill (29) or ultrasound (30), we prefer to remove the bone under direct vision so as not to damage the nasal mucosa. The lacrimal fossa consists of the frontal process of maxilla anteriorly and the lacrimal bone posteriorly. There is a suture line between the two bones. We use a small instrument (Traquir periosteal elevator, Dixey Instrument, London) (see Fig. 5), which is a small 90° instrument to push through the lacrimal bone at the anastomotic junction. Then the instrument can be used to gently push the mucosa posteriorly and to separate and obtain a cleavage plane between the bone and the nasal mucosa. This is an atraumatic procedure and gives one direct access to the proper surgical plane for bone removal (Fig. 12). It is not necessary to remove bone posterior to the suture between the lacrimal bone and the frontal process of maxilla. When the sac is open, it is important that the poste-

rior flap of the sac lies in a flat plane and not ride up over any bone. This can be achieved by removing just the anterior half of the bone of the lacrimal fossa and not removing bone more posteriorly, certainly not as far posterior as the posterior lacrimal crest at the posterior lip of the lacrimal fossa. Then using Kerrison (Storz) punches (see Fig. 5), starting with a small one and then moving to larger punches, the bone may be removed anteriorly (medially), superiorly, and inferiorly. The superior bone of the medial aspect of the nasolacrimal canal should be removed to ensure that a "sump syndrome" will not develop, and if stones are present, that they may be seen within the nasolacrimal canal. The removal of the bone is performed by sliding the inner blade of the punch in the plane between the bone and the mucosa and then extracting the bone with the punch held firmly in the hand of the operator (Fig. 12). The punch should be sharp so that there are no torsional motions when the bone is being removed. This might cause an incomplete removal of the bone with a subsequent spiral fracture up to the cribriform plate of the ethmoid and potential CSF leak. The cribriform plate lies 25 mm from the common internal punctum and, if damaged, is probably damaged by rotational forces from the bone punch.

What Should the Size of the Opening Be?

The opening should be big enough and placed in the proper position so that all of the sac can be anastomosed to the nasal mucosa. This would mean that the inferior aspect of the opening should go down to the roof of the nasolacrimal canal and in fact some of the medial wall of the nasolacrimal canal should be removed. It is important not to remove any of the bone of the nasolacrimal

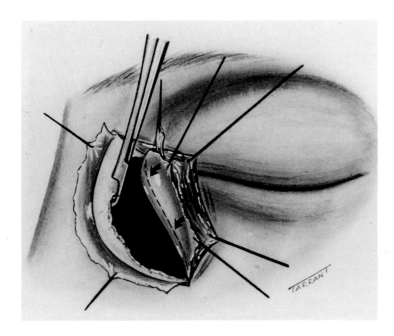

FIG. 12. Artist's diagram of bone being removed by Kerrison punches anteriorly, inferiorly, and to a lesser degree superiorly. Sac incision—*dotted line* (*arrows*). (Courtesy of Mr. Terry Tarrant, London, UK.)

canal laterally because this gets close to the origin of the inferior oblique muscle. The superior aspect of the osteotomy need not, and should not, go above the roof of the lacrimal fossa. If one leaves approximately half the medial canthal tendon intact, it is difficult to get too high. The osteotomy must not be enlarged superiorly in a posterior direction as one could get close to the suture line between the lacrimal bone and the ethmoidal bone where they meet the frontal plate, the location of the anterior ethmoidal artery (Fig. 13). This could lead to a tremendous amount of bleeding, which might be difficult to control. Aggressive posterior enlargement may encroach upon the nasofrontal duct (Fig. 14) or, more posteriorly, the ethmoidal and maxillary sinus openings (Fig. 15). There is no point in going more superior than the roof of the lacrimal fossa because there is no sac to anastomose higher up, and the risks outweigh the benefits.

The anterior aspect (medial) of the osteotomy should be far enough forward onto the frontal process of maxilla

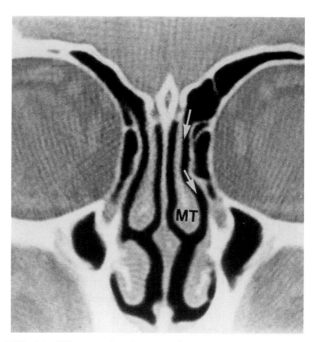

FIG. 14. CT scan showing nasofrontal duct draining frontal sinus and exiting under middle turbinate (*MT*). (From Stammberger and Hawke, ref. 82, with permission.)

including the anterior lacrimal crest, but not so far as the suture line between the frontal process of maxilla and the nasal bone. There are rich blood vessels in this suture line that may cause a lot of bleeding, and there is always the risk of affecting the architecture of the nose if the nasal bone has been somewhat removed. The sac itself measures 12 mm in height and 4 mm of this is above the medial canthal tendon. The sac conforms to the shape of the lacrimal fossa and is approximately 4 to 8 mm in an anterior posterior measurement, and almost the same in

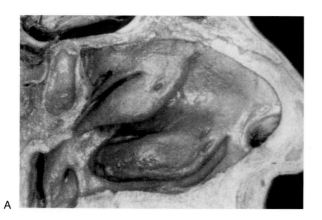

A

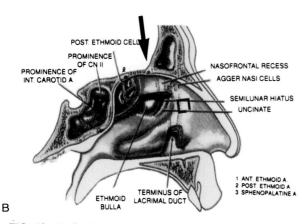

B

FIG. 13. A: Cadaver. **B:** Diagram. Relationship of the anterior ethmoidal artery (*arrow*) to the DCR site (*square*). (From Stammberger and Hawke, ref. 82, with permission.)

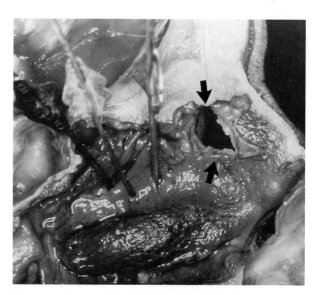

FIG. 15. DCR opening (*arrows*) relationship to anterior ethmoidal openings (probes) and the middle turbinate.

width. The osteotomy opening should be at least 12 mm in diameter according to Pico (23), but it is especially important that the osteotomy be far enough forward on the nose so that not only can the flaps of the sac be opened up, but the anterior flap should be able to be tented anteriorly over the posterior flaps to increase the diameter of the soft tissue opening between the sutured flaps. We feel it is important to preserve the nasal mucosa when one is removing the bone because we want to use the nasal mucosa for creating flaps. Also, shredding the nasal mucosa will cause more bleeding and make the procedure more difficult. The opening should be just anterior to the anterior tip of the middle turbinate (Fig. 15).

Creating Sac Flaps

The puncta are dilated and a probe is placed through one canaliculus (usually the lower) into the sac. The opening of the sac is greatly facilitated by having a probe within the sac, upon which one can cut down. Usually one can see the medial wall of the sac "tent up" when one pushes the probe in. If the punctum is tiny, it may be better identified by placing a drop of blood from the DCR site onto the lower eyelid. The blood will pass into the punctum by capillarity, and a red "dot" representing the punctum may be seen. Failing this, a #25 needle may be used to open the punctum, which can then be dilated. A "light pipe" placed within the sac can transilluminate the sac through the skin and the DCR opening (Fig. 16). It must be re-emphasized that there are actually two linings overlying the probe—the periosteum and the sac mucosa. One can then use a curved knife (we prefer a #12 Bard-Parker tonsil knife) to cut down on the probe

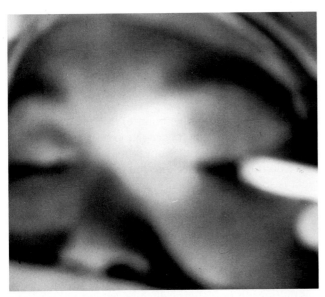

FIG. 16. A "light pipe" placed within the canaliculus can transilluminate the sac through the skin and through the DCR opening.

about 1 to 2 mm anterior to the most medial tenting of the sac by the probe. When one does this, one can identify the probe within the sac. With the probe held in the sac, curved scissors (Stevens or Werb) can be used to enlarge the sac opening. This is done in a vertical fashion with the inner blade of the scissors being placed inside the flap and then the sac cut superiorly, the scissors turned 180°, and the inferior aspect opened. We prefer to make very small relieving incisions of the sac on the posterior flaps at the most superior and inferior aspects of the incision. This allows the posterior flap to lie flat pointing toward the nasal mucosa. There may be small anterior relieving incisions made in the anterior flap at the superior and inferior aspects of the incisions. We then prefer to place traction sutures (one, two, or three) on the anterior flap to pull the anterior flap laterally and give exposure of the common internal punctum. We use a 5-0 Dexon (Davis and Geck) suture on a #23 needle. These sutures will be used later to be sutured to the anterior nasal mucosa flaps. If one is not able to see the probe tenting the sac forward, one may inject sodium hyaluronate tinted with fluorescein into the sac. Then when one opens the sac, one can be sure of being inside the sac when one sees the Healon liberated (Fig. 17; see Colorplate 9 following page 142). The other advantage is that the fluorescein will stain the cut edges of the mucosa (31). A probe should be placed through the upper punctum and canaliculus to ensure that the upper system is normal. It is useful to make sure that the probes come out at the common internal punctum together. One must take great care in avoiding a false passaging by the probes. We have been impressed that with dacryocystography we have always been able to see a common canaliculus. We feel that reports from surgical observations that the canaliculi may enter separately into the sac may be due to false passaging of one or both canaliculi on probing of the canaliculi, and the probes may enter not through the common canaliculus but may go through the lateral sac wall into the sac and give one the false impression that the canaliculi enter the sac separately. The common canaliculus is usually located more anteriorly and superiorly than one would expect. If one has trouble passing the probe, an irrigation and bubble technique (32) can be used. This is useful to show the common internal punctum without having to probe. However, we prefer to make sure that the probes pass through the common internal punctum. At this point, we follow Jones' dictum and try to ensure that there is 5 mm of bone-free area around the common internal punctum opening. If there is not, we prefer to enlarge the rhinostomy at this point. Care must be taken on removing bone once the sac has been opened so that the flaps are not excised in the punch (Fig. 18). If there is mucus or pus within the sac, especially if there has been a dacryocystitis, we take a culture.

When the sac is open one should look carefully at the

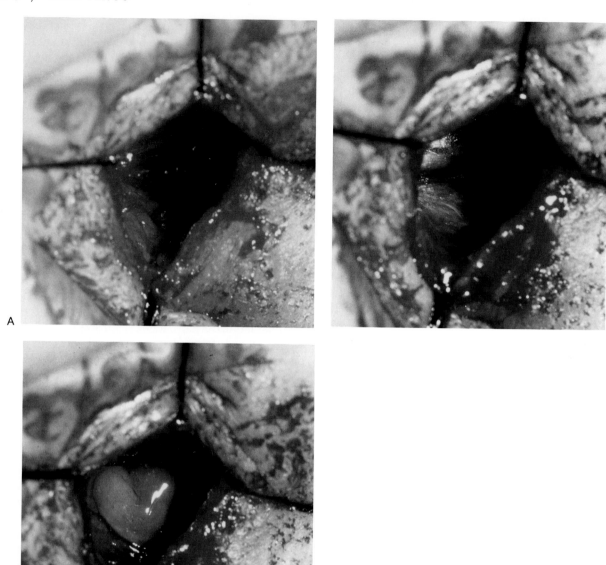

FIG. 17. A: DCR open, sac exposed. **B:** Sodium hyaluronate injected into sac. Sac distended. **C:** Sac incised, sodium hyaluronate liberated, fluorescein tints cut edges of mucosa. (From Hurwitz and Nik, ref. 31, with permission.)

mucosa to see if it is normal or if there is any question of a tumor. As well, one should look carefully for stones within the sac, common canaliculus, and into the nasolacrimal canal. If one has inadvertently incised too far lateral into the sac, one may see some orbital fat prolapse into the sac. We feel that this is not necessarily a reason to insert tubes, and we treat the fat prolapse by shrinking it with bipolar cautery, the same as we might shrink fat in a blepharoplasty. We have found that this causes adequate fat retraction, does not damage the mucosa, and if a tube was not needed without the fat prolapse, we would not put one in. Also, the ease of passage of the probe through the common internal punctum should be assessed. If it does not pass easily or if there is a membrane

overlying the probe, one must excise the membrane (common internal punctoplasty) and be prepared to put in a temporary indwelling stent tube.

We do not feel it is necessary to biopsy the sac unless there is some abnormality in the mucosa, or unless the patient is known to have a condition such as sarcoidosis or Wegener's granulomatosis.

Ethmoidal Air Cells

Anterior ethmoidal air cells may extend inferiorly to extend to the posterior wall of the lacrimal fossa in 14% of patients, as far as the suture between the two bones in

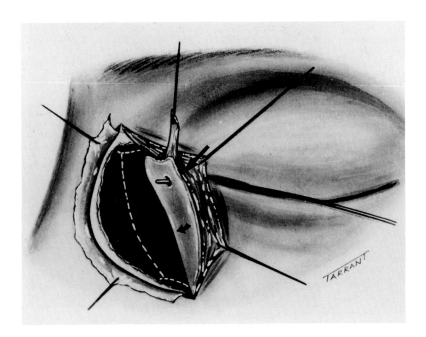

FIG. 18. A probe has been placed through the lower canaliculus into the sac through the common internal punctum. The sac has been opened. Anterior (*big arrow*) and posterior (*small arrow*) flaps are visible. The *dotted line* shows the nasal mucosa to be incised later. Of note is that the traction suture on the anterior limb of the medial canthal tendon is not mandatory. (Courtesy of Mr. Terry Tarrant, London, UK.)

the fossa in 32%, and completely across the fossa in 54% (33). For this reason, in most DCRs there will be some ethmoidal air cells between the sac and the nasal mucosa (Fig. 19). These may be handled easily and removed using an artery forceps. Some of the fine eggshell-thick bone fragments can and should be removed if they will lie in the way of the flaps. Sometimes one sees some of the ethmoidal air cells going quite far posteriorly, and it is not necessary to remove these. In patients who have had sinus problems in the past, there may be some nasal polyps present (Fig. 20). These may be removed easily using a Wilde forceps. If no Wilde forceps is present, one may use an artery forceps, although the polyp often slips through the teeth of these instruments. There may be some bleeding from the ethmoidal air cells, but this can usually be handled with cautery. If there is a significant amount of bleeding, one may use small pieces of reconstituted collagen (Surgicel), and these can be placed in the area of the ethmoids (34). However, it is rare that we have found these necessary. As stated, the further posterior one goes in removing ethmoidal air cells, the more bleeding, and the more potential for involvement of the anterior ethmoidal artery.

Before removing the bone, there may be some bleeding coming from the incisural foramen (sutura notha), which is an opening in the bone just anterior to the anterior lacrimal crest. This opening contains an emissary vein coming from vessels either regionally or posteriorly. It is not necessary to cauterize or pack vessels coming from this area. We find that when the bone is removed, including the sutura notha, the bleeding usually stops because of retraction of the vessel. It has only been the occasional time that it has not stopped, and we have used a small piece of Surgicel to help in hemostasis. If a small ethmoidal air cell cyst exists, rather than removing it one

can use bipolar cautery around the cyst and flatten it with the heat. This is useful because it works well and also helps in hemostasis.

Incising the Nasal Mucosa

We take blunt scissors and insert them into the nose after removing the patties. The scissors can be slid up along the septum, and while one is observing externally, one can locate the position of the turbinates. When the blunt scissors are slid superiorly, one can see the indentation of the nasal mucosa where the incision is to be made. If one slides the scissors more posteriorly, then one can feel the location of the turbinates. The same curved knife (#12 blade) is used to incise the nasal mucosa. We prefer to start at the inferior aspect of the opening, where there are few ethmoids, and cut down on the scissors as the incision is made vertically. The scissors protect the nasal mucosa and give accurate localization of the incision. Once an opening has been made, the suction that is being held in the other hand can be placed between the anterior and posterior flaps of the nasal mucosa where the incision has been made, and the incision can be extended inferiorly (Fig. 21). Then the scissors are turned 180° and the incision can be extended superiorly. If ethmoidal air cells are present, these can be stripped from the nasal mucosa (usually on the posterior flap superiorly) and handled appropriately. A small relieving incision anteriorly will help to mobilize the anterior flap. One may also make a small relieving incision in the posterior flap superiorly to mobilize the posterior flap. Occasionally one will find that there is a large turbinate preventing the flap from falling laterally. This is usually the anterior tip of the middle turbinate. The middle turbi-

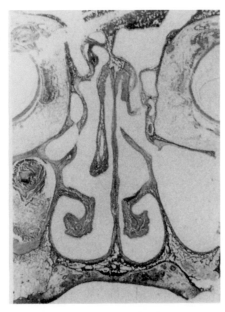

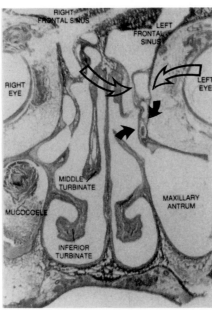

FIG. 19. Relationship of DCR opening (*black arrows*) to ethmoidal air cells (*white arrow*). (From Hawke, ref. 84, with permission.)

nate has an L-shaped configuration, and one may be able to gently mobilize the posterior flap, including the anterior tip of the middle turbinate, and "out fracture" the turbinate toward the sac. This will mobilize the turbinate and thereby mobilize the flap. This maneuver also enlarges the nasal ostium, and it is interesting that many patients state that after the DCR, they can breath better through the nostril(s).

The opening of the nasofrontal duct lies approximately 4 mm posterior to where the standard bony osteotomy is performed (35) (Fig. 22; see Colorplate 10 following page 142). Wesley (36) has stressed that in

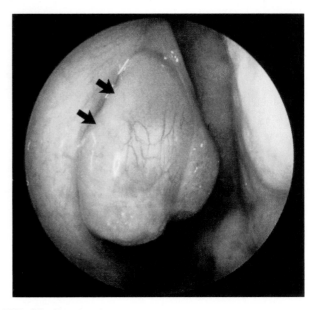

FIG. 20. Nasal polyps may present in the nose in a patient undergoing DCR, especially if there has been previous history of ethmoidal problems or polyps. (From Hawke, ref. 84, with permission.)

performing procedures on the middle turbinate one must be very careful because of the close proximity between the DCR opening and the opening of the nasofrontal duct. The nasofrontal duct drains the frontal sinus via a funnel-shaped opening. It drains behind the uncinate process onto the opening of the hiatus semilunaris underneath the middle turbinate (Fig. 23). The mobilization of the vertical part of the anterior tip of the middle turbinate in a lateral direction should do little to interfere with the drainage through the nasolacrimal funnel into the hiatus semilunaris. However, Wesley points out that excision of the anterior tip of the middle turbinate, if performed, should not extend too far superiorly, and certainly not too far posteriorly for fear of interfering with the opening of the nasofrontal duct. He also suggests that electrocautery to remove the middle turbinate

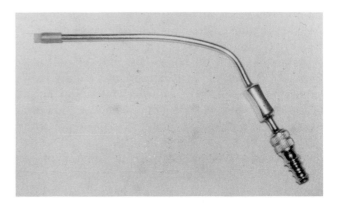

FIG. 21. Suction used in the nose. A small rubber sleeve may be placed over the tip of the suction tightly to decrease potential injury to the mucosa.

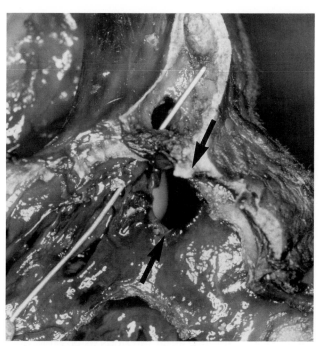

FIG. 22. Relationship of the nasofrontal duct (probe) to the DCR opening (*arrow*). (Courtesy Drs. D. Avram and J. J. Hurwitz, Toronto, Canada.)

may cause transmission of heat to the area of the duct with subsequent scarring. If the duct closes the patient may develop frontal sinusitis postoperatively (37). These patients with frontal sinusitis did not require surgical decompression and resolved with antibiotics and occasionally steroids.

If there is any question of the position of the middle turbinate, one must use a nasal speculum to examine the position of the turbinate both from inside the nose but also simultaneously through the DCR opening. If it appears that the septum is shifted toward the side of the

DCR opening, we agree with Wesley that it is difficult to perform an adequate submucous resection of the septum in the area higher up in the nose that is formed from ethmoid bone rather than the cartilage lower down, and we prefer to perform a turbinectomy to increase the size of the opening.

Occasionally one will find that the opening must be made in the nasal mucosa at the junction of the nasal mucosa and the turbinate. In this situation, the lacrimal sac flap can be sutured to the tip of the turbinate. To give good fixation of the suture, we use the sharp CE-23 needle of a 5-0 Dexon (Davis and Geck), which can be passed through the turbinate and gives some fixation to the mucosal flaps by the bone. This seems to be successful and has not compromised our success rate with the DCR.

Flaps

Although some surgeons have suggested that no flaps need be sutured, or that the anterior flap can be sutured and the posterior flap removed, or that the posterior flap can be removed and the anterior flap suspended to periosteum, we prefer to suture both posterior flaps and anterior flaps. As mentioned, we feel that this gives the greatest chance of producing an epithelial lined tract. The suturing of the posterior flaps as well as giving an epithelial lined tract tends to produce a barrier anterior to the ethmoidal air cells and one might expect that it would decrease the amount of granulation tissue growing into the DCR site from the ethmoids. We prefer to suture the posterior flaps with three (or four) sutures, and we use a 5-0 Dexon suture. The CE-23 needle swedged onto the 5-0 Dexon suture is ideal for DCR surgery. The needle is stainless steel, and is a ⅜ circle with a reverse cutting edge. The needle length is 13 mm and the radius is

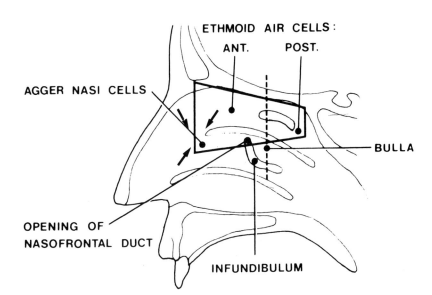

FIG. 23. Lateral wall of the nose showing relationship of the DCR opening (*arrows*) to the middle meatal structures.

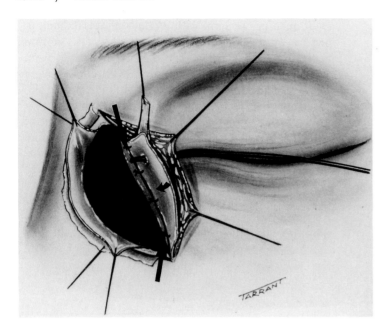

FIG. 24. Posterior flaps of sac (*small arrow*) and nasal mucosa (*large arrow*) being sutured using 5-0 Dexon sutures. (Courtesy of Mr. Terry Tarrant, London, UK.)

4.7 mm. The wire size is 0.43 mm (needle manufactured by B.G. Suizle, Inc., Syracuse, NY). The needle is strong, rigid, and does not bend easily. It is sharp enough and firm enough so that it may be passed through more solid structures such as turbinates, if needed.

We suture from the sac toward the nasal mucosa. These longer curved needles allow the surgeon to pass the needle through both flaps in one bite. To allow counter pressure while one is pushing the needle through the flaps, the suction is placed inside the nose and then moved toward the sac as the needle is passed through the flaps. The sutures are tied in a "granny knot." In tying, one takes the needle driver, securing the free end of the suture, and passes it into the nasal opening so that the knot becomes tight on the flaps. A suture is placed in the middle of the flaps, one as far inferiorly as possible, and one as high up as possible (Fig. 24). One then inspects the opening and the sac to see if tubes are necessary. The anterior flaps are sutured using three or four 5-0 Dexon sutures in a similar fashion to the suturing of the posterior flaps (Fig. 25). We prefer to tie the superior suture of the anterior flaps after the knot has been tied, to the periosteum on the superior aspect of the anterior edge of the rhinostomy, or to some remnant of medial canthal tendon. When this is tied it will "tent up" the anterior flaps and keep them well away from the posterior flaps. We do not like to fasten this to the orbicularis, even though it will keep the flaps apart, because it may potentially cause some subcutaneous contraction and "bow stringing" of the incision.

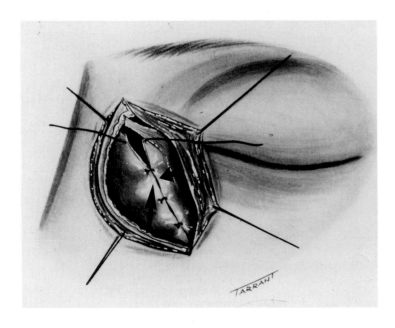

FIG. 25. Anterior sac flap (*small arrow*) and anterior nasal mucosal flap (*large arrow*) being anastomosed with 5-0 Dexon sutures. The medial canthal tendon is not reattached and just draped back over the lacrimal sac. (Courtesy of Mr. Terry Tarrant, London, UK.)

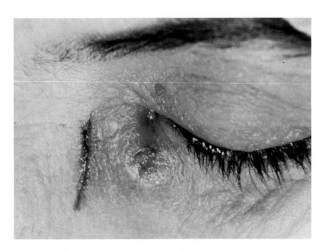

FIG. 26. The DCR is completed. Orbicularis sutures are usually not necessary because the edges of the wound usually fall into position and the skin can be sutured with three interrupted nylon sutures.

Occasionally we find that the posterior flap (or even the anterior flap) is too large. If the posterior flap is too large, we prefer to slide the blunt Stevens scissors up the nose, grasp the posterior flap with the forceps, and amputate it in the nose. It is mandatory that the posterior flaps when sutured lie flat and there are no elevations within the line of the posterior flaps. It is much less usual that we excise anterior flaps because we like the anterior flaps to form a dome overlying the common internal punctum.

Closure

The medial canthal tendon does not have to be resutured. The bone where the medial canthal tendon is usually attached is removed at the time of DCR surgery and, therefore, the reattachment could not possibly be at the right place. Faulty reattachment might pull the punctum

out of the lacrimal lake and cause postoperative tearing. As well, the posterior limb of the medial canthal tendon and the superior vertical limb of the tendon, which have not been transected, hold the inner canthus in place. We have not had a patient with telecanthus following partial disinsertion of the anterior limb of the medial canthal tendon and when the tendon had not be resutured.

We have tried closing with sutures in the orbicularis and without sutures in the orbicularis (Fig. 26). We find that the orbicularis sutures are not necessary unless the patient has had previous surgery or radiation, that is, we have not found that the wound separates. Even though special suturing and wound closure techniques have been described (38), we have not found them necessary and we close the wound with three 6-0 nylon sutures that we remove in one week (Figs. 26 and 27).

Tubes

There is a difference of opinion as to whether stents should be placed in the lacrimal system at DCR surgery. It would seem that if a proper epithelial lined tract can be created, there should be little chance of closure of the anastomosis, and a tube should not be necessary. Others feel that even with suturing anterior and posterior flaps that a stent tube should be inserted. Certainly, those advocating suturing of only one flap or not suturing of any flaps generally feel that a stent should be inserted so that hopefully epithelialization will occur around the stent. As mentioned above, it is our feeling that if one is hoping for epithelialization, it is theoretically best achieved by the suturing of flaps, rather than hoping that epithelialization will occur along a stent tube, which unfortunately will move somewhat with eyelid movement.

Silastic and silicone material seem to be the least reactive within the lacrimal system, but certainly complications of these tubes have been described. There may be significant surface reaction on the tube that can incite

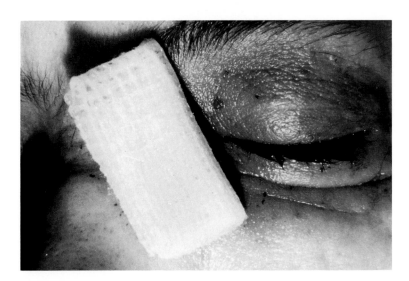

FIG. 27. After closure of the wound with three nylon sutures. A gauze impregnated with antiseptic is placed over the wound and then a patch placed on the side of the nose for 1 day. The nose is not packed unless there has been excessive bleeding.

significant inflammation (39). Inflammatory masses may occur on Silastic tubes (40). Tubes may also slit the canaliculus, and even though a slit will not usually cause a problem (41), they may potentially interfere with apposition of the puncta to the opposing lids. In fact, some authors suggest that a DCR might fail because of the intubation (42). Therefore, tubes should be inserted as stents only if absolutely necessary. However, when tubes are indicated in a DCR (especially if canalicular stenosis coexists), a stent tube may salvage the case, that is, the value of the stent outweighs the few possible complications (infections, granuloma, induced failure) (43).

Types of Intubation in DCR

Sac Stents

A tube may be placed in the nose with it passing through the anastomosis and into the sac. It is held in place by a suture through the tube and is sutured to the skin over a bolster (Fig. 28). This is usually left in place for a few weeks (44). This has the advantages of not violating the canalicular system and keeping the flaps apart. An inflatable catheter may also be used in the same manner (45). In difficult cases where one desires both a sac stent and a canalicular stent, a double stent may be used (46). These tubes are left in place for 2 to 3 weeks and are removed through the nose by cutting the suture, which is held over a bolster on the skin, and pulling the tube out the nose.

Canalicular Stents

A bicanalicular stent is the standard method of inserting a tube in the canalicular passages. The standard technique is that of the Crawford tube (47). However, in a situation where one wants to keep the canalicular passages open, it might be desirable to insert a tube that has a larger diameter than the Crawford tube. When we feel tubes are necessary, we place a Silastic tube with a 0.94-mm outer diameter through the system. There is a sleeve with a 1.57-mm inner diameter and a 2.41-mm outer diameter that holds the two free ends of the tube together. This technique is simple to perform, and the cost of the tubing is less than 10 cents. Its advantage is that the tube is fed in with a probe and there is no need to pull metal tubes through the system as one has to do with Crawford tubes.

Indications for canalicular tubing in a straightforward DCR would be:

1. where it is impossible to get 5 mm of clearance around the common internal punctum
2. where there is a major problem with the suturing of flaps
3. where there is a problem at the common canalicular level with the common canalicular being edematous or with an unexpected membrane that must be excised
4. in a situation where there is a tiny sac and large flaps can not be obtained.

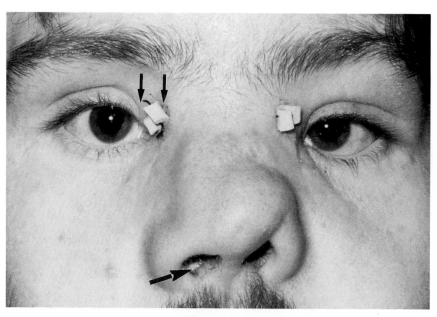

FIG. 28. Patient with a sac tube. The tube is seen within the nose (*arrow*) and passes through the DCR opening to the fundus of the sac. It is held in place by a suture placed through the top of the tube and going through the skin held in place over a rubber bolster (*two arrows*). (From Hurwitz et al., ref. 85, with permission.)

Insertion Technique (Fig. 29)

About 3 mm from each end of the smaller Silastic tube, an oblique cut is made halfway through the tube's diameter. A #0 lacrimal probe is fit snugly into this cut and inserted 2 mm into the lumen toward the end of the tube. After suturing the posterior flaps of sac and nasal mucosa, the inferior punctum is dilated and the tubing with the probe positioned inside the lumen is carefully passed into the punctum through the canaliculus until it is visualized as it passes through the common internal punctum. The tube is held with an artery forceps, the probe pulled back through the punctum, and the end tag easily pulled off. The other end is similarly passed through the superior punctum and canaliculus. Then a 1- to 1.5-cm length of larger Silastic tube is cut as a sleeve and stretched over the jaws of the artery forceps. The two ends of the smaller tubing are passed directly through the larger tube. Then the sleeve is adjusted around the smaller tube close to the common internal punctum. The eyelids are held apart so that the tube is not stretching the canaliculus and the larger sleeve within the nose is close to the common internal punctum. If the eyelids have to be stretched apart to visualize the tube, it is probably too tight and the sleeve should be loosened. The two free ends of the canalicular tubing are tied together so

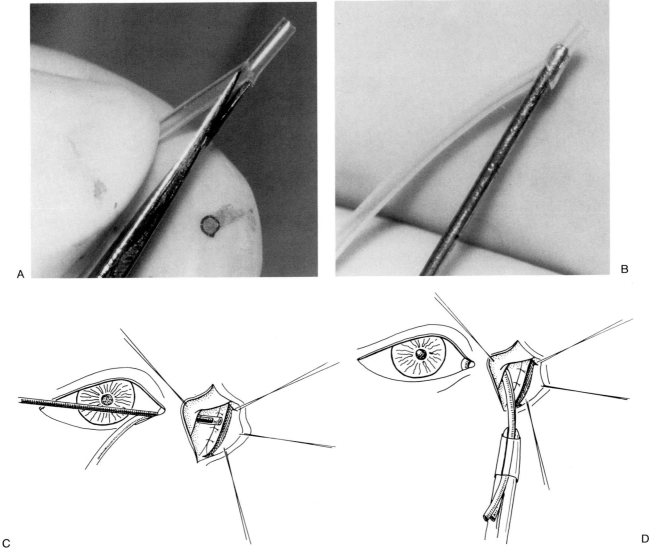

FIG. 29. A: A small Silastic tube is cut partial thickness with scissors. **B:** A #0 Bowman's probe is placed into the tube through the cut with 1 mm of tube distal to the end of the probe. **C:** Artist's diagram showing the tube inserted through the lower punctum and canaliculus into the sac. The other end of the tube is similarly inserted through the upper canaliculus and into the sac. **D:** The tubes are drawn through the DCR opening and a larger tube placed around the arms of a snap, which are separated so that the free ends of the smaller tube go through it.

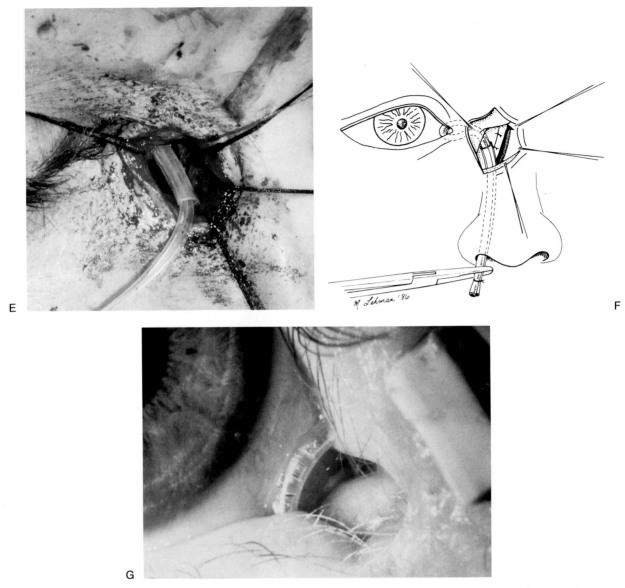

E

F

G

FIG. 29. (*Continued.*) **E:** The sleeve is passed up the nose to sit close to the common canaliculus and separate the anterior and posterior flaps. The tension of the tube at the inner canthus must be checked to ensure that the larger tube is not too closely approximated to the common canaliculus for fear of slitting the punctum. **F:** The two free ends of the tube are pulled into the nose and outside the nostril after a 4-0 black silk suture is placed around the free ends of the tube. The tube is cut and allowed to retract within the external naris so it is not visible. (Courtesy of Ms. Maria Lehman, Toronto, Canada.) **G:** Appearance of tube sitting loosely at the inner canthus, not pulling on the lids when the eyelids are separated. (Figs. A–F from Archer and Hurwitz, ref. 86, with permission. Fig. G from Hurwitz et al., ref. 85, with permission.)

that they rest about 5 mm from the external naris and can be visualized easily when it is time to remove them. We usually leave these tubes in place for approximately 2 months if they are needed in conjunction with a DCR. If the tubes are tied too tightly, the tubes may migrate in along the canaliculi and form a slit. As well, there may be "symblepharon" formation between the two puncta because of inflammatory reactions related to the tubes if the tubes are too tight (48). The sleeve on the tube is useful because it tends to hold the anterior flaps well away

from the posterior flaps, as well as being a canalicular stent. There is also with any Silastic bicanalicular intubation the potential problem of the inner canthal loop coming out into the palpebral aperture (49). The sleeve tends to eliminate this complication. On removal, the tube is cut at the inner canthus when one is sure that the nasal end is visible. If the nasal end is not visible, the patient is asked to blow the nose forcibly so that the end of the tube can be seen. It is difficult to extract the tube if one cannot see it in the nose. If it is not possible to see the tube in the nose after blowing of the nose, the patient is sent away to use some Naphazoline nasal spray approximately four times a day for 4 days, and then brought back to remove the tube. We have not had a problem seeing and removing the tube when the nose has been decongested. It is not sufficient to cut the tube at the inner canthus and have the patient blow the nose because the tube will often not come out. We do not like the idea of telling a patient we are going to remove the tube and then not being able to find the tube to remove it. This certainly can cause some consternation for the patient. When a tube is in place we tell the patient that he may have some tearing. The tube is meant only to hold the passage open and not to drain the tears. Whether the patient tears or not with a tube in place is not a yardstick as to whether the DCR will work or not. One can only tell whether the DCR will work once the tube comes out. There may be some percolation of tears around the tube and tearing symptoms will be minimized. We do like eventually to remove the tubes but there are some patients who like having the tubes in and do not have any tearing or reactions from the tubes, so one can make an argument for leaving these tubes in for the long term (50). However, leaving the Silastic tubes in long term is the exception rather than the rule.

Other forms of "stents" have been described that have been used in the nose to hold the passages open and to prevent adhesions between the lateral wall of the nose and the septum. One may insert a stent in the nose to decrease symblepharon formation between the septum and the lateral wall of the nose. The philosophy of keeping the lateral wall tissues away from the septum is indeed a good one, and one must try to avoid violating the septal mucosa, which would increase the chances of symblepharon formation during the DCR. Vegh (51) used sodium hyaluronate to act as a space stabilizer and bleeding inhibitor in DCR surgery. The Healon would also decrease the chances of synechia formation between the lateral wall of the nose and the septum, and would also help to keep the DCR open. Leone suggested using Gelfoam-thrombin packs as a DCR stent (52). This would be useful as a stent in keeping the lateral wall of the nose and the septum apart, and keeping the anterior and posterior flaps of sac and nasal mucosa apart. It would also help with hemotasis. We have not used this technique and we prefer, if possible, not to leave a volume of nonvital material in the surgical site because there is the possibility of inflammation and a subsequent risk of infection (53). There are some excellent agents to facilitate clotting such as oxidized regenerated cellulose (Surgicel), thrombin (Thrombostat), and an absorbable gelatin sponge (Gelfoam). Even though all these agents may be used as a stent, which decreases bleeding, they are all foreign materials and they do run the risk of infection and inflammation. The same may be said of bone wax, which we rarely use to stop bleeding coming from the bone.

POSTOPERATIVE MEASURES

We do not patch the eye so that the patient can report any visual changes. We do not routinely pack the nose unless at the end of the operation there is profuse bleeding. In this scenario, we will pack the nose while the patient is on the table and use a Vaseline-soaked gauze. We prefer not to use Gelfoam at the time of the first packing because these fragments cannot be removed, and we are worried about any inflammation at the DCR site. It is extremely unusual that we will pack a DCR after the procedure. The patient is instructed to put ice on the side of the nose and not to blow the nose for 2 weeks. The blood pressure is checked postoperatively and should be maintained at the preoperative level. A vaporizer is used in the recovery room and on the ward until the patient goes home. For those patients done in the outpatient department, it is necessary for the patient to have transportation and a support network at home is mandatory. The patient is told not to take any ASA if there is any pain, but acetaminophen is fine. If there is any purulent material or a mucocele at the time of the surgery, if there has been previous trauma and surgical repair, or if there has been a sinus infection, the patient is put on 250 mg of cloxacillin every six hours for 1 week. The patient is given a prescription for some gentamicin ointment to put on the sutures once the patch comes off the next day, and to use the ointment twice a day. The patient returns in 1 week to have the sutures removed.

The patient is not irrigated on the first visit unless there are complaints of tearing. If there are complaints of tearing and the system is open, the patient is given some decongestant eyedrops to use for a few days. If the system is stenotic, we tend to place the patient on a steroid-antibiotic combination. If there is some congestion in the nose, a steroid-nasal spray is used three times a day for 2 weeks. If there are no symptoms of tearing, we do not irrigate the duct until the second or third week after the surgery. We feel that during the first week there can be some retraction of the clots with subsequent bleeding, and we do not want to instrument the system while this process might be evolving. This is why we prefer not to irrigate the system unless absolutely necessary during the first 2 to 3 weeks postoperatively. The patients are given no nasal decongestants postoperatively.

DCR IN SPECIAL SITUATIONS

Abnormal Anatomy

In those unusual situations where there is severe damage to the middle meatus due to infection, trauma, cicatrizing disease, or congenital malformation, one is often not able to perform a standard anastomosis of the sac through the bony opening to the nasal mucosa. The lacrimal surgeon must be creative so that a new functional passage can be fashioned.

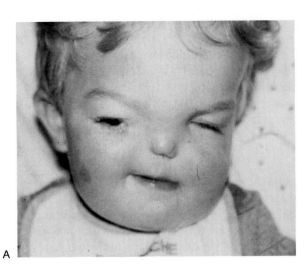
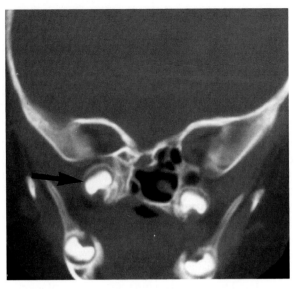

FIG. 30. A: Baby with hemifacial atrophy on the right side with a lacrimal sac mucocele. **B:** CT scan of the patient shows a deficient nasal cavity and maxillary antrum. A tooth is resting against the inferior aspect of the orbit (*arrow*). A dacryoantrorhinostomy was performed. (From Hurwitz, ref. 87, with permission.)

Patients who have had severe congenital malformations, often following reconstructive surgery (Fig. 30), those having sustained trauma and reconstructive surgery, and those having had tumors in the nose (Fig. 31), sinuses, and nasolacrimal canals may present challenges to the lacrimal surgeon to create an epithelial lined tract. Similarly, massive extirpations of basal cell carcinomas from the mid-face may destroy some of the lacrimal system (Fig. 32). In these patients it is helpful if a radiologic assessment is performed to determine how much of the system is left in order to perform a reconstruction.

When the surgeon feels that a DCR is necessary and the middle meatus is obliterated, the surgeon may simply perform a dacryocystotomy or dacryocystectomy to temporarily relieve the dacryocystitis. In an older patient this will help dramatically because these patients have decreased tear secretion even though the tear duct is blocked, and epiphora may not be a problem (Fig. 33). However, in younger patients it is desirous to drain the sac into the nose. In performing reconstructive lacrimal surgery where there is no middle meatus, the sac may be drained into the nose but sutured to the turbinate mu-

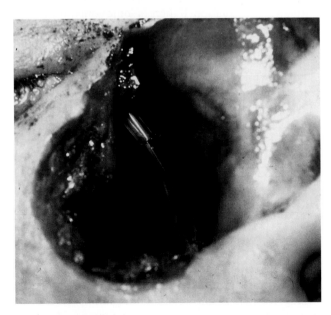

FIG. 31. Patient having had a neuroesthesioblastoma removed from the nose. The lacrimal system was reconstructed using a Silastic tube.

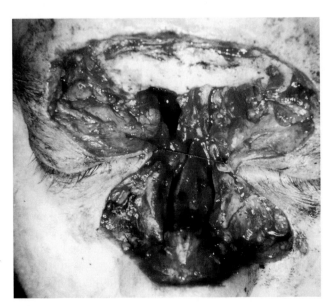

FIG. 32. Patient having had a huge resection of a midfacial basal cell carcinoma. Reconstruction was undertaken using a temporary Silastic tube bilaterally.

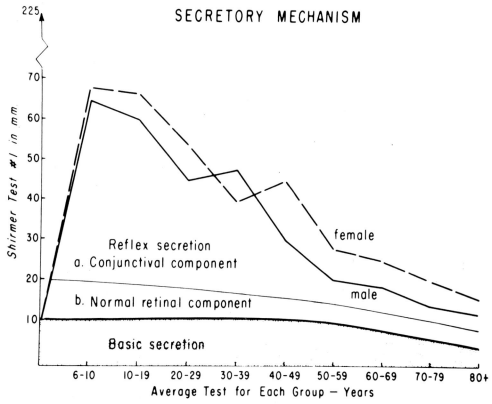

FIG. 33. Graph to show that the secretion of tears decreases as one gets older. The tear secretion at age 80 years is approximately 20% what it is at age 20 years. (From Jones and Wobig, ref. 88, with permission.)

cosa to create a posterior epithelial lined flap. This is useful, and the success rate is usually no less than that with a standard DCR. However, if there is no middle meatus present at all, the surgeon may anastomose the sac into the sinuses, usually the antrum (or the ethmoids), but it is also necessary to drain the sinuses into the nose to produce an epithelial lined tract. Merely to drain the sac into the ethmoids (dacryoethmoidostomy) usually will not eliminate the tearing but only give the patient an ethmoidal mucocele in many cases (54). The frontal sinus mucosa can probably be used in the same fashion if necessary. We have had one situation where an opening had to be made through the septum into the nasal cavity on the other side. If one is to do this, one must be careful while going through the septum so that the perpendicular plate of the ethmoid is not unduly mobilized. If it is, there is a potential of damaging the cribriform plate with a resulting CSF leak. In these difficult cases, it is probably useful to insert an indwelling temporary stent tube to keep the passages open while healing is taking place.

If there is absolutely nothing to suture the sac to, a sac marsupialization of one or both flaps may be the only recourse.

We have performed dacryocystroantrorhinostomies in patients who have had their middle meatus passages obliterated by osteopetrosis, nasal pemphigoid, severe trauma, congenital hypoplasia of the mid-face and max-

illary antra, Crouzon's disease, and following extensive surgical excisions of a significant portion of the mid-face.

Lacrimal Sac Diverticula and Cyst

When the sac is open, one may find that there is a large diverticulum or cyst that is full of pus and/or stones. In this situation, an incision may be made over the sac on the lateral aspect of the sac and the diverticulum can be excised. The DCR is then performed to drain the sac. We do not insert tubes merely because a diverticulum has been present. If an orbital cyst is present and it is of lacrimal sac origin, we prefer to approach the cyst through a lower lid crease incision to remove the cyst. If the sac is blocked one can do a DCR, but we prefer to do this through a separate skin incision via our standard DCR approach. We have tried to do perform a DCR through a lower lid crease incision, but we have not been happy with the exposure.

Wegener's Granulomatosis

In patients who have a history of Wegener's granulomatosis, or this condition is expected because of the appearance of the mucosa, a DCR in these patients may be a real challenge. The antineutrophil cytoplasmic antibodies (ANCA) test is extremely useful in making the diagnosis (55). We prefer to perform a DCR on these patients with blocked sacs, rather than a dacryocystectomy. Many of these patients are in the younger age group and although a dacryocystectomy may temporarily remove the infected debris in the sac, there is certainly the possibility of recurrence and the expectation that the patient would complain of a watery eye. We have not been impressed with wound necrosis postoperatively. It is mandatory in these patients that the orbicularis be tightly closed overlying the anterior flaps, and that the skin be closed with a suture such as silk that will cause some reaction. We have not had a problem with the wound not healing if these steps are taken. It is useful that if these patients are not on immunosuppressives, one could institute therapy before the DCR and keep the patients immunosuppressed for a while postoperatively.

Sarcoidosis

If sarcoidosis is suspected or if the diagnosis has been made preoperatively, we usually do our standard DCR. However, if there is any swelling of the mucosa, we will put in a temporary stent to keep the mucosal flaps away from each other. We will often treat these patients with steroids postoperatively. A confirmatory sac biopsy is useful in these patients.

COMPLICATIONS OF DCR SURGERY

POST-DCR Hemorrhage

Hemorrhage after DCR surgery may be divided into three groups: (a) intraoperative, (b) immediate, and (c) delayed.

1. The *intraoperative* bleeding may be controlled with a Vaseline gauze pack at the end of the case. If the patient has left for the recovery room and begins to bleed, the blood pressure must be checked and the level of excitation of the patient assessed. Often the bleeding can be stopped conservatively by giving the patient some sedation (antihistamines) systemically, or if the blood pressure is high, some antihypertensive medication. Local measures such as ice and pinching the nose usually will control the bleeding.

2. *Immediate.* This would be within the first 24 hours while the patient is either an inpatient or outpatient. In these situations, the patient might return to the ward having had no excessive bleeding at the time of surgery or in the recovery room and start to bleed. This may be a consequence of the blood pressure, which had been low during the procedure, returning to normal levels, and bleeding occurring through friable vessels. This would seem to be more of a potential for patients who had been operated on under hypotensive anesthesia. We do not feel that to do a DCR a patient needs hypotensive anesthesia, and we prefer if possible to keep the blood pressure during surgery at the patient's normal preoperative level. The exception to this might be if a difficult canalicular dissection had to be performed, and maximum visualization (with less bleeding) was indicated.

3. *Delayed.* This occurs when the patient has left the hospital, either as an inpatient or outpatient, and has done well for the first few days postoperatively, and between days 4 and 7 postoperatively has epistaxis. This is usually due to clot retraction, which is similar to a secondary intraocular bleed following a hyphema. The patient's blood pressure must be checked and the blood pressure controlled. The patient is treated with ice and usually nasal packing is indicated. We prefer if the nose is packed to place the patient on oral antibiotics, and if the patient is to be admitted, on intravenous antibiotics. It is important that the pack not be placed too high because there is the possibility of a CSF leak. There is also the potential, if the pack is too tight, for damaging the mucosa (56). Vaseline gauze packing is our choice if nasal packing is to be performed. We prefer to pack both sides even if bleeding is only on one side so that the septum will not shift and pressure will be put in the appropriate location. The bleeding is usually due to a friable blood vessel on the nasal mucosa. Occasionally it will come from a turbinate or from the nasal septum, which has been traumatized. The patient should be checked for a bleeding diathesis. If the packing can control the bleeding, it should be left in for 48 hours. It is up to the surgeon whether the patient needs to be hospitalized or not. The patient will often report a dramatic loss of blood, but usually it is not quite as much as it would appear to the patient to have been. The hematocrit should be checked and the hemoglobin should be assessed 24 hours following the bleed. The hematocrit drops initially and the hemoglobin does not drop for some time afterward. Occasionally, in a recalcitrant bleed that does not stop with Vaseline gauze, we will use a Gelfoam-thrombin pack, but we are concerned about this material staying in the area of the DCR opening for a period of time. Fortunately, most nose bleeds will stop with a Vaseline gauze pack. If this does not stop the bleeding, then we prefer to use embolization of the internal maxillary artery. This is performed by an interventional radiologist, and in treating epistaxis, is usually quite successful (57,58).

In the most recalcitrant cases of delayed postoperative bleeding, the patient has to return to the operating room, and one might tie off the anterior ethmoidal artery. We have had only one situation in which we found this had to be done, and the ligation of the artery did not stop the nose bleeding. The epistaxis was ultimately stopped by embolization. The patient may have to be transfused if there is a massive acute or sustained blood loss. However, this is unusual.

The inciting cause of the bleeding is problematic. It might be due to ASA intake (although the patients have all been told to stop ASA), increased blood pressure, dryness of the nose, or any sort of activity that may have increased the blood pressure temporarily. We have had two patients with nose bleeds who were picking at the Silastic tubing within the nose to try and pull it out while they were sleeping, and this produced in each patient a massive nose bleed.

Performing the DCR under local anesthesia seems to decrease the amount of bleeding during the surgery in comparison to the amount of bleeding one has with general anesthesia, but in our experience the incidence of postoperative bleeding is not decreased.

Postoperatively, bleeding has been one reason that many surgeons are nervous about doing DCRs as outpatients. Dresner et al. (59) had some patients who had to be readmitted following hemorrhage. In our experience, any patients who have had bleeding have all been delayed, occurring after 4 days following the operation. We have not had to readmit any of our outpatient DCR patients during the first 4 days. This would suggest that even having performed inpatient DCR surgery on these patients would not have had them in hospital when the delayed bleeding occurred, because we keep our inpatients in the hospital for only 1 day following the surgery. We agree with Seiff (60), who feels that the epistaxis, while at home, could be due to the increased activity level of an outpatient. Certainly, all outpatients (inpatients as well) should be told that they should "take it easy" for at least 1 (and possibly 2) week postoperatively.

Orbital Emphysema

The patients are told not to blow the nose for at least 2 weeks following surgery. Because of the opening into the ethmoidal air cells in most patients, there may be, on forced nose blowing, some passage of air under the lids and into the preseptal orbital space. It is extremely unusual to develop air postseptally from a DCR. As well, subcutaneous emphysema of the eyelids may occur if manual ventilation was necessary after extubation (61). Should orbital emphysema become a vision-threatening problem from postseptal air (62), a needle may be placed into the air pocket and the air withdrawn (63). Orbital emphysema looks alarming, but we have not had a situation in which it caused any trouble.

Orbital Hemorrhage

Orbital hemorrhage may occur during DCR and is a vision-threatening occurrence (64). Orbital hemorrhage during a DCR may result from excision of anterior ethmoidal air cells with an abnormal branching of the anterior ethmoidal artery. Indeed, the branches of the ante-

rior ethmoidal artery might be quite variable. The anterior ethmoidal artery is a branch of the ophthalmic artery and leaves the orbit through the anterior ethmoidal canal. It supplies the medial and anterior ethmoidal air cells and frontal sinus. It then enters the cranium and dips down the side of the crista galli. It enters the nasal cavity and emerges on the dorsum of the nose between the nasal bone and the lateral cartilage of the nose. The anterior ethmoidal artery may be thought of to have four courses: an intraorbital course, an intraethmoidal course, an intracranial course, and an intranasal course. It is possible that when the anterior ethmoidal air cells are removed or if there is traction on branches of the vessel, the vessel may be torn and there may be retraction of the proximal stump into the orbit, resulting in orbital bleeding. Orbital bleeding is diagnosed by increased retropulsion of the globe, proptosis, and progressive ecchymosis. If the orbital septum is lax, the blood may pass into the lids, but if the orbital septum is tight, there may be a rapid build-up of pressure, which may be vision-threatening.

As well, one may hemorrhage from incising the sac too far laterally and involving the orbital fat on the lateral side of the sac. The sac and the surgical site should be examined to see if there is any bleeding artery, and if there is it should be cauterized. The treatment would be to explore the wound, but in the two patients who we have had that did not settle, we performed a superomedial orbitotomy through the upper lid crease to get good access to the orbital fat and the medial wall periorbita (Fig. 34). In each case we inserted a drain, and the patients had no postoperative consequences. One could have performed a canthotomy and cantholysis, but we feel that it is better to perform a medial orbitotomy through the upper lid crease to give access to the surgical site. The use of acetazolamide, mannitol, or timolol may be useful. In the worst scenario with relentless proptosis, a bony orbital decompression might have to be considered. One could also attempt to tie off the anterior ethmoidal artery. We recommend that during the DCR as a routine, from time to time, the globe be retropulsed just to ensure that the orbital pressure is normal.

CSF Leakage

It is possible that during removal of the bone, in the fabrication of an osteotomy, one may cause damage to the cribriform plate. The usual cause, should it occur, would be due to a torsional force on the bone with a spiral fracture going up to the cribriform plate. There are fine nerve endings of the olfactory nerve that come through the cribriform plate and, if this is damaged, there may be a CSF leak. The level to which the cribriform plate dips down medially is variable (Fig. 35), and if one does not excise bone at the top of the osteotomy too far superoposteriorly or superoanteriorly, it is unlikely that

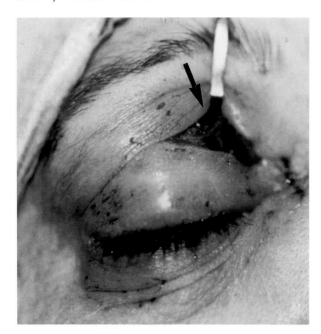

FIG. 34. Orbital hemorrhage during DCR surgery. The source of bleeding could not be found during the procedure, and with advancing proptosis, a superomedial lid crease incision was made (*arrow*) down through the orbital septum into the orbital fat and blood was evacuated. The patient did not lose any vision, and the DCR was successful. (From Hurwitz et al., ref. 64, with permission.)

one will get into the area of the cribriform plate directly. It is important to make sure that one does not put an instrument too high up into the roof of the nose, a maneuver that is not necessary. CSF leak is diagnosed by what has been described as "a double ring sign" (65). This sign is a determination of the glucose concentration of the serosanguinous fluid dripping into the operative site. CSF contains a 70% concentration of glucose as compared to the blood serum. If a drop of the serosanguinous fluid is placed on a surgical drape, there will be a large ring of CSF material around a smaller ring of blood. This is because the CSF has little protein and there is better capillarity and increased spreading of the fluid than with blood. The double ring sign may have a false positive so its appearance is not pathognomonic of a CSF leak.

If one suspects a CSF leak, the area should be packed. It is difficult to suture in this area. One can use mucous membrane, fascia lata, temporalis fascia, or muscle. The most accessible tissue seems to be local muscle, and should this happen, we advise packing the roof of the nose where the suspected CSF leak is occurring with either a flap or, failing that, a graft of muscle. Postoperatively the patient should be treated with antibiotics, the head of the bed elevated, and definitely refrain from blowing the nose. The patient should be followed for any signs of meningeal irritation, which may suggest that neurosurgical investigation is appropriate. Meningitis

following DCR surgery is rare, but may occur perhaps related to a CSF leak (66). Investigation to localize the CSF leak is advised if neurosurgical intervention is contemplated.

Infection

We do not routinely use prophylactic oral antibiotics unless there has been mucus within the sac. Despite this, postoperative infections may occur. If the DCR is patent, these infections are usually insignificant because the potential source of infection, that is the sac, would be

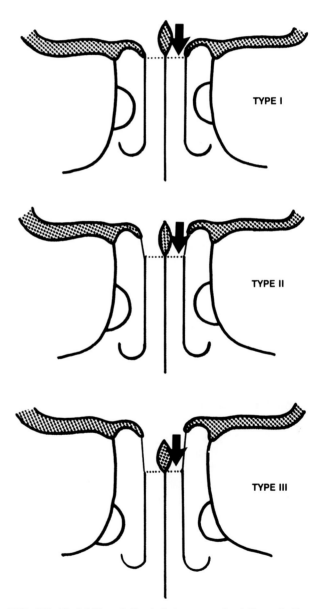

FIG. 35. Variability of the inferior aspect of the cribriform plate. Damage to the cribriform plate may cause a CSF leak and may leave the patient with a defect in the sensation of smell. (From Stammberger and Hawke, ref. 82, with permission.)

drained (directly into the nose). We have not had a postoperative wound infection, even with florid dacryocystitis at the time of surgery, that had to be treated with intravenous antibiotics.

However, soft tissue infection in the area of the wound occurs in a certain percentage of patients undergoing lacrimal surgery. Welham and Rose (67) suggest that soft tissue infection occurs in approximately 8% of patients after open lacrimal surgery. They feel that the reduction in infections can be decreased fivefold with the routine administration of postoperative antibiotics. The infections that we have experienced postoperatively have been mainly wound infections. These were much more frequent when we were putting in subcutaneous sutures. The treatment of a local wound infection is to remove the sutures and treat with hot compresses and antibiotic ointment. This usually produces prompt resolution. If the patient has not been on oral antibiotics postoperatively, we use oral antibiotics to help treat the infection. After the wound has closed and the purulent material has drained, we advise massage of the scar with garamycin ointment. We have not been impressed with unsightly scars even following infections, and they are not significantly different from the scars of those DCR patients who have not had infections postoperatively.

Problems with Silastic Tubes

Bicanalicular Silastic stent tubes may migrate in front of the cornea if no sleeve is put on them. One may grasp the tube within the nose and put a sleeve up the nose around the free ends. Alternatively, one may put a suture around the tube and hold the suture onto the side of nose with a piece of tape to hold the tube in place. Failing that, one may simply tape the loop of the tube on the side of the nose just medial to the medial canthus so that the stent will at least be in place for some period of time (Fig. 36). The tube may migrate inward and cause a slit of the canaliculus which, if the DCR is open, does not seem to cause a problem (42). If infection occurs around the tube, a dacryocystitis may develop, but this is rare. There may be crust around the tube that produces a foul discharge. Should this happen, one may toilet the nose to keep it moist and clean.

Obstruction of the Nasofrontal Duct

The opening of the duct into the middle meatus is close to the posterior opening of the DCR osteotomy. Extensive middle turbinate resection, cautery, or torsion of the rongeurs may cause damage to the duct. Frontal sinusitis may develop. There will be frontal pain, tenderness to palpation over the frontal sinus, and perhaps later on, development of a frontal mucocele (we have not seen this). The sinusitis may be confirmed on x-ray, demonstrating clouding of the frontal sinus. Antibiotics and nasal decongestants usually open the duct and allow for drainage and resolution of symptoms. Should a frontal sinus mucocele develop, sinus surgery might be necessary.

Scar Disfigurement

A hypertrophic scar occasionally develops, but this is a rare complication (Fig. 37). It is much less usual in our experience when one does not suture the subcutaneous tissues and merely sutures the skin. Routinely we have the patient massage the scar for at least 3 months postoperatively, and this tends to flatten the scar and decrease

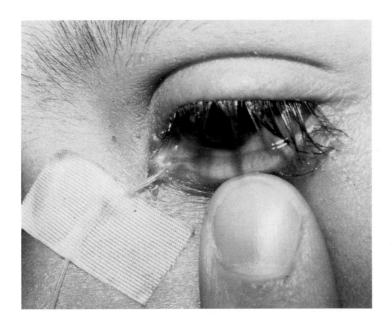

FIG. 36. A partially extruded tube. This could not be repositioned in the nose and was held with tape on the face for the duration of time that it was felt that the tube should be in place.

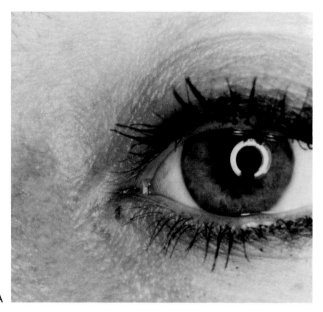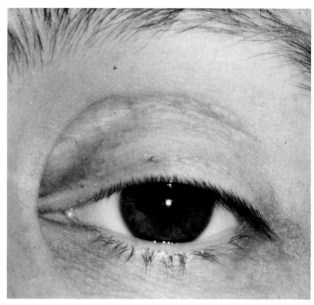

A   B

FIG. 37. A: A normal scar 3 months following DCR. **B:** A hypertrophic scar developing following a left DCR in a patient with blepharochalasis syndrome.

the contraction, and the scar usually blends into the side of the nose. Any discomfort in wearing eyeglasses because of the scar is quickly alleviated. A thick hypertrophic scar (keloid) may be treated with intralesional steroid injection of triamcinolone. However, we have had to do this very rarely. A pseudoepicanthic fold can be treated by a V-Y plasty to lengthen the scar (Fig. 38). Even after a wound infection, the scar should gradually fade (Fig. 39). We tend to massage the scar for a full year following surgery before considering scar revision.

Persistent Epiphora

Persistent epiphora may be due to DCR failure caused by complete obstruction, an incompletely anastomosed sac, or a lacrimal pump dysfunction.

Persistent Obstruction

Persistent obstruction following a DCR may be due to a closure of the anastomosis between the sac and the nasal mucosa, an obstruction of the common canaliculus, or a diversion of the sac into the ethmoids (68). It has been our experience and the experience of others that

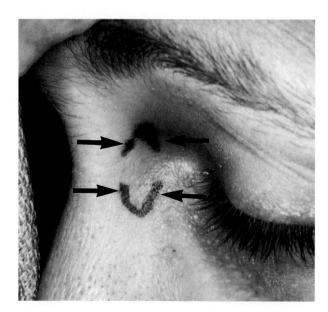

FIG. 38. Double V-Y plasty for revision of a pseudoepicanthic fold from a DCR scar. Two V incisions are undermined, and horizontal sutures at position of *arrows* decrease length of scar.

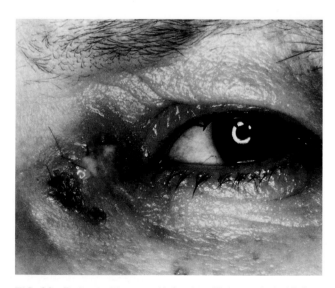

FIG. 39. Patient with wound infection. The scar faded following local antibiotics and time.

when we reoperate on DCRs that others have performed, the osteotomy is either extremely small or is not placed in the right position to effectively produce a patent epithelial lined tract. The closure of the DCR opening could be due to a number of factors. Granulation tissue growing into the opening from unanastomosed flaps could cause an obstruction, and we would agree with the conclusion of Welham and Henderson that "it can thus be seen that the principle of an accurately sutured mucosal anastomosis gives highly satisfactory results" (68).

We feel that at surgery a large osteotomy should be produced because the larger the bony osteotomy, the further separated one can place the anterior flaps from the posterior flaps. Another cause of closure may be cicatrization between the anterior flaps and the posterior flaps, presumably because the anterior flaps were not "domed up" over the posterior flaps, and that the posterior flaps were elevated and were not lying flat. One would have to assume that a large rhinostomy increases the separation of the anterior flaps from the posterior flaps. With these two principles in mind, we must consider the study done by Linberg et al. (69). These authors felt that no matter how big the DCR bony opening, the mucosal intranasal soft tissue opening closes to approximately 2 mm in diameter. They performed their study suturing only anterior flaps, but felt that even when posterior flaps were sutured as well, there was no difference. This comes as a surprise to us because we always felt, from the dacryocystogram (DCG) appearances of normal DCRs, that if most (if not all of the sac) had been anastomosed to the nasal mucosa, that the anastomosis would certainly be larger than 2 mm. We are now embarking on a study whereby we are marking the sac-nasal mucosal flaps so we can see where the anastomoses on the lateral wall actually occur. We will be able to study this with an endoscope and determine the relationship between the common internal punctal opening and the site of the anastomosed flaps. It has been our experience that it is extremely difficult to determine, after a DCR, where the anastomotic site is located because in a successful DCR the sac becomes incorporated into the side of the nose. Despite their findings, Linberg et al. suggest "while it would be foolish to suggest abandoning surgical principles that have provided a high success rate over many years, our understanding of the factors that contribute to the success rate may change" (69). It would seem, nevertheless, that one must try to keep the anterior flaps as far away from the posterior flaps in order to give as large a soft tissue opening as possible.

Bone Regrowth

It seems unlikely that failure of a DCR is due to regrowth of bone. Welham and Henderson felt that regrowth of bone was extremely unusual clinically (68).

There may be some remodeling of the bone around the DCR opening, but there is no active regrowth of bone (70). Patients who have abnormal bone in the middle meatus may have failure due to osseous causes such as an ethmoidal osteoma (71), osteopetrosis (72), Paget's disease (73), etc.

Failure Due to Tubes

It has been postulated that nasolacrimal tubes statistically increase the rate of DCR failures (43). Other materials in the nose such as packing, Gelfoam, and other foreign bodies also may be associated with increased inflammation and potential for failure.

Drainage into Ethmoids

A sac that is never anastomosed into the nose, but into the ethmoids, will not drain. Similarly, if the sac is anastomosed into the antrum, it will not drain and the antrum will fill up with fluid. If one is to drain the sac into a sinus, a rhinostomy must also be made from the involved sinus.

Common Canalicular Blockage

This may be due to an inadvertent common canaliculus block that was not diagnosed preoperatively, in which case the patient should have had either a DCR with common internal punctoplasty or a canaliculodacryocystorhinostomy (74).

The common canaliculus also may be blocked by the lacrimal surgery from surgical manipulation of the common canaliculus causing edema, sutures being put through the common internal punctum, or kinking and/or traction on the common canaliculus as the flaps are being sutured. If edema of the common canaliculus is diagnosed at the time of surgery, we suggest a bicanalicular Silastic intubation.

Lacrimal Pump Dysfunction

A lacrimal pump dysfunction, characterized by a lax lid and/or a punctal eversion, may have been present preoperatively and not diagnosed. Either this existed in conjunction with the blocked tear duct or this was the sole reason for the epiphora.

One should avoid damage to the orbicularis at the time of surgery for fear of interfering with the lacrimal pump and the lid-globe apposition. If a lacrimal pump dysfunction and/or everted punctum is the cause of postoperative tearing in a patient with a system that is 100% anatomically normal, the patient may be treated with upward massaging of the lid for a period of time. If this does not help, the everted punctum may be treated with punctal inversion, or the lax lid may be treated with a lid-tightening procedure.

MANAGEMENT OF POSTOPERATIVE TEARING

One must determine whether the system is completely or incompletely blocked. The system may be patent to syringing but there may be a stenosis within the DCR, either at the anastomotic site or at the common canaliculus.

The DCG will help to determine whether there is a large sac, a small sac, or no sac. One must carefully examine the nose to determine if there is granuloma formation or scarring at the mucosal level in the nose.

Endoscopic visualization of the nasal mucosa at the DCR site is helpful. Turbinate hypertrophy and nasal septal deviation can be diagnosed and may be the cause of failed DCRs (75). Scarring at the mucosal level and granuloma formation may be diagnosed by an endoscope and treated by simple intranasal maneuvers. One may also be able to diagnose other nasal conditions that have led to the failure, such as sarcoidosis (76). There is also the possibility of regeneration of lacrimal sac mucosa (77). This is characteristically a possibility after dacryocystectomy, but could occur after a DCR and account for some of the "granulation tissue" that is seen endoscopically.

If there is stenosis of a DCR, we prefer to do a probing in the office and see if we can pass a probe through into the nose. As the probe passes through into the nose, we move the probe in all directions to enlarge the opening. This may have to be repeated once or twice afterward, but most of our patients with seemingly unsuccessful lacrimal surgery can be rehabilitated in this fashion. It is not necessary in most cases to inject any local anesthesia to perform this maneuver. In patients who are quite sensitive, we have injected some Xylocaine with epinephrine by passing a #30 needle along the inside of a cannula and injecting at the level of the blockage. One can then probe through nicely. We initially do this without putting in any stents. Should this not work, we take the patient to the operating room and under local anesthesia pass a probe through into the nose in the same way. We use the technique that was described by Jones and Wobig (78). One should decongest the nose with cocaine preoperatively. The probe is passed into the nose to tent up the obstructed tissue. Then a Freer elevator placed intranasally is used to make a vertical cut through the mucosa down to the bone just in front of the probe. Then a small Kerrison punch can be used to remove the tissue. One can move the probe around and determine just how much of an opening has been made. We have not had to pack the nose after this maneuver except in the exceptional case. We usually pass a bicanalicular Silastic stent

tube through the small opening that we made in an attempt to hold the passage open, and leave this in place for 3 months. If this procedure does not work, the DCG that has been previously obtained is useful. If the patient has a large sac (especially if a mucocele is present), the previous procedure described may not open up the sac enough, and a repeat DCR is indicated. We approach the repeat DCR the same as we do the initial DCR and make anterior and posterior flaps (79), and we usually use a temporary bicanalicular Silastic intubation.

If a small sac or no sac exists, we find that it is difficult to locate the obstruction from an approach through the old DCR opening. We therefore elect to do a modified canaliculodacryocystorhinostomy (74). Probes are placed in the canalicular system and dissection is carried down on the probes laterally. When the probes have been identified, the scar tissue between the probes in the patent residual passages and the nasal mucosa is removed. New anterior flaps can always be obtained by increasing the osteotomy anteriorly, to give fresh anterior flaps. Posterior flaps occasionally can be obtained, but the posterior sac flap may have to be imbricated posteriorly. We attempt not to amputate the posterior flaps if at all possible, so that we can get the new tract lined both with epithelium anteriorly and posteriorly. We then are able to suture the anterior and posterior flaps of the residual sac or common canalicular tissue directly to the nasal mucosa. We insert a bicanalicular Silastic stent tube usually for 4 to 6 months.

In a failed DCR, we do not feel that one should insert a Jones bypass tube unless one has tried at least one reoperation and has not been successful (80). If canalicular obstruction exists, we will insert a Jones bypass tube more readily after a failed canaliculodacryocystorhinostomy than after a failed straightforward DCR.

The technique of balloon catheter dilatation of the soft tissue obstruction following probing is an intriguing one (81). It would seem that without open surgery and without endoscopic nasal surgery, a combination of the probing followed by dilatation of the stricture, and postoperative tubes, would give one the best chance of a nonsurgical cure of a seemingly failed DCR.

If the system is patent to syringing, the DCG may show that indeed there is a stenosis either at the junction of the sac and the nasal mucosa or at the common canaliculus-sac junction. These incomplete DCR obstructions should be treated the same as a complete obstruction as mentioned above.

A DCG may demonstrate failure due to a "sump syndrome" (79). An incompletely anastomosed sac may result in residual tearing despite the system being patent to syringing. This may be like a "retention-overflow" situation that one gets in an atonic bladder. The sump may harbor bacteria or stones. It is usually caused by inadequate bone removal, especially down to the junction of the nasolacrimal sac and the duct. It may also be due to regeneration of the sac mucosa as described by Rizk (77). The treatment is revision of the DCR to increase the size of the osteotomy and fashion larger flaps.

REFERENCES

1. Hurwitz JJ, Rutherford S. Computerized survey of lacrimal surgery patients. *Ophthalmology* 1986;93:14.
2. Veirs ER. In: Veirs ER, ed. Lacrimal disorders: diagnosis and treatment. St. Louis: CV Mosby; 1976.
3. Steinkogler FJ, Huber E, Kuchar D. Lacrimal balloon dilation. *Orbit* 1994;13:173–177
4. Callahan MA, Callahan A. Ophthalmic plastic and orbital surgery. In: Callahan MA, Callahan A, eds. *The lacrimal system.* Birmingham, AL: Aesculapius; 1979.
5. Iliff CE, Iliff WJ, Iliff NT. Lacrimal tract surgery. In: Iliff CE, Iliff WJ, Iliff NT, eds. *Oculoplastic surgery.* Philadelphia: WB Saunders; 1979.
6. Gainey SP, Robertson DM, Fay W, Ilstrup D. Ocular surgery on patients receiving long-term Warfarin therapy. *Am J Ophthalmol* 1989;108:142.
7. Hurwitz JJ, Mishkin S. Bilateral simultaneous dacryocystorhinostomy. *Ophthal Plast Reconstruct Surg* 1989;5:186.
8. Wesley RE. Intranasal procedures. In: Linberg JV. *Lacrimal surgery.* New York: Churchill Livingstone; 1988.
9. Payton KB, Hebert J, Clarke KD. Assessing and treating rhinitis. *Can Med Assoc J* 1994;15:12.
10. Hurwitz JJ, Eplett CJ, Fliss D, Freeman JL. Orbital hemorrhage during dacryocystorhinostomy. *Can J Ophthalmol* 1992;27:139.
11. Mulligan NB, Ross CA, Francis IC, Moshegov CN. The Valsalva DCR bubble test: a new method of assessing lacrimal patency after DCR Surgery. *Ophthal Plast Reconstr Surg* 1994;10:121.
12. Converse JM, ed. *Reconstructive plastic surgery*, vol 1. Philadelphia: WB Saunders; 1977.
13. Edgerton MT, Langman MW, Pruzinsky T. Plastic surgery and psychotherapy in the treatment of 100 psychologically disturbed patients. *Plast Reconstr Surg* 1991;88:594.
14. Wright MR. The male aesthetic patient. *Arch Otolaryngol Head Neck Surg* 1987;113:724.
15. Pastorek NJ. Psychological and esthetic considerations in outpatient facial plastic surgery. Presented at the annual meeting of the American Academy of Otolaryngology-Head and Neck Surgery. California, October 23, 1983.
16. Coley M, Markland A, Prin J. How to "say no" to patients who want surgery. *Plast Surg Nurs* 1991;2:17.
17. Katez P. The dissatisfied patient. *Plast Surg Nurs* 1991;2:13.
18. Hosal B, Hosal SA, Hurwitz JJ, Freeman JL. A rationale for the selection of nasal decongestants in lacrimal drainage surgery. *Ophthal Plast Reconstr Surg [in press]*.
19. Meyers EF. Cocaine toxicity during dacryocystorhinostomy. *Arch Ophthalmol* 1980;98:842.
20. Cruz O, Patrinely J, Reyna G, King J. Urine drug screening for cocaine after lacrimal surgery. *Am J Ophthalmol* 1991;11:703.
21. Nik NA, Hurwitz JJ, Chin Sang H. Mechanism of tearflow after dacryocystorhinostomy and Jones tube surgery. *Arch Ophthalmol* 1984;102:1643.
22. Harris GJ, Sakol PJ, Beatty RL. Relaxed skin tension line incision for dacryocystorhinostomy. *Am J Ophthalmol* 1989;108:742.
23. Pico G. Dacryocystorhinostomy. *Am J Ophthalmol* 1971;72:679.
24. Jones LT. The cure of epiphora due to canalicular disorders, trauma and surgical failures on the lacrimal passages. *Trans Am Acad Ophthalmol Otolaryngol* 1962;66:506.
25. Neuhaus RW, Baylis HI. Cerebral spinal fluid leakage after dacryocystorhinostomy. *Ophthalmology* 1983;90:1091.
26. Anderson RL. Medial canthal tendon branches out. *Arch Ophthalmol* 1977;95:2051.
27. Bartley GB. The role of the medial canthal tendon in external dacryocystorhinostomy. *Am J Ophthalmol* 1994;118:117.
28. Kurihashi K, Yamashita A. Anatomical consideration for dacryocystorhinostomy. *Ophthalmologica* 1991;203:1.
29. Callahan MA, Callahan A. The lacrimal system. In: Callahan MA, Callahan A, eds. *Ophthalmic plastic orbital surgery.* Birmingham, AL: Aesculapius; 1978.
30. Krasnov MM. Ultrasonic dacryocystorhinostomy. *Am J Ophthalmol* 1971;72:200.
31. Hurwitz JJ, Nik N. Lacrimal sac identification for dacryocystorhinostomy:The role of sodium hyaluronate. *Can J Ophthalmol* 1984;19:112.
32. Hecht SD. Internal common punctum during dacryocystorhinostomy. *Arch Ophthalmol* 1973;89:124.
33. Whitnall SE. The relations of the lacrimal fossa to the ethmoidal cells. *Ophthal Rev* 1911;30:321.
34. Jordan DR. Avoiding blood loss in out-patient dacryocystorhinostomy. *Ophthal Plast Reconstr Surg* 1991;7:261.
35. Avram D, Hurwitz JJ. Location of sinus ostia relative to the DCR opening. University of Toronto Research Day. 1986; Toronto.
36. Wesley R. Intranasal procedures. In: Linberg JV. *Lacrimal surgery.* New York: Churchill Livingstone; 1988
37. Wesley RE, Bond JB. Intranasal procedures for successful lacrimal surgery. *Ophthal Plast Reconstr Surg* 1986;2:153.
38. Sisler HA. Wound closure after lacrimal sac surgery. *Ann Ophthalmol* 1971;3:1357.
39. Ruby AJ, Lissner GS, O'Grady R. Surface reaction on silicone tubes used in the treatment of nasolacrimal drainage obstruction. *Ophthal Surg* 1991;22:745.
40. Dresner SC, Codere F, Brownstein S, Jouve P. Lacrimal drainage system inflammatory masses from retained silicone tubing. *Am J Ophthalmol* 1984;98:609.
41. Hurwitz JJ. The slit canaliculus. *Ophthal Surg* 1982;13:572.
42. Allen K, Berlin AJ. Dacryocystorhinostomy failure: association with nasolacrimal silicone intubation. *Ophthal Surg* 1989;20:486.
43. Walland MJ, Rose GE. The effect of silicone intubation on failure and infection rates after dacryocystorhinostomy. *Ophthal Surg* 1994;25:597.
44. Iliff CE. Simplified dacryocystorhinostomy. *Trans Am Acad Ophthalmol Otolaryngol* 1954;58:590.
45. Vila-Coro A, Gutierrez MA, Rodriguez-Bermejo MC, Vila-Coro A. Inflatable catheter for dacryocystorhinostomy. *Arch Ophthalmol* 1988;106:692.
46. Hurwitz JJ, Archer KF, Gruss JC. Double stent intubations in difficult post-traumatic dacryocystorhinostomy. *Ophthal Surg* 1988;19:33.
47. Kraft SP, Crawford JS. Silicone tube intubation in disorders of the lacrimal system in children. *Am J Ophthalmol* 1982;94:290.
48. Jordan D, Nerad J. An acute inflammatory reaction to silicone stents. *Ophthal Plast Reconstr Surg* 1987;3:147.
49. Burns JA, Cahill KV. Management of complications associated with Silastic tube intubation of the nasolacrimal drainage system. In: Bosniak SL, Smith BC, eds. *Advances in ophthalmic plastic and reconstructive surgery of the lacrimal system.* Elmsford, NY: Pergamon Press; 1984.
50. Veloudios A, Harvey JT, Philippon M. Long term placement of silastic nasolacrimal tubes. *Ophthal Surg* 1991;22:225.
51. Vegh M. Healon as space stablizer in dacryocystorhinostomy. *Orbit* 1989;8:133.
52. Leone CR. Gelfoam-thrombin dacryocystorhinostomy stent. *Am J Ophthalmol* 1982;94:412.
53. Hatt M. Hemostasis in oculoplastic surgery. *Orbit* 1985;4:135.
54. Goto T. Dacryocystoethmoidostomy. *Am J Ophthalmol* 1968;65:68.
55. Kalina PH, Lie JT, Campbell RJ, Garrity JA. Diagnostic value and limitations of orbital biopsy in Wegener's granulomatosis. *Ophthalmology* 1992;99:120.
56. Gonnering RS. Dacryocystorhinostomy and conjunctivo-dacryocystorhinostomy. In: Dortzbach RR, ed. *Ophthalmic plastic surgery prevention and management of complications.* New York: Raven Press; 1994.
57. Elder L, Montanara W, Terbrugge K, Willinsky R, Las Jaunias P, Charles D. Angiographic embolization for the treatment of epistaxis. A review of 108 cases. *Otolaryngol Head Neck Surg* 1994;111:44.

58. Cowen D, Terbrugge K, Hurwitz JJ. The treatment of post-DCR hemorrhage by embolization. In: Proceedings of European Society of Dacriology Toronto. Milan: Ghedini, 1994.

59. Dresner SC, Klussman KG, Meyer DR, Linberg JV. Outpatient dacryocystorhinostomy. *Ophthal Surg* 1991;22:222.

60. Seiff SR. Outpatient dacryocystorhinostomy. *Ophthal Surg* 1991;22:481.

61. Wojno PH, Walter K. Subcutaneous emphysema of the eyelids after dacryocystorhinostomy. *Am J Ophthalmol* 1993;115:671.

62. Jordan DR, White GL, Anderson RL, Phiese SM. Orbital emphysema: potentially blinding complications following orbital fracture. *Ann Emerg Med* 1988;117:853.

63. Hunts JH, Patrinely JR, Holds JB, Anderson RL. Orbital emphysema—staging and acute management. *Ophthalmology* 1994;101:960.

64. Hurwitz JJ, Eplett CJ, Fliss D, Freeman JL. Orbital hemorrhage during dacryocystorhinostomy. *Can J Ophthalmol* 1992;27:139.

65. Neuhaus RW, Baylis HI. Cerebral spinal fluid leakage after dacryocystorhinostomy. *Ophthalmology* 1983;90:1091.

66. Beiran I, Pikkel J, Gilboa M, Miller B. Meningitis as a complication of dacrycystorhinostomy. *Br J Ophthalmol* 1994;78:417–418.

67. Welham RAN, Rose GE. Soft tissue infections after open lacrimal surgery. *Ophthalmology* 1994;101:608.

68. Welham RAN, Henderson P. Failed dacryocystorhinostomy. *Trans Am Acad Ophthalmol Otolaryngol* 1974;78:824.

69. Linberg JV, Anderson RL, Bumsted RM, Barreras R. Study of intranasal osteum external dacryocystorhinostomy. *Arch Ophthalmol* 1982;100:1758.

70. Hinton P, Hurwitz JJ, Cruickshenk B. Nasolacrimal bone changes in disorders of the lacrimal drainage system. *Ophthal Surg* 1984;15:516.

71. Sternberg I, Levine MR. Ethmoidal sinus osteoma—a primary cause of nasolacrimal obstruction and dacryocystorhinostomy failure. *Ophthal Surg* 1984;15:295.

72. Orengo SE, Patrinely JR. Dacryocystorhinostomy and osteopetrosis. *Ophthal Surg* 1991;22:396.

73. Hurwitz JJ. Failed dacryocystorhinostomy in Paget's disease *Can J Ophthalmol* 1979;12:291.

74. Doucet TW, Hurwitz JJ. Canaliculodacryocystorhinostomy and the management of unsuccessful lacrimal surgery. *Arch Ophthalmol* 1982;100:619.

75. Allen KM, Berlin AJ, Levine HL. Intranasal endoscopic analysis of dacryocystorhinostomy failure. *Ophthal Plast Reconstr Surg* 1988;4:143.

76. Weingarten R, Goodman EF. Late failure of a dacryocytorhinostomy from sarcoidosis. *Ophthal Surg* 1991;12:343.

77. Rizk SNM, Dark AJ. Sac regrowth following dacryocystectomy. *Trans Ophthal Soc UK* 1967;87:695.

78. Jones LT, Wobig JL. Preoperative and postoperative management of lacrimal problems. In: Jones LT, Wobig JL, eds. *Surgery of the eyelids and lacrimal system.* Birmingham, AL: Aesculapius; 1976.

79. Welham RAN, Henderson PH. Results of dacryocystorhinostomy analysis of causes for failure. *Trans Ophthal Soc UK* 1973;94.

80. Welham RAN. Canalicular obstructions and Lester Jones tube. What to do when all else fails. *Trans Ophthal Soc UK* 1973;93:623.

81. Becker BB, Berry FD. Balloon catheter dilatation and lacrimal surgery. *Ophthal Surg* 1989;20:193.

82. Stammberger H, Hawke M. *Essentials of functional endoscopic sinus surgery.* St. Louis: CV Mosby: 1993.

83. Freeman MS. Incision planning and bosie soft tissue surgery. *Otolaryngol Clin North Am* 1990;23:865.

84. Hawke M. *Pocket atlas of diseases of the bone and paranasal sinuses.* Astra Pharmatek, 1993.

85. Hurwitz JJ, Archer K, Gruss JS. Lacrimal intubations in posttraumatic dacryocystorhinostomy. *Orbit* 1988;7:329.

86. Archer K, Hurwitz JJ. An alternative method of canalicular stent tube placement in lacrimal drainage surgery. *Ophthal Surg* 1988;19:510.

87. Hurwitz JJ. Dacryocystorhinoplasty. In: *Lacrimal system.* Milan: Ghedini, 1994.

88. Jones LT, Wobig JL. Lacrimal system. In: *Surgery of the eyelids and lacrimal system.* Birmingham: Aesculapius, 1976;65.

CHAPTER 37

Canaliculodacryocystorhinostomy

Jeffrey Jay Hurwitz

The operation of canaliculodacryocystorhinostomy was described in the British literature by Jones and Corrigan in 1959 (1).

The same term was used by Tenzel (2) to refer to a membrane overlying the common internal punctum on the inside of the sac. He recommended excising the membrane, doing a dacryocystorhinostomy (DCR), and inserting stent tubes. We will refer to this procedure as a DCR plus common internal punctoplasty (DCR-CIP). We will not use the term "canaliculodacryocystorhinostomy" in describing this procedure.

The common canaliculus is a definitive structure that we have been able to identify routinely radiologically with dacryocystography (DCG) (3). As well using microscopic anatomical analysis, Kurihashi and his coworkers have been able to identify the fact that the common canaliculus is a structure that was present on every one of their dissection specimens. Although it may vary in length and have variable projections and folds within its lumen, it did exist as a structure routinely (4). It is our feeling that the canaliculi pass into the common canaliculus before passing into the sac and any alterations in this pattern must indeed be considered as the extreme exception to the rule.

Therefore, the common canaliculus, measuring between 1.2 and 5.0 mm, is a definitive structure and can be operated on if necessary.

The term "canaliculodacryocystorhinostomy" can refer to two separate situations (Fig. 1) (Table 1):

1. obstruction within the common canaliculus (not at the mucosal junction with the sac)
2. obstruction of the individual canaliculi close to the junction of the lateral common canaliculus

J. J. Hurwitz: Oculoplastics Program, Mount Sinai Hospital; and Department of Ophthalmology, University of Toronto Faculty of Medicine, Toronto, Ontario M5S 1A8, Canada.

We will refer to the first situation as "a common canaliculo-DCR" and the second one as a "canaliculo-DCR."

COMMON CANALICULO-DCR

Indications

1. Lateral common canalicular obstruction
2. failed DCR surgery with a residual sac that is small or with no residual sac
3. following dacryocystectomy where there is no sac
4. following extrusion of a Jones tube if it is found there is sufficient patent common canaliculus for reanastomosis

Investigation of Patients for Common Canaliculo-DCR

A DCG will identify those patients who have an obstruction within the common canaliculus. These patients would be found on syringing to have total reflux through the upper canaliculus when irrigation is performed through the lower canaliculus, and would be found to have clinically a "soft stop" on probing. With a DCG, an obstruction will be found within the common canaliculus.

Technique of Common Canaliculo-DCR

A standard DCR incision is made and the orbicularis muscle and subcutaneous tissues are separated and retracted. In this procedure, it is necessary to identify the anterior limb of the medial canthal tendon and reflect the inferior half of the tendon laterally (Fig. 2). The tendon is held in place with a traction suture. Probes are then placed within the canaliculi and the level of obstruction within the common canaliculus noted (Fig. 3). We

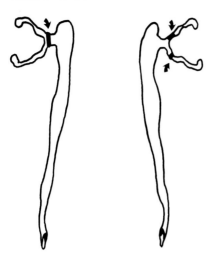

FIG. 1. Obstruction on the right side at the lateral aspect of the common canaliculus where the upper and lower canaliculi join the common canaliculus. This patient would be treated with a common canaliculo-DCR. On the left side there is an obstruction of the individual canaliculi proximal to the common canaliculus. This patient would be treated with a canaliculo-DCR. (From Doucet and Hurwitz, ref. 5, with permission.)

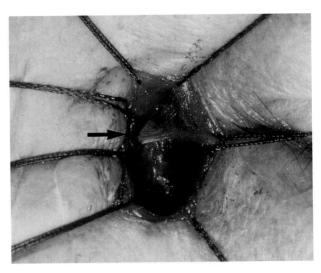

FIG. 2. The anterior limb of the medial canthal tendon (*arrow*) is cut along its lower 5 mm and a suture is put through it to reflect it laterally. (From Doucet and Hurwitz, ref. 5, with permission.)

use loupes rather than an operating microscope in performing this surgery. We feel that the operating microscope limits the mobility of the surgeon so, for the past number of years, we have used loupes when performing this procedure.

The medial canthal tendon is reflected laterally and a traction suture is used to hold the medial canthal tendon in a lateral position. We only disinsert the lower half of the medial canthal tendon. Probes are placed within the canalicular system, and using a sharp dissection with a sharpened Rollet's periosteal elevator, we cut down on the most medial aspect of the probes (Fig. 4). With a common canalicular obstruction the probes can be seen to be coming through a common lumen. Scar tissue be-

tween the obstructed common canaliculus and the lacrimal sac is then excised. A Silastic tube is then placed through each punctum and these tubes exit through the newly formed but shortened common canaliculus (Fig. 5). The tubes are then retracted laterally. Attention is then focused on the sac and a standard rhinostomy is performed. We tend to enlarge the anterior aspect of the rhinostomy slightly more in this procedure than in the standard DCR to ensure that adequate nasal mucosal flaps will be obtained. This is important because the sac is usually normal in these patients, and the sac flaps are not as big.

The sac is then opened medially. This is slightly more difficult because it is not possible to put probes into the sac because of the common canalicular obstruction. Flaps are created anteriorly and posteriorly on the me-

TABLE 1. *Management of canalicular obstruction based on site of obstruction*

Site of obstruction	Other factors	Recommended surgery
Medial common canaliculus only		DCR with common internal punctoplasty
Lateral common canaliculus only		Canaliculodacryocystorhinostomy
Lower canaliculus only, more than 8 mm from punctum	Upper canaliculus patent	DCR
	Upper canaliculus obstructed	Canaliculodacryocystorhinostomy
Lower canaliculus only, less than 8 mm from punctum	Upper canaliculus patent	DCR
	Upper canaliculus obstructed	Conjunctivodacryocystorhinostomy
Upper canaliculus only, more than 8 mm from punctum	Lower canaliculus patent	Surgery usually not needed
	Lower canaliculus obstructed	Canaliculodacryocystorhinostomy
Upper canaliculus only, less than 8 mm from punctum	Lower canaliculus patent	Surgery usually not needed
	Lower canaliculus obstructed	Conjunctivodacryocystorhinostomy
Combined upper/lower canalicular obstruction	Either canaliculus patent for more than 8 mm from punctum	Canaliculodacryocystorhinostomy
	Neither canaliculus patent for more than 8 mm from punctum	Conjunctivodacryocystorhinostomy

DCR, dacryocystorhinostomy.
From Rodgers and Hurwitz, ref. 6, with permission.

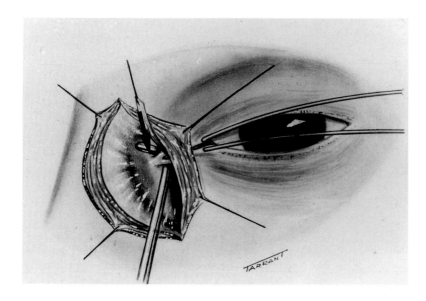

FIG. 3. Probes are placed within the canaliculi. It is now possible to open the common canaliculus (*arrow*) and dissect down on the probes. (Courtesy Mr. Terry Tarrant, London, UK.)

dial aspect of the lacrimal sac as one would for a standard DCR. Nasal mucosal flaps are created, and posterior flaps of the sac and nasal mucosa are sutured using three 5-0 Dexon sutures. Once the sac is opened, it is possible to explore the lateral wall, and an opening is made in the region of the common internal punctum. Then one or two 5-0 Dexon sutures can be used in the posterior flaps of the common canaliculus to suture directly to the lateral wall of the sac. This is sometimes facilitated by making a small superior and inferior snip in the common canaliculus so that flaps can be obtained. Then the bicanalicular Silastic stent tubes are placed through the anas-

tomosis and down into the nose (Fig. 6). Having done this, the anterior flaps of the common canaliculus and lateral wall of the sac can be sutured using two 5-0 Dexon sutures. Then the anterior flap on the medial wall of the sac can be sutured with three 5-0 Dexon sutures directly to the anterior flap of nasal mucosa overlying the tubes. The skin incision is then sutured using three 6-0 nylon sutures. The postoperative care is the same as for a standard DCR (5).

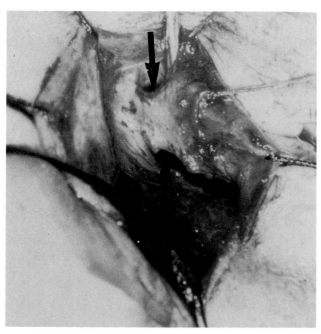

FIG. 4. The common canaliculus has been totally dissected. (From Doucet and Hurwitz, ref. 5, with permission.)

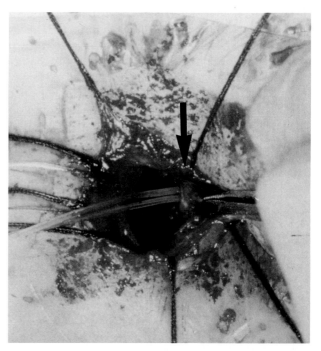

FIG. 5. The common canaliculus has been opened, silicone tubes have been passed into the canalicular system, and then the tubes can be retracted laterally. (From Doucet and Hurwitz, ref. 5 and Hurwitz and Archer, ref. 9, with permission.)

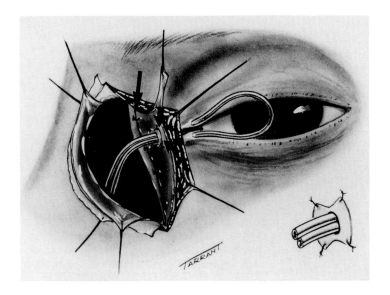

FIG. 6. The posterior flaps of sac and nasal mucosa have been sutured (*big arrow*), the common canaliculus has been sutured into the lateral wall of the sac (*small arrows*), and the tubes have been passed in through the newly created system and down into the nose. (Courtesy of Mr. Terry Tarrant, London, UK.)

Modified Common Canaliculo-DCR (6) (Fig. 7)

To prevent suturing as many flaps, one may make the initial incision in the sac for the DCR to lie on the anterolateral aspect of the sac rather than to open the sac medially as one would for a standard DCR. When this is performed, the large flap created can be mobilized toward the nasal mucosa and forms a large posterior sac flap. This may be sutured directly to the posterior flap of nasal mucosa using three 5-0 Dexon sutures. The size of the posterior nasal mucosa flap must be quite small to allow a large anterior nasal mucosal flap to be fashioned. This large nasal mucosal flap anteriorly may be brought across to join the anterior flap of the common canaliculus directly after the Silastic tubes have been placed down the system. Of note is the fact that there is only the necessity for suturing one series of anterior flaps, and it may be possible to have to suture only the one set of posterior flaps. The suturing of the posterior lip of the common canaliculus to the lateral wall of the sac is optional, but we prefer to put at least one suture to help create an epithelial lined posterior tract from the common canaliculus to the sac.

Prognosis for Common Canaliculo-DCR

When the operation is performed for the proper reason, the procedure has a success rate in the range of 75% to 80% (7). Even though these results are not universal (8), there are certain steps that can be taken to increase the success rate of this procedure.

1. the correct indication for this procedure
2. the appropriate investigation especially using dacryocystography
3. adequately removing scar tissue between the common canaliculus and the sac

4. using a large Silastic stent tube (as compared to the smaller Crawford tube diameter) to keep the epithelial flaps far apart

However, the patient must be told that the procedure sometimes will not work and they may require an insertion of a bypass tube as a secondary procedure, through an inner canthal approach.

CANALICULO-DCR

Indications

This procedure is performed when there are at least 8 mm of patent upper and/or lower canaliculus. If only one canaliculus is blocked, this procedure is not necessary, and it should be limited to those cases in which both canaliculi are blocked (9).

Surgical Technique

This procedure is performed in a similar fashion as to the common canaliculo-DCR, except that on dissection, the probes will each be found to have a separate surrounding lumen (i.e., the obstruction was "pre–common canaliculus"). An incision may be made between the two lumens to create a larger "common lumen." This may then be sutured to the sac as one does for the common canaliculo-DCR.

This procedure may be modified in the same way that the common canaliculo-DCR is modified to decrease the number of flaps (6).

Success of This Operation

When this procedure is performed for distal individual canalicular obstructions, the success rate is approxi-

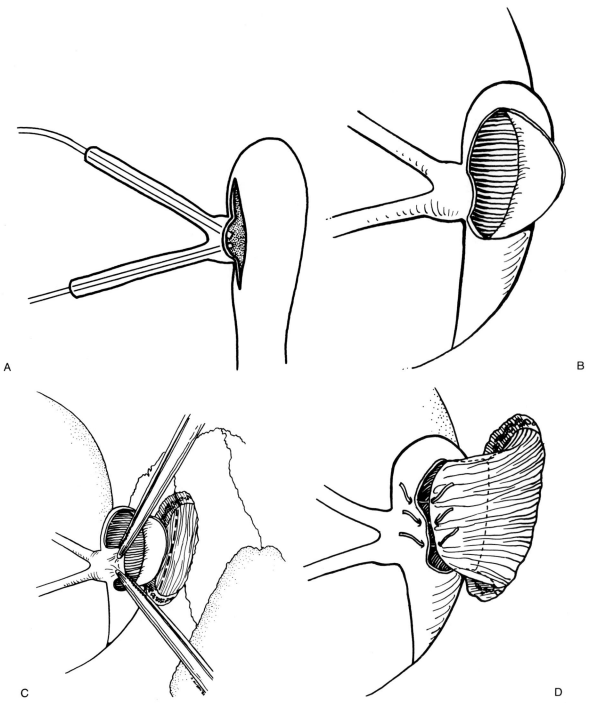

FIG. 7. A: Modified common canaliculo-DCR. A lateral incision is made in the lateral wall of the sac and the flap is reflected medially. **B:** Flap rotated medially. **C:** The common canaliculus has been opened and the newly created flap from the anterior lacrimal sac is taken all the way over to suture to the posterior flap of the nasal mucosa. This obviates the need to have an anastomosis between the posterior common canaliculus and the posterior flap of the lacrimal sac. **D:** After the tubes are inserted, the anterior flap of the common canaliculus can be sutured directly to the anterior flap of the nasal mucosa. (From Rodgers and Hurwitz, ref. 6, with permission.)

mately 50% to 60%. These patients definitely should be told that there may be a second operation necessary to insert a Jones tube at a later date if this procedure does not work. The stent tube should be left in place for 4 to 6 months. We do not prefer, in these difficult cases, to insert a Jones tube at the same time as the reconstructive surgery because, for a Jones tube to lie properly, we feel that we would run the risk of violating the canaliculi or common canaliculus, which may prejudice the reconstructive procedure from being successful.

Modifications of the Canaliculo-DCR

One may perform a canalicular (or common canalicular)-sac anastomosis without performing a DCR (10,11). However, we feel that if the sac is to be opened, then it is preferable to drain the sac through a DCR for fear of the sac scarring up at a later date.

Canaliculorhinostomy

If the sac has been excised, one may suture the canaliculi directly to nasal mucosal flaps. This situation arises occasionally after failed lacrimal surgery (12) or after removal of a tumor (13). In fact, this procedure can be performed after any indication for a dacryocystectomy (3).

We have had a few patients in whom Jones tubes had been placed by other surgeons, and the Jones tubes subsequently extruded. These patients were found to have enough residual canalicular passages that a canaliculorhinostomy could successfully be performed. We feel that in these cases of canaliculorhinostomy, the tubes must be left in for as long as possible, probably for at least 6 months. If this procedure fails, a Jones tube can always be placed secondarily.

At the time of surgery one should try to probe through the canalicular obstructions if at all possible. If there is only a small membrane, the surgeon may elect merely to probe the strictures, perform a DCR, and put in a bicanalicular Silastic stent tube. We prefer to do the DCR at the same time, so that in the eventuality that the procedure will not work, one may insert a bypass secondarily without having to open up the operative site to remove bone a second time. If one cannot probe through the obstruction, or if the probing is exceedingly difficult and inconclusive, then a full canaliculo-DCR should be performed.

CONCLUSION

This chapter outlines those situations in which patients with canalicular and common canalicular obstruc-

tions can be treated by reconstructive surgery than by insertion of a permanent life-long prosthesis such as a Jones tube. Because of the potential problems with Jones tubes (which are outlined in Chapter 38), we feel that it is important to reconstruct the lacrimal passages rather than bypass them, if this is at all possible. Indeed "nature's way" is probably the "best way" (14). These procedures are not successful in every patient, and in some cases, secondary surgery with the insertion of a permanent prosthesis is necessary. However, more often than not, these procedures work, leaving the patient grateful and the surgeon pleased. If the reconstructive procedure does not work, as with a seemingly failed DCR, we try to resurrect the situation by conservative methods such as probing, dilatation, and possibly endonasal procedures. If these do not prove successful, we usually do not repeat the canaliculo-DCR but proceed directly to the insertion of a Jones tube (15)

REFERENCES

1. Jones BR, Corrigan MJ. Obstruction of the lacrimal canaliculi. In: *Proceedings of the second international corneal-plastic conference.* London, 1967; Oxford, 1969: Pergamon Press.
2. Tenzel RR. Canaliculodacryocystorhinostomy. *Arch Ophthalmol* 1970;84:765.
3. Hurwitz JJ, Welham RAN, Maisey MN. Intubation macrodacryocystography and quantitative scintillography: the "complete" lacrimal assessment. *Trans Am Acad Ophthalmol Otolaryngol* 1976;81:575.
4. Kurihashi K, Imada M, Yamashita A. Anatomical analysis of the human lacrimal drainage pathway under an operating microscope. *Int Ophthalmol* 1991;15:411.
5. Doucet TW, Hurwitz JJ. Canaliculodacryocystorhinostomy in the treatment of canalicular obstruction. *Arch Ophthalmol* 1982;100:306.
6. Rodgers KJA, Hurwitz JJ. A simplified canaliculodacryocystorhinostomy. *Orbit* 1983;2:231.
7. Hurwitz JJ, Rutherford S. Computerized survey of lacrimal surgery patients. *Ophthalmology* 1986;93:14.
8. Naugle T. Conjunctivodacryocystorhinostomy. In: Bosniak SL, Smith DC, eds. *Advances of ophthalmic plastic reconstructive surgery.* vol 3. Elmsford, NY: Pergamon Press; 1984.
9. Hurwitz JJ, Archer KA. Canaliculodacryocystorhinostomy. In: Linberg JV, ed. *Lacrimal surgery.* New York: Churchill Livingstone; 1988.
10. Hatt M. Surgery of acquired canalicular stenosis. *Orbit* 1992;11:153.
11. Busse H, Meyer-Rustenberg HW, Kroll P. Canaliculo-dacryocystotomy. *Orbit* 1985;4:69.
12. Doucet TW, Hurwitz JJ. Canaliculodacryocystorhinostomy after unsuccessful lacrimal surgery. *Arch Ophthalmol* 1982;100:619.
13. Older JJ, Sims LM. Canaliculorhinostomy following dacryocystectomy for removal of a benign fibrous histiocytoma of the lacrimal sac. *Ophthal Surg* 1993;24:753.
14. Veirs E. In discussing the paper by Jones LT. The cure of epiphora due to canalicular disorders, trauma and surgical failures on the lacrimal passages. *Trans Am Acad Ophthalmol Otolaryngol* 1962;66:506.
15. Welham RAN. Canalicular obstruction and the Lester Jones tube. What to do when all else fails. *Trans Ophthal Society UK* 1973;93:623.

CHAPTER 38

Lacrimal Bypass Surgery

Jeffrey Jay Hurwitz

The most difficult obstructions to treat in the lacrimal drainage pathways are those located distal to the punctum but in the proximal canaliculi. Typically, canalicular reconstructive surgery is problematic at the best of times for obstructions in this location. Attempts at probing, and with the insertion of tubes to hold the passages open (1), has been problematic in the treatment of acquired obstructions. Attempts to diathermize canalicular membranes have not had great success in the past, but with newer diathermy equipment with insulating electrodes (2) the treatment may have some promise in the future.

Present-day investigative techniques are by and large inadequate to determine the status of the system distal to the obstruction. We have not had much success in trying to inject either methylene blue into the tear sac, performing dacryocystography via injection into the tear sac, performing surgical cut down on the canaliculus to assess the proximal canaliculus and sac, or retrograde probing along the common internal punctum and common canaliculus once the sac is opened. There have been only a small handful of patients who we have been able to reconstruct without using a permanent bypass tube (Jones) for proximal canalicular obstructions, where one of these techniques was found to be of use.

Articles will occasionally appear in the literature describing a technique for treating these proximal canalicular obstructions. We have not been sufficiently pleased with the results of any of these procedures, other than a bypass tube.

If a proximal canalicular obstruction exists we usually treat the patient with a DCR and insertion of a bypass tube. It is our feeling that a bypass tube should be inserted only if it is unfeasible or unrealistic to reconstruct the existing pathways, that is, if it is impossible to render the patient epiphora free on the long-term basis without a permanent prosthesis.

Other techniques of total bypass of the lacrimal system, with the insertion of grafts, mucosal grafts, and skin grafts between the conjunctiva and the nose, have not withstood the test of time and have not had acceptable success rates for the relief of epiphora. Canalicular transplantation has been attempted, but it has not been routinely performed on a wide scale (3).

We feel that the best chance of success is the insertion of a drainage tube between the inner canthus and the nose, and that lining the track is not necessary (4).

INDICATIONS FOR BYPASS TUBES

1. *Less than 8 mm of residual canaliculi.* When the canaliculodacryocystorhinostomy (canaliculo-DCR) operation was first described by Jones in 1960 (5), he suggested that if there was as little as 5 mm of remaining patent proximal canaliculi, that a canaliculo-DCR could be performed. We have technically found it difficult to perform this operation if there were less than 8 mm of patent canaliculi remaining and, therefore, we and others (6) suggested this procedure has a higher success rate if there are at least 8 mm of remaining canaliculi. The Moorfields group, headed by Welham, and our group have been able to reproduce the results initially described by Jones, which is to reconstruct the lacrimal passages with a canaliculo-DCR so that there would be long-term patency in most patients, but only if 8 mm or more of patent canaliculus remains.

The exception to the rule would be in a situation where there was severe trauma to the canalicular region and even though 8 mm of patent canaliculi remained, there was such extensive scarring that the prognosis for a successful canaliculo-DCR would be lessened. In these cases, we suggest inserting a bypass tube.

J. J. Hurwitz: Oculoplastics Program, Mount Sinai Hospital; and Department of Ophthalmology, University of Toronto Faculty of Medicine, Toronto, Ontario M5S 1A8 Canada.

2. *Punctal agenesis.* If it is felt that both puncta exhibit a complete agenesis and there are no punctal papillae, then one usually finds that the canaliculi, and even the sac, are maldeveloped. We have not had much success in injecting methylene blue into the sac, doing dacryocystography with a sac injection, or cutting down on the canaliculi medially to determine how much residual canaliculus remains distally. We insert Jones tubes in these patients.

3. *Severe trauma to the upper and lower canaliculi proximally.* The distal canalicular obstructions are usually treated by a canaliculo-DCR. If attempts at reconstruction of combined proximal upper and lower canalicular lacerations fail, we prefer to insert a Jones tube.

4. *Following unsuccessful canaliculo-DCR (but not after an unsuccessful DCR).* We prefer to attempt a reconstructive procedure should a DCR fail.

5. *Following canalicular obstruction after canaliculitis involving both canaliculi where the canaliculi become obstructed, or the canaliculi stay patent but do not function properly.*

6. *Lid-globe malposition.* In patients with an anterior location of the punctum relative to the lacrimal lake (centurion syndrome, discussed in Chapter 25). If eyelid and medial canthal reconstruction is not successful, a bypass tube may help to drain the tears.

In patients with facial nerve palsy, we have not been happy with inserting Jones tubes to try and remove the tears. The reason for this is that the tearing is usually related to an eyelid pumping dysfunction due to a residual orbicularis weakness. We have shown that a Jones tube will not function properly if there is not a normally functioning lacrimal pump and orbicularis (7).

7. *Tumors of the inner canthi.* When a dacryocystectomy and canaliculectomy have been performed because of a tumor, we do not re-establish drainage into the nose until we are sure that there will be no recurrence of the tumor. At a secondary procedure, later on, if there are no canaliculi we will insert a bypass tube to drain the tears.

8. *Failed bypass tube.* We will assess the system and if there is enough residual canalicular tissue remaining, we will attempt a reconstruction. However, if there is not we will reinsert a bypass tube.

9. *Canalicular stenosis.* Repeated dilatation of a stenotic canaliculus may lead to a complete obstruction (8). One may try temporary stenting of the passages but if this does not work, then a bypass tube is usually indicated.

DCR AND BYPASS TUBE

Philosophy

Many attempts have been made in a patient with complete canalicular obstruction to produce an epithelial lined tract between the conjunctival cul-de-sac and the lacrimal sac. Flaps of conjunctiva have been pulled toward the lacrimal sac, flaps of lacrimal sac have been pulled toward the conjunctiva, and ethmoidal and antral mucosa have been pulled into the surgical ostium. As well, grafts of veins, mucosa, and epidermis have been placed in the ostium to attempt to produce an epithelial lined tract. Even though these passages will often stay open, the patients will usually not be free of epiphora because the lacrimal pump function has been totally circumvented. Jones (8) conceptualized that the insertion of a bypass tube that had capillary action into the ostium would drain tears from the palpebral aperture into the nose. When he first described that in 1962, there were some skeptics, and indeed there are still some skeptics. The eventual success rates of this procedure vary from 41% (9) to 100% (10). We stress the term "eventual" because to achieve the success rates, more than one operation is often necessary. We agree with Jones that it is not necessary to line the outer tract of the tube with any mucosa. In fact, it is probably better that there is some scar tissue contraction around the tube to hold it in place.

Once the tube is in place, it should be considered to be a life-long prosthesis. Any surgeon who had at one time hoped that the tubes could be removed usually found that the tubes, when they are removed or when they extrude, left the patients with a recurrence of symptoms of epiphora and the openings closed. It is our experience that there are only rare cases, that is, when there has been radiation to the area or multiple severe trauma to the area, that the opening may indeed stay open. Even if the opening does stay open, it will often leave the patients with some epiphora because of the loss of the tube's capillarity.

It was also hoped that the epithelium would migrate to line the ostium around the Jones tube, so that if it did come out, the ostium would be lined with epithelium. We have biopsied a few channels when the Jones tube had extruded, from shortly after the insertion to periods up to 3 years following the insertion, and we did not find any patient in whom the tract was lined with epithelium. The tracts were all lined with scar tissue. This would suggest that epithelium does not migrate around the tube, and that the tube is indeed necessary to stay in the ostium to drain the tears into the nose.

There have been many attempts at creating tubes to lie in the inner canthus and drain into the sac (11,12). As well, tubes have been implanted within the sac to drain into the nose (13). However, we agree with Jones that for the best functioning and maintenance of an artificial tube, both the ocular and the nasal end must be able to be visualized clinically, and must be able to be serviced.

An external conjunctivorhinostomy has been described by Murube del Castillo (14). These silicone tubes with a short Pyrex cylindrical tube fastened superiorly would sit at the inner canthus and then would pass under the skin along the side of the nose to drain posteriorly beneath the inferior turbinate into the nose. These tubes would have the potential indication for insertion when there was no hope for any aperture within the inside of the nose in the area of the middle meatus for an insertion of a Jones tube. The results of long-term patency, however, are problematic (Murube del Castillo, personal communication).

The ideal tube should be straight rather than curved, because from basic principles of fluid dynamics, there is better drainage along a straight tube than a curved tube. The tube should also not be porous and should be hydrophobic, so that no tears (and hopefully no salts from the tears) stick to its surfaces. The tube must also have some rigidity so that it does not collapse. The ideal tube also must sit firmly in place and hopefully cause no reaction in the surrounding tissues.

The Pyrex glass tube developed by Jones (Gunther Weiss Glass Blowers, Portland, OR) seems to be the closest to the ideal tube. This tube is not perfect, and may cause some potential problems (which will be listed below), but has withstood the test of time.

Tubes of other material such as polyethylene (8), silicone (12), polypropylene (15), and Teflon (16) have all been designed, but it would still seem that the Pyrex glass gives the best drainage of all.

Because of the variable success rates in the bypass tube surgery, some surgeons have devised other techniques to relieve the epiphora in conjunction with the insertion of a Pyrex glass bypass tube. Putterman and Epstein (17) performed a bicanalicular Silastic tube insertion in conjunction with a Jones tube insertion so that if one procedure did not work, perhaps the other one would. Also, Bosniak and Smith (18) suggested performing a palpebral lobectomy (19) in conjunction with a Jones tube insertion. They felt that if a Jones tube insertion did not eliminate the tearing, then perhaps a palpebral adenectomy would. We have not performed bicanalicular Silastic tube intubation or palpebral lobectomy in conjunction with a DCR and insertion of a bypass tube. It is our philosophy that if there is a problem with the bypass tube, we would try and rectify it rather than go to another procedure.

Pyrex Glass (Jones) Tubes (Fig. 1)

These tubes have ocular flanges that drain the tears out of the palpebral aperture measuring 3.0, 3.5, and 4.0 mm. All the tubes have a gentle nasal flange. The tubes may be straight or curved, but we use only the straight tubes. The tubes have a 1.5- to 1.7-mm inner diameter and a 2.5-mm outer diameter along the shaft of the tube. Some of the tubes have suture holes at the junction of the head and neck of the tube. The tubes made by Weiss have no rough edges along the suture holes, and it is extremely unusual to have any reaction along the edges of

the suture holes, although we have had a few cases with granuloma formation with or without suture holes. Because fixation is so easy with the tubes having suture holes, the only Jones tubes we insert are those with suture holes. The tubes vary in length from 9 mm to 25 mm, but shorter ones or longer ones can be ordered upon request. We have had Pyrex glass tubes made by other glass blowers, but none of them have been able to reduplicate the expertise of those made by Weiss.

Technique of Insertion—Primary Operation

A standard DCR approach is used. An incision is made on the side of the nose, and bone is removed between the lacrimal sac and the nasal mucosa. The lacrimal sac is opened, as is the nasal mucosa. Any ethmoidal air cells between the two are superficially exenterated. It is important that for the proper functioning of a Jones tube, that it must not lie on a large turbinate (anterior tip of the middle turbinate), where the posterior flaps have been sutured.

If there is a large anterior tip of the middle turbinate, it has been advocated that this should be removed (20). However, it must be remembered that the middle turbinate does contain erectile tissue and that there can be a tremendous amount of bleeding from excising the middle turbinate. There are measures that can be undertaken to try and decrease the bleeding coming from the middle turbinate. First, the patient has been pretreated with decongestant nasal spray and cocaine packing. Along with this we use the tip of an insulated monopolar cautery to pass beneath the mucosa of the anterior tip of the middle turbinate. This causes some immediate hemostasis and we hope longer term will cause some atrophy of the erectile tissue. Instead of excising the mucosa and the head of the turbinate, we prefer to make a small incision into the surface of the turbinate mucosa after cauterizing, and then separate the bone of the turbinate from the surrounding mucosa. We then use a blunt scissors passed up the nose and cut the bony head of the middle turbinate. Then when the posterior flap of sac and nasal mucosa is sutured, the needle may pass through the cut ends of the turbinate mucosa and when the suture is secured this tends to aid in hemostasis. Also it may help in fixation of the posterior flap of sac. We agree with Wesley (21) that if one tries to cut the turbinate with a hot monopolar cautery, there can be spread of heat posteriorly to the frontal recess and the area of the hiatus semilunaris where the nasofrontal duct enters. This has been shown to cause obstruction of the duct and ensuing frontal sinusitis. One does not need to remove the posterior lacrimal crest, but only the bone of the lacrimal fossa at the time of performing the osteotomy. This helps prevent getting too far posterior to the region of the nasofrontal duct. We prefer to cut the anterior tip of the middle tur-

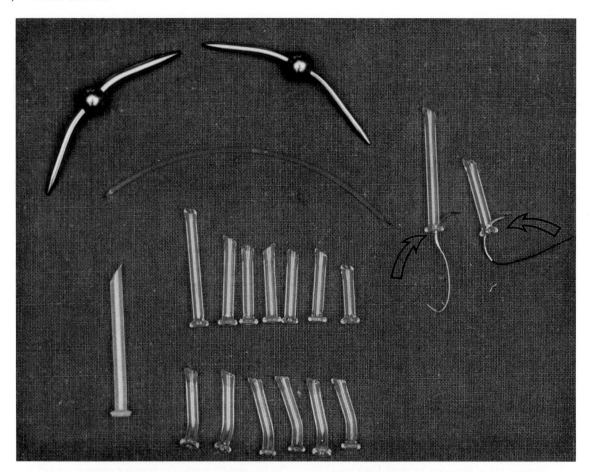

FIG. 1. Jones tube set-up. A series of curved and straight Jones tubes of varying lengths are shown. To the left of the glass Jones tube is a Jones polyethylene tube, which is larger and wider. At the right are two Jones tubes with suture holes where sutures can be passed through the lip of the tube and anchored to the inner canthal tissues. Above the tubes is a small stiff plastic bougie for cleaning the tubes. Above this are two gold dilators that can be used to keep the passage open when the Jones tubes are being changed. (From Hurwitz, ref. 4, with permission.)

binate with scissors rather than trying to lift it out with a forceps. We are concerned that since the opening of the nasofrontal duct is approximately 1 cm behind the tip of the anterior turbinate, it is unpredictable how much bone will be removed from the middle turbinate if it is pulled out. If more bone is removed than is desired, the nasofrontal duct may be damaged because one may remove some of the bone of the hiatus semilunaris (22). As well, we are concerned that if the bone is merely pulled out and not cut, there may be some disturbance of the cribriform plate with an ensuing CSF leak. It must be remembered that the middle turbinate is part of the ethmoid bone and is connected via the ethmoidal labyrinth to the cribriform plate. We have found that in treating the erectile tissue of the middle turbinate, if a unipolar cautery is not available, it is probably as effective to cauterize the surface with a bipolar cautery. However, we feel that the bipolar surface cauterization may cause some scarring of the mucosa, which would not be desirable, so we feel if one has the choice, on theoretical grounds, insertion of a unipolar cautery beneath the mucosa to destroy the erectile tissue may be most advantageous.

The posterior flaps of sac and nasal mucosa (with or without some mucosa of the turbinate) are sutured with three 5-0 Dexon (Davis and Geck) sutures.

Attention is then focused on the caruncle. A lid speculum is inserted. If the caruncle is tiny or nonexistent, we will use a bipolar cautery to touch the inner canthus for hemostasis purposes. If there is a moderate to large caruncle, in past years we would remove the caruncle, but we were concerned about the fact that if the conjunctiva was cut and there was a free surface, there would be migration of the conjunctiva to the inner canthus and this might cover the tube. We therefore now use bipolar cautery to the caruncle to shrink it, in a similar fashion to shrinking orbital fat in a blepharoplasty. Much to our delight, we found that we could shrink and atrophy even the largest caruncle without damaging the conjunctiva. This gave us good access to entry at the medial canthus, without violating the conjunctiva. The incidence of overgrowth of the tube by conjunctiva or plica tissue is tremendously reduced since we have been doing this maneuver. Therefore, after bipolar cautery, a #18 needle is passed through the caruncle about 2 mm posterior to mucocutaneous junction (Fig. 2). The needle is directed toward the common canaliculus but perhaps slightly inferior to it so that the tube ultimately would lie in a more vertical orientation than horizontal. We feel that this is important because we have shown that more vertically orientated Jones tubes tend to drain better than more horizontally orientated Jones tubes (7).

It has been described that one can three-snip the canaliculus and put the tube along the canaliculus horizontally into the sac and into the middle meatus. We have tried this but have abandoned this procedure for a few reasons. First, the tube lies too horizontally. Second, we cannot get the tube to get a good snug inner canthus fixation, and third, there is too much "dead space" inferior to the tube in the nose. Once the #18 needle has been placed from the inner canthus into the nose, one gets a small canaliculus knife and passes this through the inner canthus and into the sac along the side of the needle (Fig. 3). The needle can then be withdrawn. Using the sac as a fulcrum, the knife can be moved inferiorly and then superiorly at the inner canthus to enlarge the opening. A special corneal trephine has been described by Henderson (23), but we have not used this instrument because we have not found it a problem in producing the desired opening at the inner canthus. Once this has been performed, we take two large probes and pass them through the opening at the inner canthus so they hit upon the septum. We then inspect the probes hitting the septum using a nasal septum to make sure that there is adequate

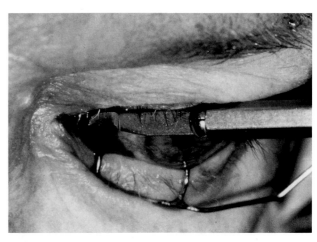

FIG. 3. A Graefe knife is inserted along the side of the needle into the nose. When the tip is in the nose, the needle is withdrawn.

clearance of the middle turbinate. We push one probe against the septum and then grasp it at the inner canthus with a snap. We then measure this distance. We would like the tube to sit approximately 2 to 3 mm away from the septum so we subtract 2 to 3 mm from whatever distance we measured. We then select from our inventory of Jones tubes the appropriately sized tube. We then put a 6-0 nylon suture through the suture hole in the tube and place a #2 Bowman's probe down the shaft of the tube. We place the Bowman's probe at the inner canthus and into the nose (Fig. 4). Then we can push the Jones tube through the opening into the nose. We then like to look in the nose and see where the Jones tube is lying. If it is satisfactory we can withdraw the probe and pass the

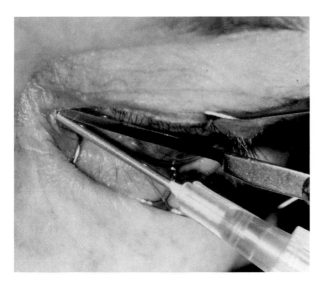

FIG. 2. A #18 gauge needle (below) is placed through the cauterized caruncle anterior to the anastomosed sac and nasal mucosal posterior flaps and into the nose. The Graefe knife (above) passes along the needle.

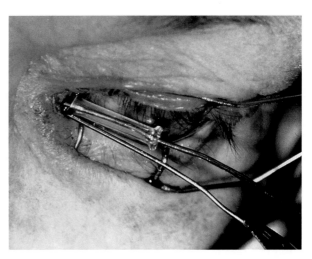

FIG. 4. Two probes are placed into the opening and pushed against the septum. An artery forceps grasps one probe at the inner canthus, is withdrawn, and the distance from the inner canthus to the septum is measured. A Jones tube slightly shorter is inserted using a probe in its lumen as a guide.

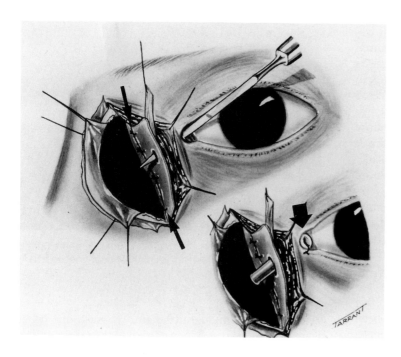

FIG. 5. Artist's diagram showing suturing of posterior flaps (*big arrows*) and insertion of Graefe knife to create an opening. In the *lower diagram*, the Jones tube has been inserted and is fastened in place at the inner canthus (*short arrow*). (Courtesy of Mr. Terry Tarrant, London, UK.)

suture through the tissues at the inner canthus for about 3 or 4 mm and tie the suture (Fig. 5). A drop of saline is placed on the inner canthus and it should flow without any suctioning directly through into the nose. It is important to inspect the tube in the nose to make sure it is lying free. One may use a suction at the nasal end of the tube to make sure that the fluid is indeed going through the tube (24). If the patient is awake, the patient can be asked to open and close the eyes and if one looks in the nose, the mobility of the tube should be observable. This means that the tube is not abutting against the septum, and it is probably lying in a good position (25). As well, we like to push a cotton-tipped applicator against the ocular end of the tube and push the tube toward the nose. If it does not move and the nasal end of the tube abuts on the septum, the tube is probably too long and a smaller one should be put in. If the tube is not passing beyond the posterior flaps or beyond the anterior tip of the middle turbinate, or is deflected by the anterior tip of the middle turbinate, the tube should be removed, more of a turbinectomy may have to be performed, and a longer tube may have to be reinserted. We prefer to do this at the time of surgery because if we are not happy with the tube at the time of surgery, we definitely will not be happy with it afterward. The anterior flaps of the sac and nasal mucosa are then sutured over the tube and the skin is sutured with 6-0 nylon sutures (Fig. 6).

We feel that it is important to suture posterior flaps and to suture anterior flaps. The suturing of the flaps definitely helps with hemostasis. The sutured flaps will also not lie redundantly in the area of the tube and will not cover the nasal end of the tube. If the flaps are su-

tured there will be less of a tendency for granulation tissue to grow into the region between the flaps, and perhaps form granulomas that may press on the tube and deflect its position. Postoperatively, the patient is not treated with any ointment because we do not like the

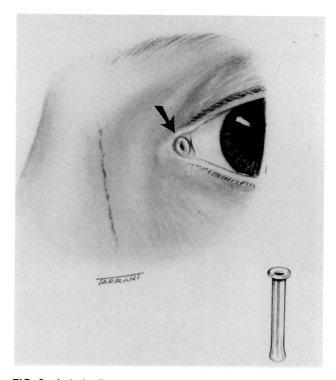

FIG. 6. Artist's diagram showing the wound sutured and the Jones tube in place (*arrow*). (Courtesy of Mr. Terry Tarrant, London, UK.)

idea of ointment getting into the tube and potentially blocking it. We like to use some steroid eyedrops, preferably a water-soluble steroid that is not particulate, three times a day to shrink the tissues at the inner canthus so they will not hypertrophy and potentially block the tube. However, if steroid is to be used, it is mandatory that the surgeon eliminate the possibility of the canalicular obstruction having been caused by a herpes simplex infection. If there has been a lot of congestion in the nose, allergic rhinitis, etc., we will treat the patient with a glucocorticoid nasal spray for approximately 2 weeks postoperatively.

Anesthesia

The same criteria for determining whether a patient should be operated on under a general or local anesthesia is used as for a DCR. The main advantage for local anesthesia is so that one can check for the "rocking phenomenon" (25).

Care of the Tube (Fig. 7)

Before the operation the surgeon must have a satisfactory interview with the patient, who will be aware of the fact that this tube will be in place forever, and if the tube does come out that the tearing will undoubtedly start again. The patient is to be instructed that if the tube comes out, he must either put the tube back in himself or, failing this, must be able to get in touch with the surgeon or a regional physician who will be able to reinsert it. If the tube comes out within 24 hours, it usually can be reinserted without a problem, but after this it is much more difficult and often further surgery is required.

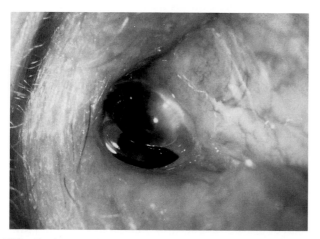

FIG. 7. Jones tube sitting in good position at the inner canthus.

The patient must be instructed that if he is to blow his nose, he must either close the eyes tightly and/or place his finger over the inner canthus, because theoretically the tube can be blown out. As well, the patient is told that whenever he is wiping his eye, he must pat it gently *toward* the nose because theoretically wiping the tube outward may cause traction on the tube and it may be pulled out. It must be emphasized that on wiping the eye *toward* the nose, that it must be done gently because theoretically the patient may push on the tube and the tube may slide down into the opening between the inner canthus and the nose.

To keep the tube clean the patient is told to splash some water on the inner canthus and then, while holding the other nostril, to snort water down into the tube and into the nose. He is told to do this every morning and every night for the rest of his life. We agree with Weil (26) that the patient should not be instructed to stick anything into the tube to clean it. We feel that most patients are not able to do this, and we have been happy with having the patients clean the tubes with water. If there is a lot of discharge of mucus within the tube, we tell the patients that they can use some decongestant eyedrops from time to time (naphazoline), and or use some naphazoline nasal spray occasionally (but only a maximum of 3 days at a time).

We warn the patients that we may occasionally have to change the tubes, but in our practice this is very rare. We see the patients 1 week after the surgery to remove the sutures, 2 to 3 weeks after to irrigate the tubes, and after the next 3-month visit we see them every 6 months. At the 6-month visits, we have them Valsalva to see if they can blow air out of the tube. If they can then this means that the tube is open. We usually confirm this by irrigation, but this may not be necessary. It is helpful that the surgeon look in the nose and check the "rocking phenomenon" and hopefully see the end of the tube and where it is related to the nasal septum. We prefer to slide the tube out slightly and clean the outer edge of the tube while it is still sitting within the opening. If one wants to remove the tube totally (this in our experience is very unlikely), we use the Weiss gold dilator (see Fig. 1) that we insert at the inner canthus. We clean the tube and then we reinsert the tube once we remove the dilator. Usually the tubes slide out nicely and are easy to replace in this fashion. We also check the size of the tube at the inner canthus. We usually insert the tube with the largest ocular diameter (4.0 mm) because this has the least chance of sliding down the opening. However, with patients who have narrow palpebral apertures, we insert a 3.5-mm tube routinely. We must check and see if the tube is irritating the inner canthus and if a 4.0-mm tube is irritating the inner canthus, we will remove it and put in a 3.5-mm tube. We have not yet seen a situation where a 3.5-mm tube, even in a teenager, interfered with the closure of the eyes and/or caused irritation. We do not routinely put in a 3.0-mm tube because, with the outer diameter of the tube at the ocular end being only 2.5 mm, we are fearful that the tube will slide inward through the opening and be lost in the nose.

Occasionally one will find that the tube has slid down the opening. The first time we saw this we were extremely concerned and, in fact, it was not until we looked up the nose that we actually could see the tube. We found this first patient, and three subsequent patients, to have the tubes fixated in the opening by the tissues, and fixated in the nose draining tears for up to 7 years that we have followed these four patients. It would seem that there may be some contraction of the soft tissues within the opening around the lip of the tube that would hold it in place. In none of these four patients have we found it necessary to replace the tube. Therefore, if the tube is not visible at the inner canthus, it may be lost totally, or it may still be sitting in the nose. The inner canthus also should be checked for granulation tissue. If granulation tissue exists, one may treat it with topical steroids and it may involute, or it may simply be snipped away with Vannas scissors. There may be some bleeding because there is often a vascular base, but we prefer not to cauterize near the opening of the tube unless absolutely necessary, and the bleeding usually stops with a bit of pressure in the office.

We usually remove the suture holding the tube in place at approximately 6 to 8 weeks after insertion. When we do this, we remove the suture at the slit lamp and then have the patient blow the nose forcibly. If the tube starts to extrude we put another suture in place. This is extremely important in patients who have had radiation damage to the inner canthus and a subsequent Jones tube because these patients seem to have much poorer soft tissue contraction around the tube and are at much greater risk for an extrusion once the suture is removed. We have had some patients with radiation in whom we have left the sutures in for more than 1 year without a problem. The patients *must* be told that after the operation when they blow their nose that they will blow air back into their palpebral aperture area. The patient may have some complications on flying in an airplane and/or scuba diving. Even though it has been reported that there may be problems for a pilot flying an aircraft, such as pressure breathing difficulties and difficulty performing a Valsalva maneuver (27), we have had three pilots who have had their Jones tubes in place for as long as 12 years without a problem. As well, we have had two scuba divers who can clear their masks by closing their eyes tightly. One will temporarily use a little plug in his Jones tube to help him when he has to clear his mask forcibly.

The need for follow-up examinations and ongoing maintenance of the tube is important, and the patient must realize that. A study done by Rosen et al. (28) showed that 11.6% of patients who had functionally successful operations were not satisfied with the results, the most common because of this need for frequent examinations and maintenance of the tube.

IMPLANTATION AFTER DCR SURGERY

If a patient has already had a DCR, and if the bony opening is large enough, one may be able to insert a bypass tube without opening up the incision and recreating new flaps. The presence of a bony opening may be assessed by ultrasound, but we feel that if we really want to know the size of the bony opening, we will use a computerized tomography (CT) scan. A reformatted CT scan, or a three-dimensional CT scan, is even better for this purpose.

If it is our own patient in whom we performed the initial osteotomy, we do not investigate the size of the opening because we know that we make a large bony opening and that it should be adequate to take the passage of a Jones tube. However, we do investigate the patients if someone else has performed the osteotomy because we want to make sure that the osteotomy has been placed in the right position, as well as being the appropriate size.

Jones stated (8) that even after an extrusion of a tube, if the opening has closed one can merely, in the office, apply some local anesthesia and use a knife to create a new passage. We have found this difficult to do, and we would agree with Weil (26) that this procedure is probably best done in an operating room because there may be a significant amount of bleeding.

The Jones tube insertion is performed by inserting a sharp dilator through the inner canthus into the nose if a previous Jones tube had been in place. If there had been no previous Jones tube the caruncle must be cauterized as in a primary procedure and a #18 needle passed through the inner canthus into the nose. Then a probe can be placed through the inner canthal opening just created into the nose along to the septum. It is again mandatory that the nasal mucosa be decongested. Then the length of the probe is measured and another probe with a tube on it is placed into the opening and slid nasally. Again it is mandatory that the length of the tube be at least 2 to 3 mm (preferably 3–4 mm) less than the measured length from the inner canthus to the septum. It must be emphasized that the septum and mucosa have been decongested, and one would expect that when they return to their nondecongested state, that the opening of the tube might be closer to the septal mucosa. This is why we give some margin for error when measuring the length of the tube and its proximity to the septum. However, it is also mandatory that the tube pass beyond the posterior flaps and the tip of the middle turbinate. Water is then placed on the inner canthus and if it flows nicely into the nose, then the suture through the suture hole can be tied after it is passed through the inner canthal tissue.

COMPLICATIONS OF JONES TUBE INSERTION

Hemorrhage

Bleeding is the same problem after a Jones tube insertion as after a DCR. In each operation, one may treat (or excise) the anterior tip of the middle turbinate, with the surgeon usually being more aggressive in the Jones tube procedure. Therefore, bleeding may be more likely. It is important that if the nose is to be packed postoperatively, that pressure not be placed up against the Jones tube because this may dislodge the tube. Also, if the packing pushes on the tube at its nasal end, the ocular end may be forced laterally and may strike the cornea and produce corneal damage. We prefer to try to prevent the bleeding, especially from the tip of the middle turbinate. It is also useful to use some Gelfoam or small pieces of Surgicel to place on the tip of the middle turbinate if it has been resected and if there is bleeding from it. However, we must emphasize that any of these artificial hemostyptics can cause some inflammation as they absorb. If at the end of the operation there is some bleeding, rather than packing the nose, we prefer to use some Gelfoam to place into the middle meatus just inferior to where the tube is coming into the nose. This tends to hemostase the cut edge of the middle turbinate. We also do not like to place a lot of Gelfoam here because again we are concerned about causing reaction in the area of the hiatus semilunaris where one finds the opening of the nasofrontal duct. This is the main difference in the management of epitaxis immediately after Jones tube insertion, as opposed to standard DCR. The patient should be warned postoperatively that there may be some bleeding from the nose, but it may appear that "the eye is bleeding," as blood passes from the nose through the tube and out the ocular end. This warning will tend to relieve some of the anxiety of the patient.

Patient Dissatisfaction

Rosen et al. (28) showed that 18% of patients with Jones tube procedures were dissatisfied, 6.5% because the operation did not work and the rest because of problems such as difficulty with long-term follow-up, tearing in the recumbent position, fogging and spraying of the eyeglasses, and esthetic considerations. It is indeed frustrating for the patient when the surgeon feels that the operation has worked and the patient has concerns. Therefore, we feel that it is important that the patient should be told preoperatively that the Jones tube is not perfect, but it is "the best we have." They also found that there was a lower rate of compliance in children than in older patients. This certainly has been our experience, and we prefer not to place Jones tubes in children who would not be able to (with supervision if necessary) properly maintain them.

Extrusion

Most series will suggest that the most common complication of Jones tubes is extrusion (29–33). In fact, Rose and Welham felt that if patients with Jones tubes lived long enough, virtually all of them would have extrusions (30).

Extrusions may occur during the immediate postoperative period (6 weeks), or may be late (after 2 years). The immediate extrusions are usually due to problems with the positioning of the tube, the size of the tube, or hypertrophy of the middle turbinate and/or septal mucosa. The hypertrophy of the mucosa may be treated by decongestants in the short term, but it is often necessary to perform a turbinectomy at a later sitting. We do not feel that a septoplasty has much to add, and we prefer to use a shorter length tube, hopefully in a more vertically oriented position.

If the tube has extruded, we ask the patient to return immediately, hopefully with the tube. If there is an opening at the inner canthus, we attempt to insert the Weiss gold dilator to dilate the opening. If we can do this, then we put the tube over a probe and insert it into the opening and secure it with a suture. If we cannot dilate the opening wide enough, we have used a smaller diameter Teflon canalicular tube (16) at the inner canthal position, and even though it is smaller than the Jones tube inner diameter, some patients will be relieved of epiphora. Because the outer wall of the Teflon tube is softer, one may scallop the outer wall with a scalpel. This will form a rough edge around the tube and will increase the adhesiveness between the soft tissues and the tube. We have not had one of these smaller tubes extrude. The Teflon tubes do not drain as well as glass, and they tend to form more concretions inside the tubes. Therefore, they have to be cleaned more frequently than do the glass Jones tubes (a similar situation would be the need for cleaning soft contact lenses more frequently than hard contact lenses).

If there is no opening at all, then usually we will take the patients back to the operating room electively. If the patient has not been able to find the tube, we will try if there is an opening present to insert a probe through toward the nose and measure the size of the tube appropriately. Hopefully, one will be able to retrieve the operative note and find out the exact length of the tube, and from the inventory of tubes be able to replace the identical tube. However, when the identical tube has been replaced, one must do an examination to determine why that identical tube would have been extruded the first time, that is, was there a problem with the septum and/or the turbinate? If the tube seems too long, one could put in a smaller tube at the time.

We are not sure why delayed extrusion occurs. Perhaps the channel around the tube comprised of fibrous soft tissue stretches with time and the tube is not held in place. We would think that if the tract is lined with any sort of epithelium (vein graft, mucosa, epithelium), that the extrusions would be greatly increased. Therefore, we prefer not to line the tract with mucosa because we feel it is important to have some fibrous, nonepithelialized tissue to hold the tube in place. We realize that it is probably easier to replace a tube with an epithelial lined tract, but with our technique (essentially only slightly modified from Jones' original technique), we have only rarely had the need to replace an extruded Jones tube. We treat our late extrusions that same as our early extrusions. Veirs (13) has described putting a hole in the nasal end of the tube and putting a suture through this and holding it in place at the external naris. We have tried this in two patients. It worked well in one patient but in the other patient he pulled on the suture and the tube was pulled down through the opening into the nose and had to be

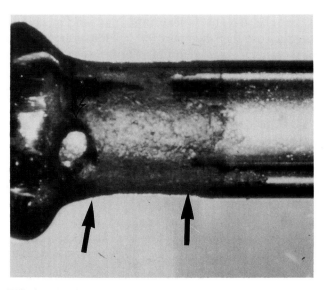

FIG. 9. Modified Jones tube with a 4-mm area roughened up by a miniature grinder in an attempt to promote soft tissue contraction around the tube to keep it in place. *Black arrows* outline roughened area. *Clear arrow* shows suture hole.

replaced. We therefore try to treat extrusions by modifying the tube at the ocular end.

With repeated extrusions, specially designed Jones tubes have been manufactured. Gladstone and Putterman (31) designed a tube that had a second flange 3 to 6 mm from the ocular flange. They reported an increased success rate of holding the tubes in place. Another report from the same center (32) suggested that modifying the tube to increase its diameter and/or putting on a flange in the area of the soft tissue would decrease the extrusion rate.

We have tried modifying the neck of the tube in a similar fashion to Putterman's group, by putting a small piece (3–4 mm) of silicone around the neck of the tube so that the soft tissues would fit snugly around each edge of the silicone (33). One must dilate the passage widely so that the silicone does not slide on the glass while the tube is being positioned. This technique seems to work reasonably well and does not require a specially designed glass tube (Fig. 8).

We have tried to modify the outer surface of the Jones tube in contact with the soft tissues to make it rougher so as to increase the adhesion between the tube and the tissues (34). We use a miniature grinding wheel and roughen the outer edges of the tube 4 to 5 mm from the neck of the tube along the shaft. We have placed the tube in four patients so far, and the tubes have not extruded (follow-up time, maximum 8 months) (Fig. 9). One might expect granulomas around the roughened edges of the Jones tube, but these have not occurred. However, to determine whether this technique helps in the delayed extrusions (after 2 years), long-term follow-up is mandatory.

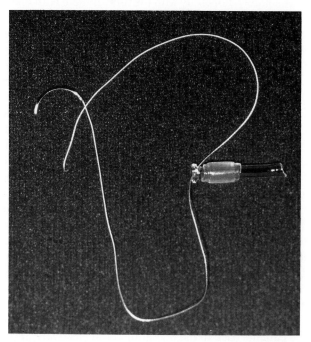

FIG. 8. A modified Jones tube to help treat an extrusion. A 4-mm piece of silicone tubing is fit around the body of the tube. Soft tissue contraction around the edges of the silicone seems to help prevent the tube from extruding. A suture through the suture hole is also used to snug the tube tightly at the inner canthus. (From Corin et al., ref. 33, with permission.)

Breaking of the Jones Tube (35,36)

Breaking of the Jones tube is extremely rare and is usually due to increased instrumentation. Theoretically, it would be easier to break the tube via instrumentation through the suture hole in the neck of the tube because potentially it would be weaker here. However, we think this is extremely unlikely because it is so rare to see broken Jones tubes (37). We have seen one patient having been operated on in a different center who was sent to an outlying area and told to have her Jones tube irritated routinely. She presented with a conjunctival reaction due to the irritation from the tube at the site of the breakage and a watery eye. We removed the tube and replaced it with another tube.

Migration of the Tube

The tube may migrate in many different directions:

1. *Inward.* The tube may migrate into the nose, especially if too small a lip size has been used. This will cause a gutter at the inner canthus, which may be cosmetically disfiguring. The tube, however, usually will keep functioning, unless the tube slides all the way down the nose and the opening closes off. If this presents a cosmetic problem, the tube can be removed, a canthoplasty can be performed on the gutter with sutures, and the tube replaced.

2. *Superior migration of the tube.* If the tube migrates superiorly at its ocular end, it often means that there is something pushing the tube inferiorly at the nasal end. A reposition of the tube is usually necessary.

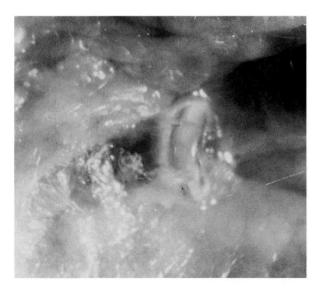

FIG. 10. Lateral migration of Jones tube. The tube is not functioning, and the patient has epiphora. (From Hurwitz and Howcroft, ref. 29, with permission.)

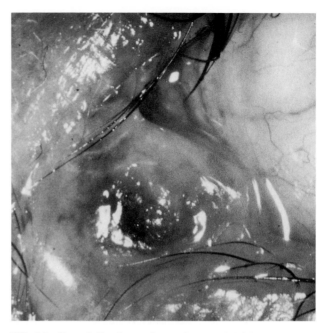

FIG. 11. Granulation formation at the mouth of the tube compromising drainage. The granuloma may be snipped away and the base cauterized. (From Hurwitz and Howcroft, ref. 29, with permission.)

3. *Inferior migration.* The ocular end migrating inferiorly is usually due to the nasal end migrating superiorly, almost always due to hypertrophy of the anterior tip of the middle turbinate. One can try and decongest the anterior tip of the middle turbinate and reposition the tube, but it is our experience that usually this must be treated with diminution of the turbinate either by cryotherapy or ultimately turbinectomy.

4. *Lateral migration of the tube* (Fig. 10). This may be due to the septum pushing the tube laterally (in which case a shorter tube is necessary), or the tube being too short and the turbinate pushes the tube laterally (decongestion of the turbinate, plus or minus turbinectomy is indicated). Scar tissue at the medial canthus medial to the tube may push the tube laterally. The scar tissue may be excised and the base cauterized. As well as the tube not functioning and the patient tearing in this situation, this is a more potentially serious situation as the tube may irritate the cornea and cause epithelial abrasion and/or a corneal ulcer.

Plugging of the tube. Mucus build-up may occur within the tube. This may be because of irritation of the tube or may be due to the same inflammatory process that may have caused the canaliculi to be blocked in the first place. When this happens we make sure that the patient has been adequately looking after the tube. Then we may use some decongestant nasal spray from the ocular and/or nasal end for a short period of time. It is important for the ophthalmologist at this point to clean out the tube with a probe, and it may be necessary if this happens frequently to remove the tube, give it a good cleaning, and reinsert it in the office.

Granulation formation. Granulation tissue may form at the ocular end of the tubes coming from the caruncle, the plica, or the conjunctiva (Fig. 11). If there is a small granuloma, one may simply snip this with a scissors at the slit lamp. Occasionally a granuloma may develop at the site of the hole in the nasal end of the tube, but this in our experience has been unusual.

Membranes may grow over the whole ocular end of the tube and it may be difficult even to determine from the ocular examination whether the tube is present (Fig. 12). This is more frequent in patients with Stevens-Johnson syndrome. The pressure of the tube can obviously be confirmed by looking in the nose. If one pushes on the medial canthal area with a firm instrument, such as a probe, one may feel the tube in place. It may be possible at the slit lamp with a sharp cataract knife to clean the scar tissue off the medial canthus so that the tube can be viewed. If one can see the tube, then one can usually extract the tube from the scar tissue, put a suture through the suture hole to hold it in the proper position, and the problem will usually be solved. If one cannot find the tube and there is too thick scar tissue, the patient usually needs to have some local anesthetic injected into the area, and an incision made down to the medial canthus and the tissue excised. Silver nitrate cauterization is also helpful, but it is mandatory that the silver nitrate does

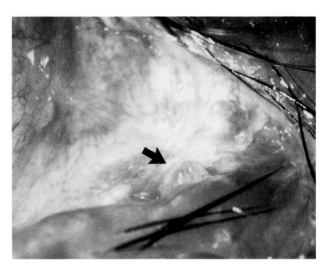

FIG. 13. Polypropylene tube (canalicular tube) inserted through punctum and canaliculus into the nose. (From Hurwitz, ref. 15, with permission.)

not get close to the cornea. We use the 0.5% silver nitrate sticks that one uses for nasal cauterization, but we make a point at the end of the stick so that there is minimal chance of the silver nitrate spreading in the area. If this procedure is unsuccessful, the patient should be given a general anesthetic to revise the operative site.

Drug toxicity. Drug toxicity may occur from medication put into the eye passing down to the nasal mucosa where it is quickly absorbed. This has been reported with phospholine iodide (37). We have also seen ocular toxicity from a patient who was "snorting" cocaine, so that when he was under the influence of cocaine, the cocaine passed up his Jones tube into the eye and anesthetized

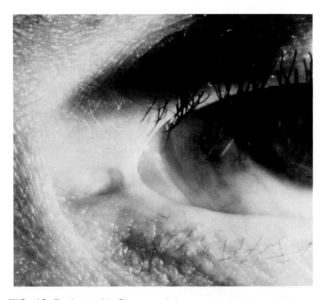

FIG. 12. Patient with Stevens-Johnson syndrome and Jones tube. The tremendous reaction at the inner canthus has not only caused the Jones tube to be totally occluded by a membrane, but symblepharon formation between the upper and lower lids has developed.

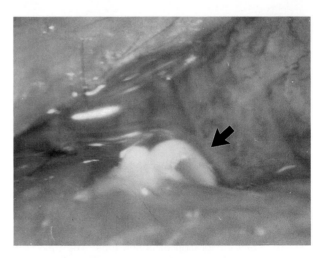

FIG. 14. Canalicular Teflon tube inserted through the punctum and canaliculus and into the nose. (From Hurwitz, ref. 16, with permission.)

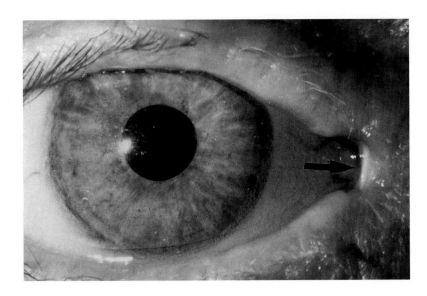

FIG. 15. Teflon tube in patient with artificial eye inserted at inner canthus and going into the nose. Tube has been in place for 5 years with no problems. (From Hurwitz, ref. 16, with permission.)

the eye. While he was rubbing his eye, the Jones tube irritated the cornea and gave him a corneal ulcer, and the deep scar in his cornea remains to this day.

Diplopia. Diplopia may occur after Jones tube insertion and is probably due to conjunctival tension bands from the region around the Jones tube so that when the patient abducts the eye, there is limitation (38). We feel that this complication may have something to do with the way the caruncle was treated. We have seen this complication in our earlier days of Jones tube insertions when we removed the caruncle (and probably some conjunctiva). However, since we have been shrinking the caruncle with bipolar cautery, we have not seen this complication develop.

Patient dissatisfaction. A patient may have a functioning Jones tube, but the tube may cause irritation and foreign body sensation. We have had this happen in a very small number of patients, and often it is due to a larger ocular lip. We have been able to help by putting in a tube with a smaller ocular lip. We have had two patients in our experience who had to have the Jones tubes removed because of chronic irritation in spite of drops, etc. Both of these patients had tearing after removal of the tubes, but one patient asked to have the tube reinserted, and said he would "live with the irritation," but he did "not want to live with the tearing." Some patients may complain of being able to blow air back in front of the eye, especially if they smoke (37). We are aware of another patient who had had a Jones tube inserted in another city, and had to have constant positive pressure oxygen treatment. This patient ultimately developed a severe dry eye problem because of the air constantly blowing up the Jones tube. The patient's ophthalmologist is now treating this patient with an intermittent punctal plug to be placed within the lumen of the Jones tube.

CONCLUSION

For canalicular obstructions, if possible, we advise reconstructing the system rather than inserting a permanent artificial prosthesis. However, when all else fails and when nothing else is possible, the Jones Pyrex glass tube, in our hands, has a success rate of 75% to 80% after the initial operation and up to 85% to 90% after a secondary revision (excision of a membrane, reinsertion, turbinate management). Many surgeons, including our group, search for the "ideal" tear duct tube. We have developed polypropylene tubes (15), (Fig. 13) and Teflon tubes (16) (Figs. 14 and 15), placing them at the inner canthus and along the canaliculus. However, the Jones Pyrex glass bypass tube has withstood the test of time and is the "gold standard" against which all other tubes must be measured.

REFERENCES

1. Crawford JS. Intubation of obstruction in the lacrimal system. *Can J Ophthalmol* 1977;12:289.
2. Hurwitz JJ, Johnson D, Howarth D, Molgat Y. High frequency radio-waves: full thickness electrosection of eyelid tissues. *Can J Ophthalmol* 1992;82:28.
3. Hiti H, Schuhmann G, Fachinger C, Tutz W. Die patielle caniculus transplantation. *Klin MBL Augenheilk* 1981;179:524.
4. Hurwitz JJ. Tear duct bypass tubes. *Transplantation* 1986;3:6.
5. Jones BR. The surgical care of obstruction in the lacrimal canaliculus. *Trans Ophthal Soc UK* 1960;80:343.
6. Welham RAN. Canalicular obstructions in the Lester Jones tube. What to do when all else fails. *Trans Ophthal Soc UK* 1973;93:623.
7. Nik NA, Hurwitz JJ, Chin Sang H. Mechanisms of tearflow after dacryocystorhinostomy and Jones tube surgery. *Arch Ophthalmol* 1994;102:1643.
8. Jones LT. The cure of epiphora due to canalicular disorders, trauma, and surgical failures on the lacrimal passages. *Trans Am Acad Ophthalmol Otolaryngol* 1962;66:506.
9. Lisman RD, Smith B, Silverstone P. Success rate of conjunctivo-dacryocystorhinostomy. Presented at the 17th meeting of the

American Society of Ophthalmic Plastic and Reconstructive Surgery. New Orleans, Louisiana. November 11, 1986.

10. Jones LT. Lacrimal surgery. In: Tessier P, Callahan A, Mustarde JC, Salyer KE, eds. *Symposium on plastic surgery in the orbital region.* St. Louis: CV Mosby; 1976.

11. Chandler AC, Wadsworth JAC. Conjunctivo-dacryocystorhinostomy. *Am J Ophthalmol* 1974;77:830.

12. Reinecke RD, Carroll JM. Silicone lacrimal tubing implantation. *Trans Am Acad Ophthalmol Otolaryngol* 1969;73:75.

13. Veirs ER. *Lacrimal disorders: diagnosis and treatment.* St. Louis: CV Mosby; 1976.

14. Murube del Castillo J. Conjunctivo-rhinostomy without osteal perforation. *Arch Ophthalmol* 1982;100:310.

15. Hurwitz JJ. New polypropylene tube to stent or bypass the lacrimal system. *Can J Ophthalmol* 1984;19:261.

16. Hurwitz JJ. Teflon tubes for stenting and bypassing the lacrimal drainage pathways. *Ophthal Surg* 1989;28:55.

17. Putterman AM, Epstein G. Combined Jones tube—canalicular intubation and conjunctivo-dacryocystorhinostomy. *Am J Ophthalmol* 1981;91:513.

18. Bosniak SL, Smith BC. *Advances in ophthalmic plastic and reconstructive surgery. The lacrimal system,* vol 3. Elmsford NY: Pergamon Press; 1984.

19. Taira C, Smith B. Palpebral dacryoadenectomy. *Am J Ophthalmol* 1973;75:461.

20. Kulwin DR, Tiradellis H, Levartiovsky S, Kersten RC, Shumrick KA. The value of intranasal surgery in assuring the success of a conjunctivo-dacryocystorhinostomy. *Ophthal Plast Reconstruct Surg* 1990;6:54.

21. Wesley R. Intranasal procedures. In: Linberg JV, ed. *Lacrimal surgery.* New York: Churchill Livingstone; 1988.

22. Avram D, Hurwitz JJ. Proximity of the sinus orifices to the DCR opening. Presented at the Annual Departmental Research Day. Dept of Ophthalmology, University of Toronto, 1985.

23. Henderson P. A trephining technique for the insertion of Lester Jones tubes. *Arch Ophthalmol* 1971;85:448.

24. Kartchner MJ, Mather TR, Dryden RM. Interoperative monitoring of Jones tube function. *Ophthal Plast Reconstruct Surg* 1989;5:192.

25. Nagashima K. Rocking phenomenon of Jones tube in place. Its clinical importance. *Arch Ophthalmol* 1984;102:116.

26. Weil B. The Lester Jones operation: conjunctive dacryocystorhinostomy with permanent prothesis. In: Yamaguchi M, ed. *Recent advances on the lacrimal system.* Japan: Asahi Evening News; 1978.

27. Markin BG, Tredici TJ. Aeromedical complications of conjunctivo-dacryocystorhinostomy. *Am J Ophthalmol* 1969;67:593.

28. Rosen N, Askenazi I, Rosner M. Patients dissatisfaction after functionally successful conjunctivo-dacryocystorhinostomy with Jones tube. *Am J Ophthalmol* 1994;117:636.

29. Hurwitz JJ, Howcroft MJ. Use of Lester Jones tubes: a review of 40 cases. *Can J Ophthalmol* 1981;16:176.

30. Rose GE, Welham RAN. Jones' lacrimal canalicular bypass tubes: twenty-five years experience. *Eye* 1991;8:13.

31. Gladstone TJ, Putterman AM. A modified glass tube for conjunctivo-dacryocystorhinostomy. *Arch Ophthalmol* 1985;103:1229.

32. Migilori ME, Putterman AM. Recurrent Jones tube extrusion successfully treated with a modified glass tube. *Ophthal Plast Reconstruct Surg* 1989;5:189.

33. Corin SM, Hurwitz JJ, Tucker SM. A simple technique for the prevention and management of Jones bypass tubes extrusion. *Can J Ophthalmol* 1988;23:322.

34. Hurwitz JJ, Cowen D. Prevention and management of Jones tube extrusion. The lacrimal system. In: Ghedine, ed. *Proceedings of the European Society of Dacryology.* Toronto; 1994.

35. Pamajier JH, Henkes HE, Delecourt PW. Experiences with the Jones tube in a Rotterdam Eye Clinic. *Ophthalmologica* 1975;171:353.

36. Doucet TW, Hurwitz JJ. The broken Lester Jones tube. *Can J Ophthalmol* 1982;17:32.

37. Laping K, Levine MR. Jones tubes—How good are they? *Arch Ophthalmol* 1983;101:260.

38. Skov CMB, Maxow ML. Diplopia following Jones tube placement. *Ophthal Surg* 1984;15:932.

CHAPTER 39

Endonasal Dacryocystorhinostomy

Jeffrey Jay Hurwitz

The intranasal dacryocystorhinostomy (DCR) was first described in the beginning of the twentieth century (1). The procedure was felt to be the least traumatic approach following prior tear sac surgery that had failed because of a membrane over the intranasal ostium (2). Jones states that the main disadvantages of the procedure are that because of monocular vision, visualization may be difficult, and that bleeding may be more difficult to control than via the external route. The success rate was definitely not as good as that with an external approach, and was essentially reserved for patients with previously unsuccessful tear duct surgery or for those patients refusing to have a skin incision (2).

With the development of small diameter endoscopes and those that have angled fields of view, intranasal visualization improved tremendously, and the intranasal DCR was therefore resurrected. The endonasal procedure is used mostly in DCR revisions, but is used by some surgeons as a primary procedure. The endonasal DCR has the advantage of not producing a skin scar.

To produce a drier field at the time of endonasal DCR, a laser was introduced to decrease the amount of bleeding that one often experiences with an endonasal procedure without a laser. Also, because of the "media appeal" of having an operation performed "with the laser," patient preference may be toward that of a laser-DCR regardless of the success rate.

ENDONASAL DCR WITHOUT LASER

Endoscopic visualization of the nasal anatomy totally transformed the intranasal DCR into a procedure whereby the surgeon could have excellent visualization of the structures. Visualization of the area may be

achieved by using 4-mm endoscopic telescopes with 0° and 30° angulation. Occasionally a 70° angulation telescope is useful. Messerklinger showed that it was possible to introduce, alongside these endoscopes, surgical instruments that may be used to perform surgical resections (3).

Before this, surgeons had attempted to use a microscope for binocular visualization within the nose (4). However, with the microscope it is impossible to tilt it so that one can visualize all the recesses within the nose. This drawback is true even for the external DCR, and we prefer to use high power loupes rather than a microscope if increased magnification is necessary through the external approach.

The use of the endoscope in the nose requires thorough knowledge of the anatomy of the nose and the surrounding structures. Certainly, there are a number of complications to the orbit, lacrimal system, or optic nerve that have been described following the use of the endoscope within the nose and sinuses (5). As well, "the learning curve for video endoscopy is somewhat steep" (6).

INDICATIONS FOR ENDONASAL DCR WITHOUT LASER

Failed DCR

If the obstruction after a DCR can be shown to be at the level of the lining of the nose at the junction of the sac and the nasal mucosa, it may be approached via an endonasal route.

Primary DCR

The ideal candidate for a primary endonasal DCR is that patient in whom lacrimal stones and tumors can be

J. J. Hurwitz: Oculoplastics Program, Mount Sinai Hospital; and Department of Ophthalmology, University of Toronto Faculty of Medicine, Toronto, Ontario M5S 1A8, Canada.

excluded, where there is no history of previous trauma to the mid-face, and where there is a large mucocele of the tear sac. It is now generally felt that if the tear sac is large, the success rate will be much higher (7). Mannor and Millman (8) suggested that dacryocystography (DCG) should be performed before performing an endonasal DCR. If the sac is found to be large, the success rate was much higher than if there was a small sac or no sac. They felt that the lacrimal sac anatomy as determined by a preoperative DCG is an extremely important prognostic factor with respect to surgical success.

TECHNIQUE OF INTRANASAL DCR WITHOUT LASER

The nose must be adequately decongested with preoperative oxymetazoline nasal spray as well as cocaine nasal packing. The procedure may be performed under local anesthesia or general anesthesia. It is important that there is excellent surgical exposure. Therefore, it is often necessary to perform a middle turbinectomy or to remove the perpendicular plate of the ethmoid bone if there is a septal deviation, using a septoplasty (9). In some cases an intranasal ethmoidectomy may have to be performed to remove adhesions from previous surgery and open the agger nasi cells, which are in the region of the tear sac.

One disadvantage of this procedure is the need for meticulous hemostasis. Bleeding may obscure the view the surgeon has through the endoscope and make the procedure much more difficult (9).

The punctum is dilated and a probe is placed as far as the sac. Then a light pipe is placed through the canaliculus and into the tear sac. This will help to identify the location of the tear sac while looking up the nose. However, one may be able to identify the sac endonasally because the lacrimal bone is flat and it is situated at the anterosuperior aspect of the lateral nasal wall. It usually lies anterior and superior to the superior attachment of the middle turbinate (10). Then using endoscopic visualization, a curved sickle knife (#66 Beaver) is used to make two incisions in the nasal mucous membrane. The first incision goes vertically perpendicular to the bridge of the nose, just beneath the roof of the nose (0.5 cm). Then another incision is made vertically anterior to the anterior aspect of the middle turbinate. The two incisions join together superiorly and the flap created may be turned down inferiorly to overly the inferior turbinate. This will expose the bone down to the attachment to the lateral wall of the nose. Because it is difficult, if not impossible, to suture the flaps intranasally, it is probably best to excise the flap. Turning down of the flap gives good exposure of the bone. A Freer elevator may be used to break through the bone in the area of the lacrimal bone where one sees the maximum transillumination.

One may remove the bone using upbiting and downbiting sphenoidal and DCR punches. One should not remove bone posterior to the posterior lacrimal crest for fear of entering the orbit. As well, one should not remove bone superior to the fundus of the sac for fear of involving the cribriform plate. Often anterior ethmoidal air cells may have to be removed. A turbinectomy may be performed as well by this route, but removal of the anterior tip of the middle turbinate often results in a significant amount of bleeding. Strips of Gelfoam may be used to pack any areas of bleeding. It is useful to use as little Gelfoam as possible because there is the risk that when it absorbs it may cause inflammation in the area of the DCR opening. However, it is invaluable in providing hemostasis. Once the bone is removed, the soft tissues of the lacrimal sac may be visualized. A long-handled Vannas scissors may be used to open the sac as the light pipe is passed medially to tent up the medial wall of the sac. An incision may be made perpendicular to the first incision and then a flap of sac may be removed. Bicanalicular Silastic stent intubation is then performed. Nasal packing is generally not needed unless there is significant bleeding at the end of the procedure.

Even though it is generally our philosophy to try and produce an epithelial lined tract, this is technically difficult with an intranasal DCR (to suture the flaps) and, therefore, even though the obstruction is at the lower end of the sac, we temporarily intubate the system for 3 to 4 months.

This same technique may be used to provide an opening in the nasal mucosa, the bone, and the lacrimal sac, in a procedure where a Jones bypass tube is to be inserted. The procedure is performed in exactly the same way, except it may be necessary to perform a larger middle turbinate resection so the tube sits properly within the nose. The success rate using this technique may be quite high in the "easy case," with a big sac and no previous trauma (11).

REVISION DCR VIA THE ENDONASAL APPROACH—WITHOUT LASER

If a previous DCR does not stay open despite repeated probings and nasal medications, the endonasal approach may be useful in ultimately achieving patency without reopening the whole surgical site. A light pipe is placed through the canaliculi as far nasally as possible. After adequately decongesting the nasal mucosa, with the use of endoscopic visualization, a Howarth elevator with its sharp end may be passed into the nose. The sharp end cuts a window around the light pipe and then, using a long-necked Vannas scissors, a window can be excised. Bleeding may be controlled using Gelfoam pieces. A bicanalicular Silastic intubation is then performed, and the nose packed if there is any excessive bleeding. The tubes are kept in place for 3 to 4 months. The success rate of an endonasal revision is comparable to that following a full reoperation via the external route (9).

LASER DCR

Endonasal DCR Using Laser

The use of the laser not only to make an opening in the nasal and lacrimal mucosa but also to cut a hole in the bone arose from an attempt to eliminate the need for intranasal punches and knives, and also for a need to decrease the amount of bleeding. It was hoped that the lateral heat spread with laser energy would be enough to cause hemostasis of the adjacent tissues, but not to cause damage to the surrounding important structures of the lacrimal system and the orbit (12). Early procedures described using a high-powered Argon blue-green laser coupled to a 300 μm quartz fiberoptic catheter to create the opening.

To improve on the visualization, the adjunctive use of an endoscope was described (6). These authors described the use of a carbon dioxide laser, and later a potassium titanyl phosphate laser. To decrease the amount of lateral heat spread, Yag lasers were used (13).

The use of the laser alone was often not adequate to provide a large enough opening in the bone, and often the use of the laser was augmented with punches (14), drills, bone curets (10), or other standard DCR instruments. The use of these adjunctive instruments decreases the need for higher laser power that might be necessary to cut through the bone. Using this technique, no flaps are made, and to keep the opening patent, a bicanalicular Silastic intubation is mandatory, usually for a period of 4 to 6 months.

Technique of Endonasal Laser DCR

This procedure may be performed under local or general anesthesia. The nose is decongested with oxymetazoline nasal spray and cocaine. If under local anesthesia, one may inject Xylocaine via an infratrochlear and a para-infraorbital nerve block, as well as locally onto the side of the nose. The punctum is dilated and a probe placed into the sac. Then a light pipe is placed into the sac to illuminate the inside of the nose. With endoscopic visualization, the laser (the type of laser to be used depends on the surgeon) (12–16) is placed up the nose toward the light pipe and, using pulsed bursts of laser energy, ablation is performed. If necessary, the laser may be used to ablate the middle turbinate. The ablation should be in the area of the thin lacrimal bone. The light pipe may then be pushed medially, and often if laser ablation has also produced a hole in the sac, the light pipe may be passed into the ostium. The rhinostomy may be

"cleaned up" using a small DCR bone punch. A bicanalicular Silastic stent tube is inserted and left in place for 6 months. The area can be packed with Gelfoam strips, or if there is significant bleeding, the nose can be packed with a Vaseline gauze pack.

Expected Success Rate

The expected success rates using this procedure vary from 50% to 80% or more, depending on the study. However, none of these studies has a large number of patients; even though most failures occur within the first 4 months following surgery (14), a long-term follow-up study with many patients is necessary to determine the true success rate of this procedure.

Complications

Hemorrhage

Even though it is felt that a real advantage of this procedure is a decrease in bleeding, the risk of bleeding even with this technique has not been eliminated (15).

Failure Rate

The failure rate of this procedure has not been established because long-term follow-up on a large number of cases is not yet available. However, it would seem that the success rate does not compare favorably with the success rate of the external DCR (13). Kong et al. (17) found nasal granulations in 50% of their patients at 6 weeks.

Intranasal Adhesions

These may be quite common due to inflammation from lateral heat spread and can occur in 10% of patients (17). Certainly thermal damage to surrounding tissue such as the nasal mucosa, the turbinate, the septum, and the ethmoids is possible as well. There is definitely an increased risk of atrophic rhinitis with thermal injury to the turbinate.

Equipment Failure

The equipment for this procedure is quite sophisticated, and there is certainly the possibility of the machinery not working properly so that one must have to revert to a standard DCR, either intranasal or external (7).

Laser Risks

With the use of the laser, appropriate risks must be taken to protect both the patient and the surgeon from laser damage (7). As well, there is the risk of spread of either neoplastic or viral material from the smoke plume (7).

Complication of Tubes

Because it is mandatory that tubes be placed in the system for an extended period of time (6 months), the potential for inflammatory complications of tubes becomes a real possibility (see Chapter 36).

Inadvertent Discovery of Tumor or Stones

If a tumor or stones are found within the sac, the procedure cannot be completed, and one must revert to a standard external DCR.

TABLE 1. Comparison of DCR techniques

	External	Endonasal	Laser
General features			
Outpatient possibility	Yes	Yes	Yes
Local anesthesia possibility	Yes	Yes	Yes
Surgical time	30–40 min	30–40 min	40–60 min (increased set-up time)
Cost of technology	Very low	Low (endoscope)	High
Reliability of technology	High	Reasonably high	Variable
Success rate	High (93–95%+)	70–80% (selected cases)	50–80% (selected cases)
Media appeal	Nothing special (but high success)	Good: no scar	High (use of laser)
Surgical bleeding	Controllable	Usually controllable	Decreased (not always)
Surgical creation of mucosal lined tract	Yes	No	No
Need for tubes to keep passage open	Usually not	Yes	Yes
Specific features			
Skin incision	Yes	No	No
Resultant skin scar	Yes (often invisible)	No	No
Orbicularis dissection	Yes (fibers spread, not cut)	No	No
Increased difficulty if small sac	Negligible	Yes	Yes
Handling of stones	Easy	Difficult	Difficult
Risk of "sump"	Negligible	Higher	Higher
Damage to mucosa	Negligible	Minimal	High
Sac tumor	Manageable	May be missed	May be missed
Handling of common canaliculus obstruction	Easy	Difficult	Difficult endonasally
Potential for common canalicular damage	Low	Low	Higher (energy spread)
Good for re-ops	good	good	uncertain
Nasal features			
Value in Jones tube surgery	Valuable	Valuable	Valuable
Potential atrophic rhinitis	Low	Low	Higher
Potential obstruction of nasofrontal duct	Low (depends on osteotomy size and position)	Low (depends on osteotomy size and position)	Higher (also factor of energy spread to duct)
Handling of ethmoids	Easy (remove)	Quite easy (remove)	More difficult (burn through)
Handling of turbinate	Easy (SMR)	Quite easy (remove)	More difficult; try to burn through
Conclusion			
No. of decades available	9	8 (1 with endoscope)	1
Withstood test of time	Yes	Without endoscope: no With endoscope: not yet	Not yet
Author's preference: primary DCR	99%	1% (if patient requests no scar and does not object to second operation)	0% (percentage will increase with improved technology and decreased morbidity)
Revision DCR	–Second choice if sac-nasal mucosal obstruction –First choice if common canaliculus block	First choice if sac-nasal mucosal obstruction	Not used
Revision Jones tube surgery	First choice if tube loss or tube displacement not due to turbinate	First choice if turbinate hypertrophy or granuloma	Not used

DCR, dacryocystorhinostomy; SMR, submucous resection.

Damage to Orbital Fat

Kong et al. (17) found a very high rate of orbital fat herniation using laser. They advocate using the laser less, and radiosurgical or bone instruments as a replacement.

Laser DCR: Transcanalicular Route

A laser may be introduced through the canaliculus to burn through the lacrimal sac, bone, and nasal mucosa (18). The Argon blue laser may not have enough energy to penetrate the thick bone, and increased energy using this laser may have undesirable side effects whereby the surrounding tissues may be damaged. Use of the THC: Yag laser in a pulsed fashion is able to ablate the tissue without causing as much surrounding tissue damage (19). Mitomycin was also suggested in an attempt to keep the opening patent. Bicanalicular Silastic intubation is also necessary.

The Holmium Yag laser can be used to cut a 1-mm diameter channel through the canaliculus and into the nose. Intubation is mandatory for approximately 6 months (20). The success rate of this procedure should be judged following a long-term follow-up after the tubes have been removed to see if the system remains open and functional.

AUTHOR'S PHILOSOPHY ON ENDONASAL AND LASER-ASSISTED DCR SURGERY

The real advantage of performing endonasal DCR surgery is to eliminate the need for a scar on the skin, and also hopefully to decrease bleeding. However, as mentioned in Chapter 36, techniques may be used to minimize the size of the incision and decrease the resulting scar. The intraoperative and postoperative bleeding following a laser-DCR may not necessarily be any different than after a standard external DCR. The reliability of the technology for the laser-DCR is variable, the cost is much higher, and certainly initially the surgical time is much longer. Both the laser-DCR and the external DCR can be performed under local or general anesthesia and as either an inpatient or outpatient. The success rate certainly as of this writing is significantly higher with an external DCR, which has withstood the test of time.

It has always been our philosophy that with a DCR, one is trying to produce an opening lined with epithelium that can be fabricated at the time of an external DCR but not at the time of an intranasal DCR. With the improvement in diagnostic modalities, such as canaliculoscopy (see Chapter 18), and nasal endoscopy (see Chapter 17), those cases that would benefit by intranasal surgery may be able to be better identified.

There is no question that intranasal surgery has undergone some exciting advancements, and we will be hearing much more regarding developments in this field. There already seems to be a trend away from endoscopic endonasal DCR surgery with a laser—either a Ho:Yag or a contact Nd:Yag, and instead to use other endonasal techniques (15,17). In the meantime, the external DCR is our preference in almost all circumstances for a primary DCR, but the intranasal revision DCR (without laser) in our hands has an ever-increasing role in failed DCRs (Table 1).

REFERENCES

1. Mosher HP. Mosher-Toti operation on the lacrimal sac. *Laryngoscope* 1915;25:739.
2. Jones LT, Boyden B. The rhinologist's role in tear sac surgery. *Trans Am Acad Ophthalmol Otolaryngol* 1951;34:654.
3. Messerklinger W. *Endoscopy of the nose.* Baltimore: Urban and Schwarzenberg; 1978.
4. Heermann J, Neues D. Intranasal microsurgery of all paranasal sinuses, the septum and the lacrimal sac with hypotensive anesthesia. *Ann Otolaryngol Rhinol Laryngol* 1986;95:631.
5. Neuhaus RW. Orbital complications secondary to endoscopic sinus surgery. *Ophthalmology* 1990;15:12.
6. Gonnering RS, Lyon DB, Fisher JC. Endoscopic laser assisted lacrimal surgery. *Am J Ophthalmol* 1991;111:152.
7. Gonnering R. Dacryocystorhinostomy and conjunctival-dacryocystorhinostomy. In: Dortzbach RK, ed. *Ophthalmic Plastic Surgery. Prevention and management of complications.* New York: Raven Press; 1994.
8. Mannor GE, Millman AL. The prognostic value of preoperative dacryocystography in endoscopic intranasal dacryocystorhinostomy. *Am J Ophthalmol* 1992;113:134.
9. Metson R. Endoscopic surgery for lacrimal obstruction. *Otolaryngol Head Neck Surg* 1991;104:473.
10. Rebeiz EE, Shapshay SM, Bawlds JH, Pankratov MM. Anatomical guidelines for dacryocystorhinostomy. *Laryngoscope* 1992;102:1181.
11. Whittet HB, Shun-Shin GA, Awdry P. Functional endoscopic transnasal dacryocystorhinostomy. *Eye* 1993;7:545.
12. Massaro BM, Gonnering RS, Harris GJ. Endonasal laser dacryocystorhinostomy: a new approach to nasolacrimal duct obstruction. *Arch Ophthalmol* 1990;108:1172.
13. Woog JJ, Metson R, Puliafito CA. Holmium:Yag endonasal laser dacryocystorhinostomy. *Am J Ophthalmol* 1993;111:1.
14. Boush GA, Lemke BN, Dortzbach RK. Results of endonasal laser assisted dacryocystorhinostomy. *Ophthalmology* 1994;101:955.
15. Bartley GB. The pros and cons of laser-dacryocystorhinostomy. *Am J Ophthalmol* 1994;124:103.
16. Migliori ME. Contact ND:Yag laser endonasal dacryocystorhinostomy. Presented at the American Society of Ophthalmic Plastic and Reconstructive Surgeons. San Francisco, 1994.
17. Kong YT, Kim TI, Kong BW. A report of 131 cases of endoscopic laser lacrimal surgery. *Ophthalmology* 1994;101:1793.
18. Christenbury JD. Translacrimal laser dacryocystorhinostomy. *Arch Ophthalmol* 1992;110:170.
19. Silkiss RZ. THC-Yag nasolacrimal duct recanalization. *Ophthal Surg* 1993;24:772.
20. Dutton JJ, Holck DEE. The Holmium Yag laser for canalicular reconstruction. Presented at the American Society of Ophthalmic Plastic and Reconstructive Surgeons. San Fransicso, 1994.

Subject Index